SÔTAI

SÔTAI

Balance and Health Through Natural Movement

by Keizo Hashimoto, M. D.
with Yoshiaki Kawakami, M. D.

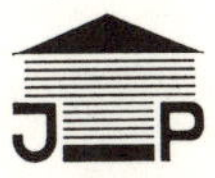

Japan Publications, Inc.

Translated by Stephen Brown and Richard Held

This book originally published in Japanese under the title of 操体法写真解説集 (Sōtai-ho Shashin Kaisetsu-shu) by Hakuju-sha Publishing Company, Tokyo, in 1979.

Published by Japan Publications, Inc., Tokyo

Distributors:
United States: *Kodansha International/ USA, Ltd., through Harper & Row, Publishers, Inc., 10 East 53rd Street, New York, New York 10022.* South America: *Harper & Row, Publishers, Inc., International Department.* Canada: *Fitzhenry & Whiteside Ltd., 150 Lesmill Road, Don Mills, Ontario M3B 2T6.* Mexico and Central America: *HARLA S. A. de C. V., Apartado 30–546, Mexico 4, D. F.* British Isles: *International Book Distributors Ltd., 66 Wood Lane End, Hemel Hempstead, Herts HP2 4RG.* European Continent: *Boxerbooks, Inc., Limmatstrasse 111, 8031 Zurich.* Australia and New Zealand: *Book Wise (Australia) Pty. Ltd., 101 Argus Street, Cheltenham Victoria 3192.* The Far East except Japan: *Japan Publications Trading Co., Ltd., 1–2–1, Sarugaku-cho, Chiyoda-ku, Tokyo, 101.*

First edition: August 1983

ISBN 8–87040–534–9

Printed in Hong Kong

FOREWORD

The human body is specially designed in order that man may live with the greatest amount of comfort on earth. Living in harmony with this design not only means that one remains free of disease, but also that one's health and vitality can be increased. The secret to conforming with this flawless design can be summarized into four basic points. They are regulation through breathing and diet and that through physical and mental activity. All these functions without exception have to be performed as the personal responsibility of each individual. Even if just one of these processes goes against natural laws, the body loses its functional balance to tip toward an unhealthy condition.

The role of medical science should be to elucidate the laws that govern these four basic processes in life, and to help individuals with physical imbalances to regain their equilibrium. There are great number of people on this earth who suffer because of war and famine, and large numbers are unable to receive the most basic of medical care. Be that as it may, even in the most advanced societies of this day, the majority of people are in an unhealthy state from physical imbalances caused by their violation of the fundamental laws of nature.

Back in 1974 Dr. Hashimoto, in order to sound a warning about the current approach to medicine, submitted a paper to the Japan Medical Association concerning distortions in basic physical structure as it relates to complaints of general malaise. The integrity in the basic structure of the human frame is maintained by the integration of the above mentioned four basic functions, but the majority of people in this modern age are unable to maintain a balance even in this most basic interaction. For this reason Dr. Hashimoto drew on his clinical experience to shed light on the laws governing the four basic functions of man. Among these, he focused on the integration of physical movement with breathing to introduce a new form of exercise. This method was named *Sōtai* and is now applied widely in Japan to treat and facilitate the recovery of those who are sick or "semi-sick," as well as to increase the level of health and vitality in "not so healthy" and healthy individuals alike.

In physiological terms *Sōtai Therapy* is exercise which brings about muscular relaxation by harmonizing the breathing and movements of the patient made within the natural limits of the range of motion. Subjectively speaking, Sōtai consists of movements which "feel good" and are easy to perform for the patient, and are movements without pain or undue strain. Thus, these are movements in which the "internal sensitivity" of the patient plays an important part and this includes sensitivity to "comfort and ease" as well as "discomfort and pain."

Sōtai is often compared to simple stretching exercises and Yoga, but its unique feature lies in being movement performed in the direction away from discomfort and pain. In Sōtai each movement is made slowly to the limit of mobility with a slight amount of resistance applied against it, and the movement is brought to a stop at the farthest point still comfortable for the patient where tension is held for about five seconds before all effort is relaxed at once with the patient's inhale. While Sōtai is similar to stretching exercises and Yoga in some respects, it is distinguished by the above mentioned features.

This manual of Sōtai Therapy is being published in the English edition on this occasion in hopes that it will contribute to the health and well-being of all people in the world. The aim of this book on Sōtai was to make it possible for even those with no specialized medical knowledge to study the photographs and the accompanying text to locate distortions in their own physical makeup and to correct these themselves according to natural principles so as to eliminate symptoms which cause discomfort and pain. Naturally, the results of these adjustments are far more pronounced when two persons use this book to perform these movements with each other's assistance.

Although Sōtai Therapy is not effective in alleviating all symptoms and conditions, it invariably proves effective in facilitating the natural healing process. Sōtai Therapy has some things in common with relaxation exercises and consequently some people are more given to it than others. Also, because Sōtai relies to a great extent on the sensitivity of each patient, this causes the results to vary. It is therefore important that both the therapist and the patient get a feel for the precise timing involved. The learning of breathing techniques for this purpose is considered to be invaluable.

It can be said that the majority of the over four billion people that populate this earth suffer from poor health caused by physical imbalances. The authors would find their greatest reward if this book could serve as a clue for such people in restoring their health. This book was compiled by the cooperative efforts of Dr. Hashimoto's students to produce a book easy to understand and put to use. The authors wish to express their appreciation to Kenzo Kase D.C. who conceived of this English edition, and the translators Stephen Brown and Richard Held, as well as the President of Hakujyu-sha Publishing Company, Mr. Nakayama, and the President of Japan Publications Inc. Mr. Yoshizaki, who all helped to make this edition possible.

CONTENTS

2. Mobility Examination and Sōtai Techniques

3. Proper Position and Hand Placement for Therapist

4. Checkpoints for Morphological Observation

5. Kinesiological Linkage and Response of Body

6. Minor Symptoms—An Enigma to Modern Medicine

7. Sōtai Exercises—Active Movement in the Comfortable Direction

8. Exercises Applying Kinesiological Principles

9. Sōtai treatment According to Symptoms

1. SŌTAI THERAPY—*Basic Forms*

The pleasant sensation elicited by movement in harmony with the slow exhalation of each breath is the essence of Sōtai Therapy. When the appreciation of such movement becomes established as a natural and constant state of being, this is called health.

Sōtai is a method enabling human beings to adapt to their environment by harmonizing respiration, ingestion, physical movements and mental activity. This book is primarily concerned with the integration of physical movements and breathing, which is herein referred to as Sōtai movements. In this chapter Dr. Hashimoto demonstrates the basic forms routinely used in Sōtai Therapy.

Sōtai Technique for Adjusting Posture Along Median Line (Elevation of Pelvis) —*Relief from abnormal tension*

Supine A

Using the shoulders, elbows and heels as support points, the patient raises her hips by arching her body upward (Figs. 1 and 2). After two or three seconds of holding her body in this position, the patient completely relaxes her efforts all at once. After the tension in the patient's body has been released in this manner, she rests for another two or three seconds and recovers normal breathing.

This movement has many objectives including the release of abnormal tension in the body, which therefore makes this movement essential in Sōtai Therapy. (Refer to page 31 for detailed instructions.)

Fig. 1 Supine A

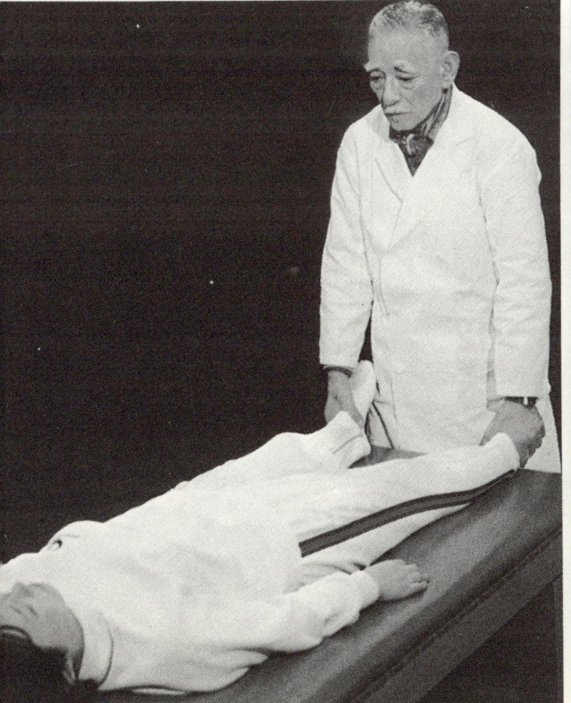

Fig. 2 Supine A

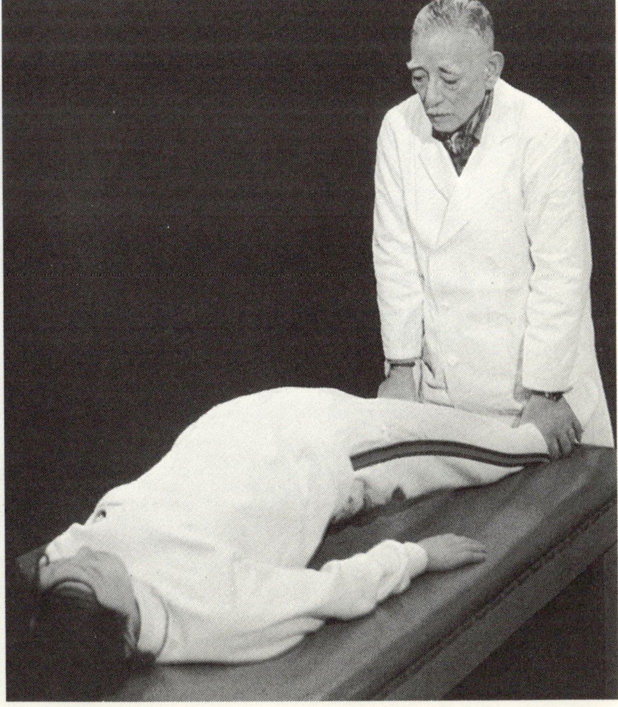

Mobility Examination and Sōtai Technique for Hip Flexion
—*Relief from coxalgia and lumbago*

Supine E

Dōshin: With both legs extended, the patient alternately raises her right and left legs (Fig. 3). Sensations of comfort and discomfort produced during the movements are noted.

Sōtai: The patient presses down, against a small amount of resistance provided by the therapist, with the leg which caused the greater discomfort when lifted (Fig. 3).

As in the movements illustrated in Figures 1 and 2, this movement also serves to remove abnormal tension. (Refer to page 42 for detailed instructions.)

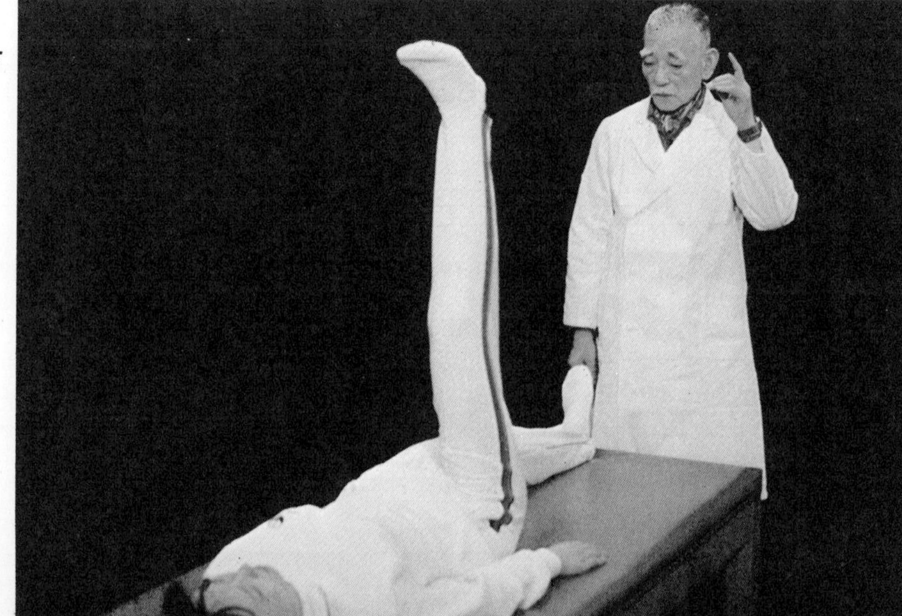

Fig. 3 Supine E

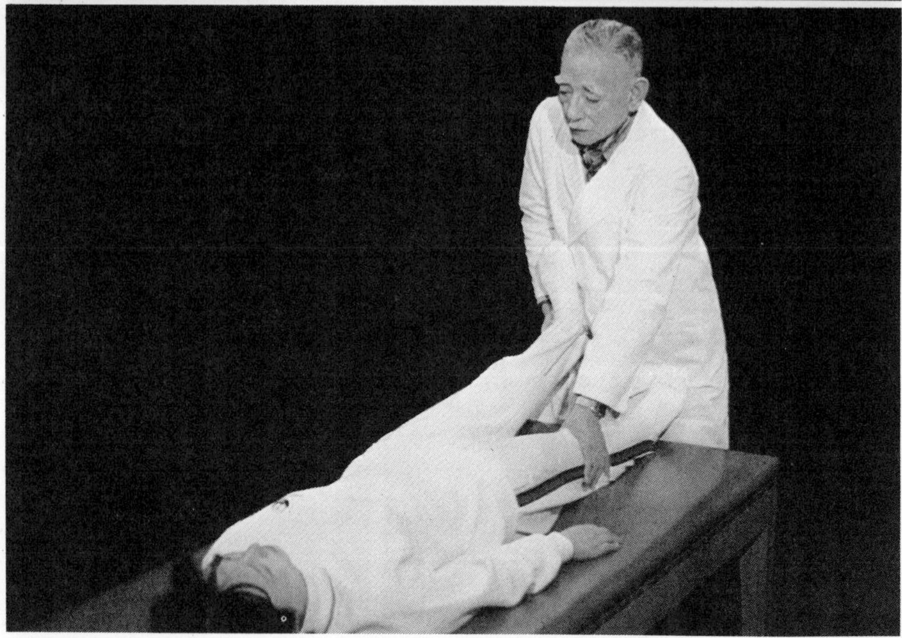

Fig. 4 Supine E

Mobility Examination and Sōtai Technique Applying Pressure Alternation on Knees—*Elimination of pain in the knee joint*

Supine F

Dōshin: The therapist alternately applies downward pressure on the right and left patellas (Fig. 5). Sensations of comfort and discomfort are noted.

Sōtai: If the patient feels discomfort in either leg upon application of pressure, she flexes (raises) that knee as the therapist gently applies resistance to this movement (Fig. 6). For the other leg, the patient raises her knee to allow the therapist to support it from below. Then the patient lowers her knee by extending her leg against light resistance provided by the therapist. (Refer to page 36 for detailed instructions.)

Fig. 5 Supine F

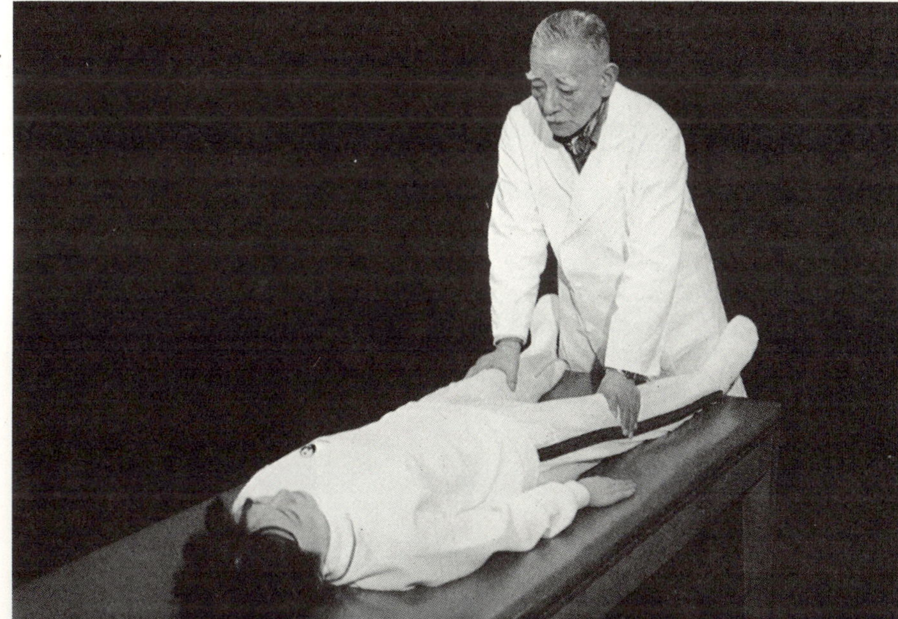

Fig. 6 Supine F

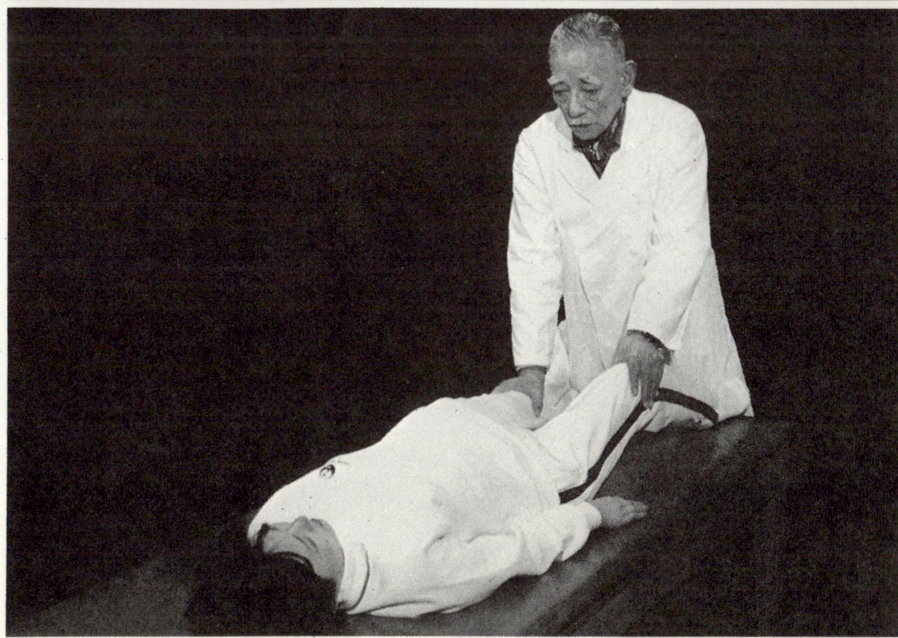

Palpation Examination of Popliteal Fossa for Abnormal Tension and Pressure Sensitivity, and Sōtai Technique for Increasing Mobility of Hip Joint (1)
—*Correction of distortions in pelvis, digestive problems, tension and heaviness of lower limbs*

Supine G

This is a palpation method for examining pressure sensitive areas as well as indurations accompanying muscle tension on the posterior side of the knee joint (Figs. 7 and 8). Pressure sensitive points may be found on the medial and lateral ends of the popliteal fossa. When these points are normalized with the Sōtai technique, subjective symptoms of discomfort will cease with amazing rapidity.

Although the extent to which symptoms can be eliminated depends partly upon the linkage relationships within the patient's joints during this movement, in some cases the effect of this technique extends as far as relieving symptoms of the lower back. At times this small movement eliminates the discomfort of lumbago so instantaneously that the patient is astonished at the quick relief provided. (Refer to page 45 for detailed instructions, also refer to page 169 in "Enigma to Modern Medicine.")

Fig. 7 Supine G

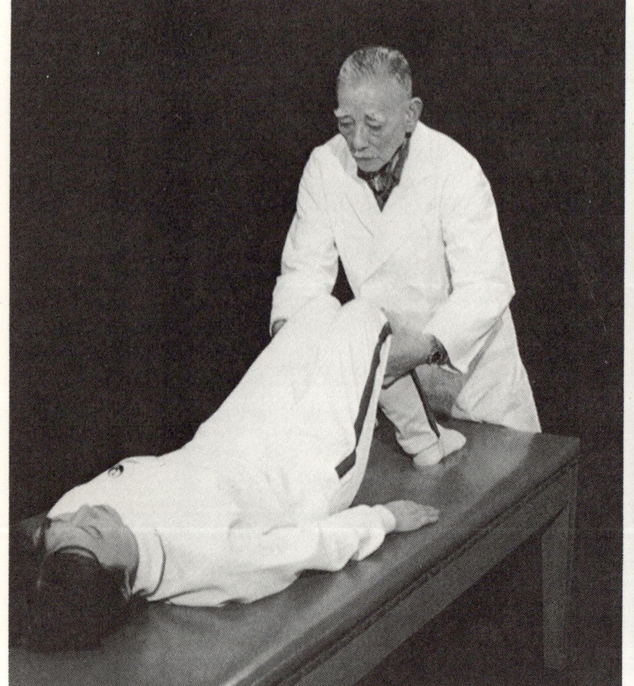

Fig. 8 Supine G

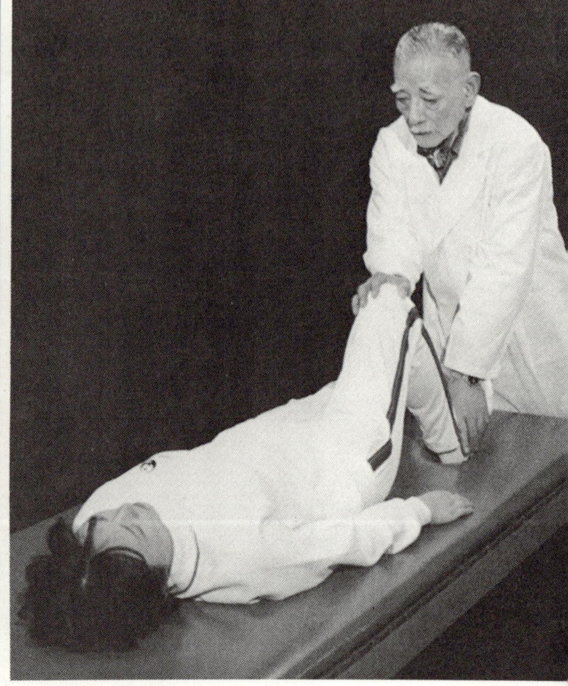

Palpation Examination of Gluteus Muscles for Abnormal Tension and Pressure Sensitivity, and Sōtai Technique for Increasing Mobility of Hip Joint (2)

Supine J

Figure 9 shows the palpation examination, and Figure 10 shows the mobility examination.

Some of these Sōtai techniques require experience to produce the exact motion specified. However, the therapist need only repeat the procedure which is the easiest to execute, two or three times. To begin with, it is best to start with the mobility examination shown in Figure 10. (Refer to page 60 for detailed instructions, also refer to page 169 in "Enigma to Modern Medicine.")

Fig. 9 Supine J-1

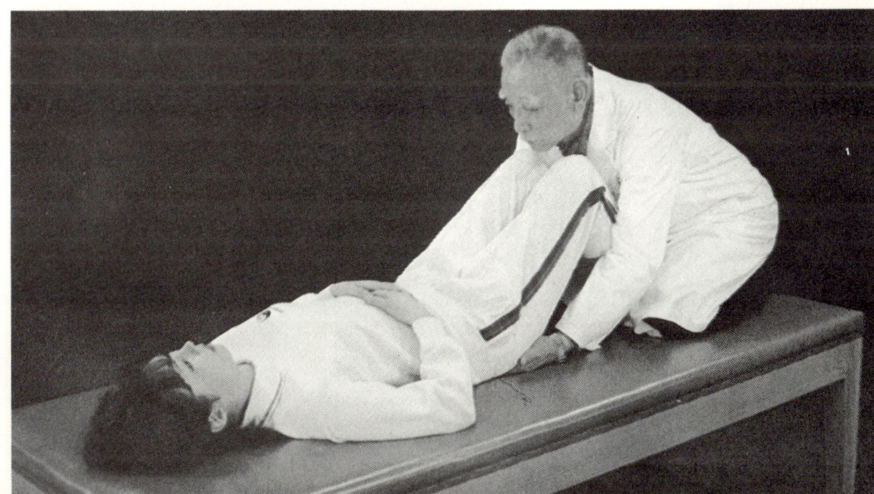

Fig. 10 Supine J-2

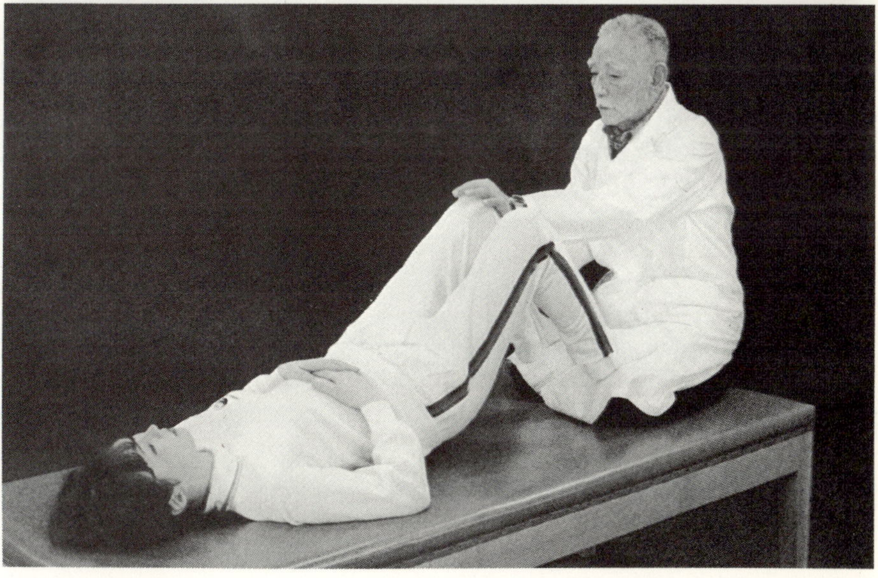

Palpation Examination and Sōtai Techniques for Pressure Sensitivity in Adductors of Hip Joint
—Improving eyesight and relieving asthenopia

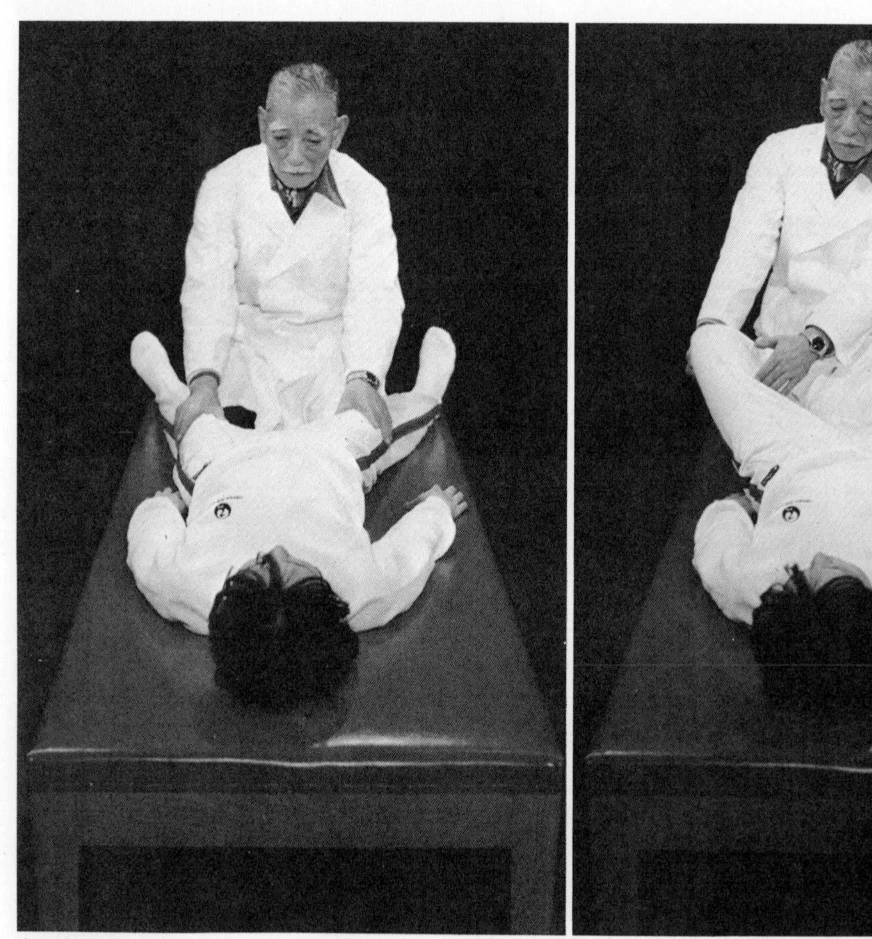

Fig. 11 Supine I

Fig. 12 Supine I

Supine I

Dr. Hashimoto discovered an extremely sensitive point on the adductor muscles while probing for pressure points on the liver meridian*, and he named this point Sei-gan (clear eyes). This Sōtai technique makes use of this meridian point to loosen tension in the adductor muscles of the thighs (Figs. 11 and 12).

Abnormal tension in the adductors not only invites the deterioration in the functioning of the lower limb, but also may be related to interferences in the ocular function. (Refer to page 55 for detailed instructions, also refer to page 172 in "Enigma to Modern Medicine.")

---

*One of the channels or pathways for the flow of vital energy in Oriental medicine.

Mobility Examination and Sōtai Technique for Hip Rotation with Knee Flexed
—*Alleviation of lumbago, rachialgia, fatigue and digestive problems*

Supine H

Dōshin: Turn the patient's flexed knees downward to the left, and then to the right, noting at this time the sensations of comfort and discomfort, as well as restrictions in mobility (Figs. 13 and 14).

Sōtai: With this Sōtai movement it is possible for the patients to obtain similar results by simply performing the movement three or four times on their own, without the application of resistance by the therapist. (Refer to page 50 for detailed instructions.)

Fig. 13 Supine H

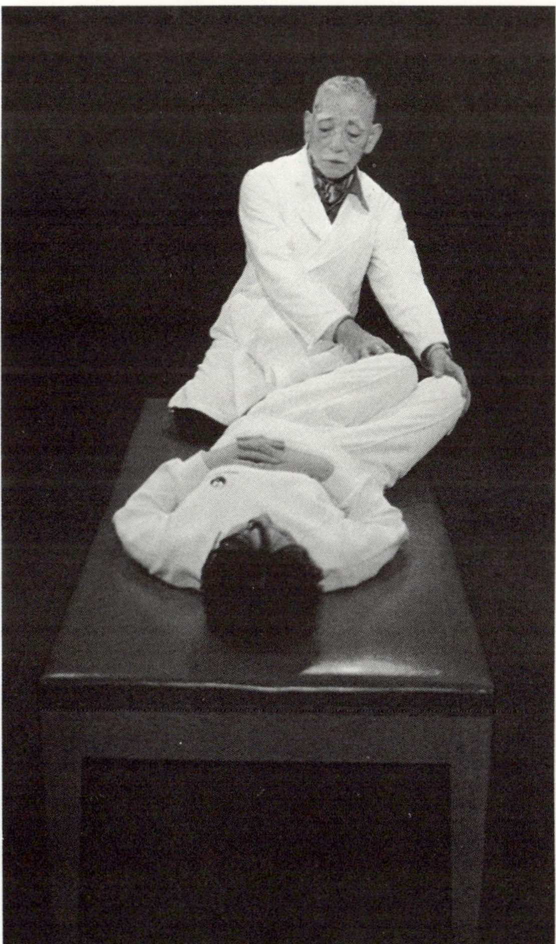

Fig. 14 Supine H

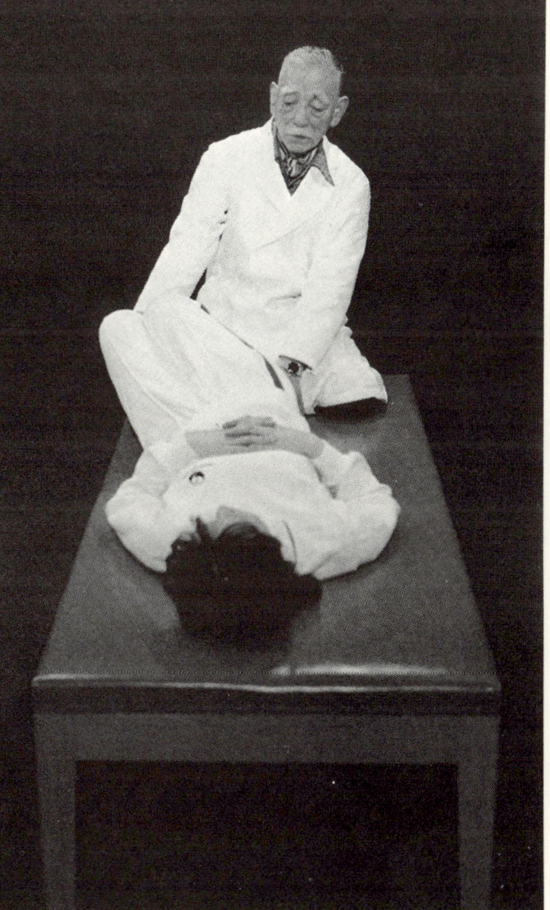

Sōtai Technique for Shoulders and Arms
—*Relief from discomfort in the neck, shoulders and arms*

Supine N
Deciding the appropriate angle at which to position the arm during the lateral and medial rotation can be fairly complicated. As a general rule, the arm is extended to the side, with the hand between the nipple and the waist, while keeping it within 30° of level (Fig. 15). (Refer to page 72 for detailed instructions.)

Palpation Examination and Sōtai Technique for Indurations and Pressure Sensitivity Along the Cervical Vertebrae
—*Alleviation of headaches, heaviness of the head, asthenopia, nasal congestion, tinnitus, and for hypertension*

Supine M
Symptoms in the cranial and facial regions brought about by distortions in the alignment of cervical vertebrae are a common occurrence. Cervical distortions, however, often result by linkage to distortions occuring in other parts of the body. (Refer to page 69 for detailed instructions.)

Fig. 15 Supine N

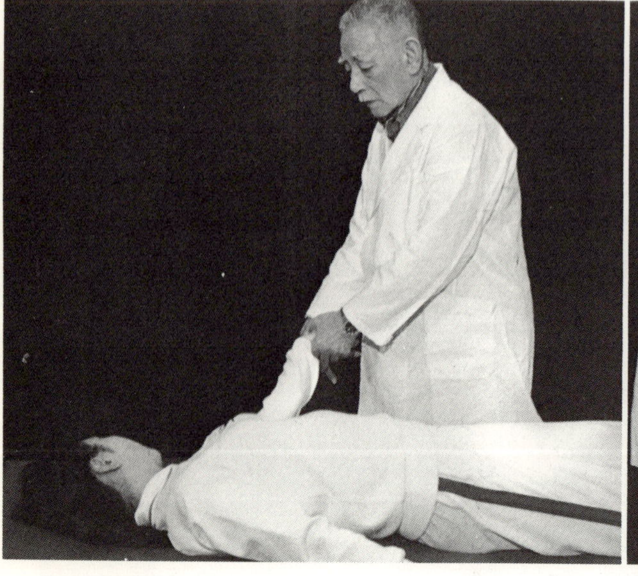

Fig. 16 Supine M

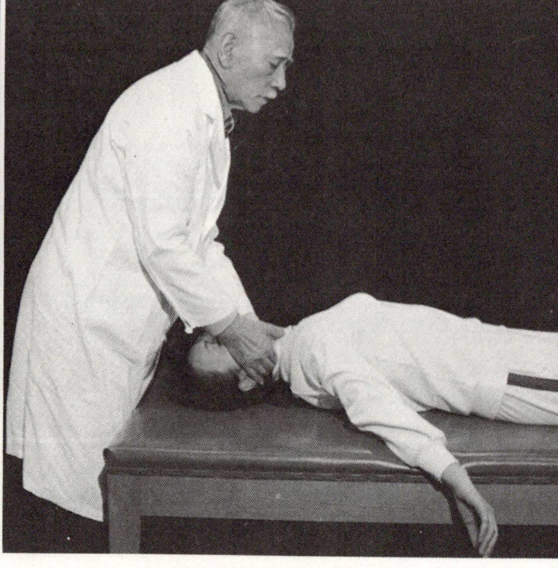

Mobility Examination of Knee Flexion

Prone A

Dōshin: In this mobility examination, the suppleness and flexibility of the knee joints are examined by alternately flexing each knee and pressing the heel to the hip (Fig. 17). The heel may not reach the hip easily in some cases due to abnormal tension in the psoas and/or the femoral muscles.

Fig. 17 Prone A

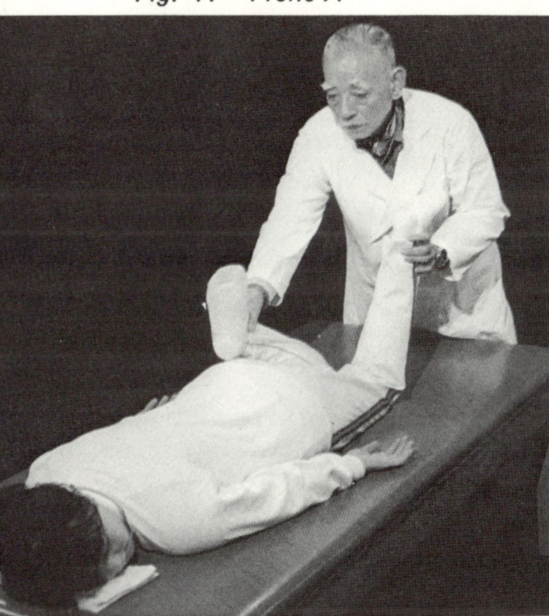

Fig. 18 Prone C

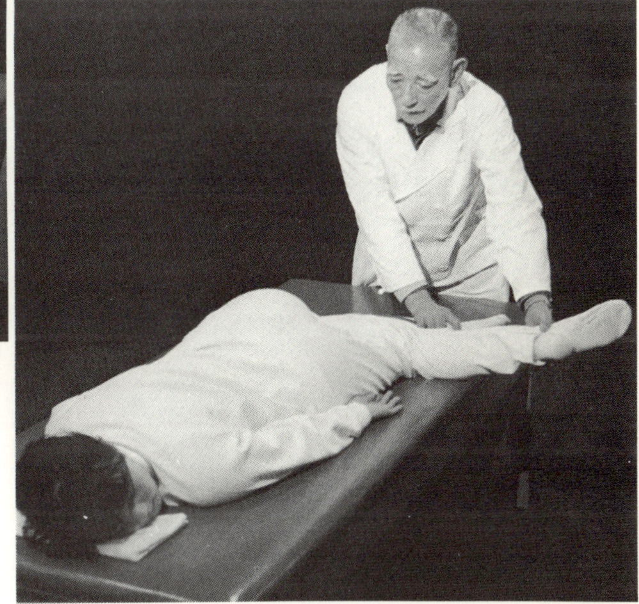

Mobility Examination of Hip Rotation with Knees Flexed

Prone C

Dōshin: In this mobility examination, difficulties or problems in movement are investigated by slowly rotating the lower limbs together, to the right and left with the knees flexed (Fig. 18). It is more difficult to rotate the legs to one side compared to the other when abnormal tension exists in the psoas muscles.

Sōtai Technique for Removing Abnormal Tension in Muscles of the Back, Hips and Thighs
—Eliminating pain and fatigue in the back and lumbar areas

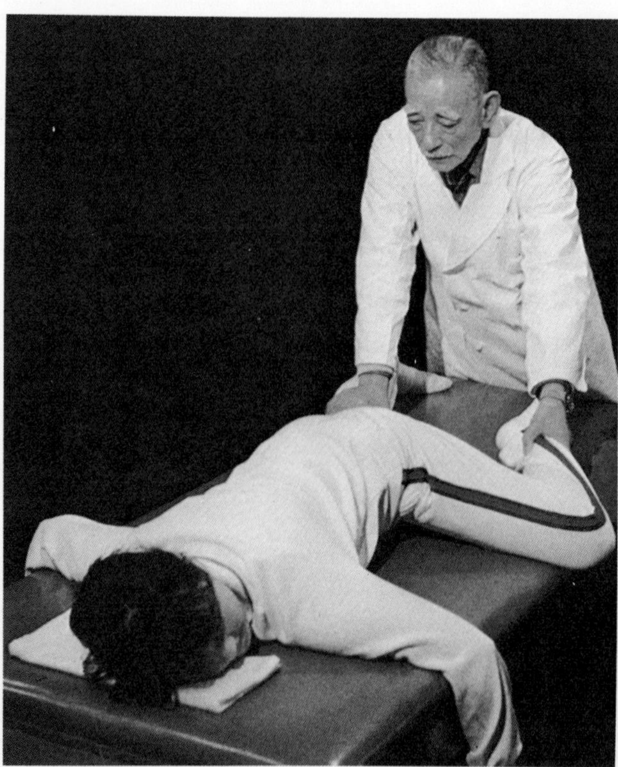

Fig. 19 Prone A

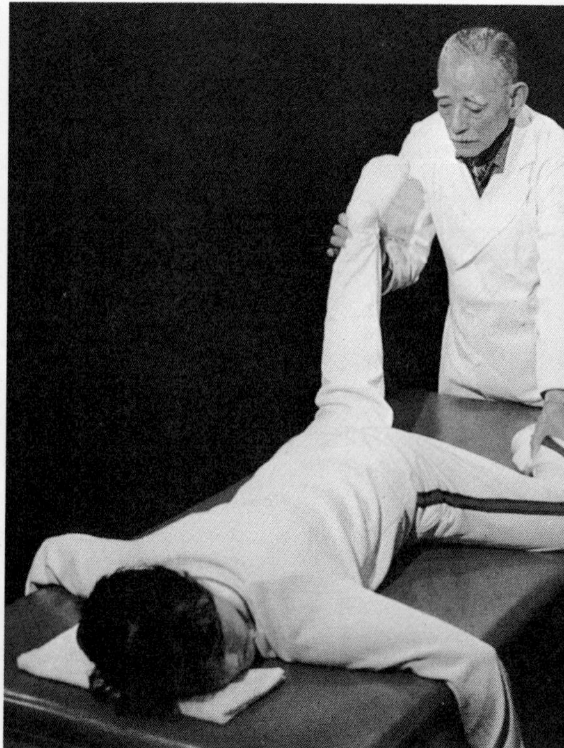

Fig. 20 Prone A

Prone A

This technique is a combination of the knee flexing mobility examination and the Sōtai Prone Position C mobility examination. In cases where the heel does not reach the hip with the knee flexion, the limb is extended. After the more comfortable direction has been determined by the Prone Position C mobility examination, the patient draws the more comfortable limb up toward her side (Figs. 19 and 20).

Since there is a certain "knack" involved in performing this particular technique, refer to Chapter 2 and study the directions thoroughly. In these examinations, it is important to test each movement in a slow and steady manner without any strain or use of excessive force. (Refer to page 74 for detailed instructions.)

Mobility Examination and Sōtai Technique for Alternately Flexing Hip Joints
—*Alleviation of low back pain and fatigue, lateral displacement of pelvis, and abnormal tension in the thighs*

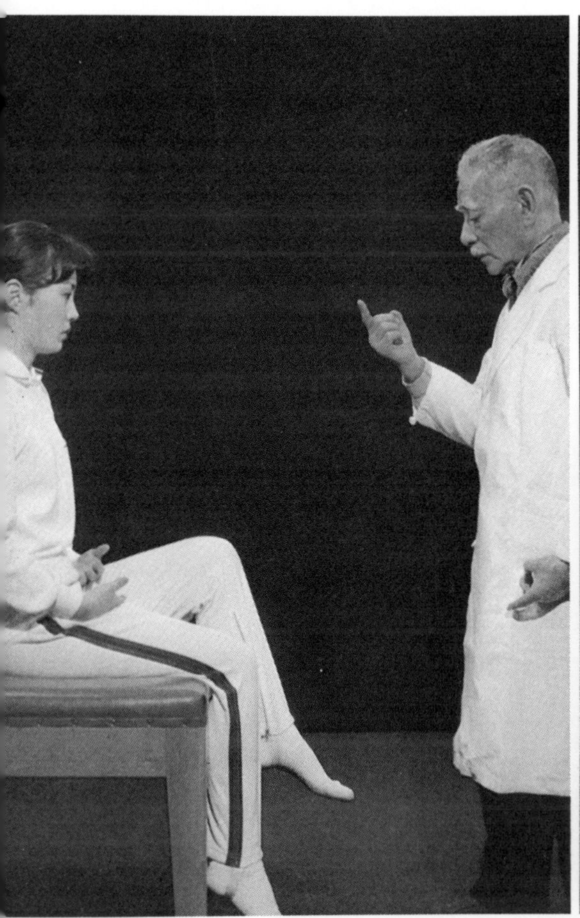

Fig. 21 Seated A

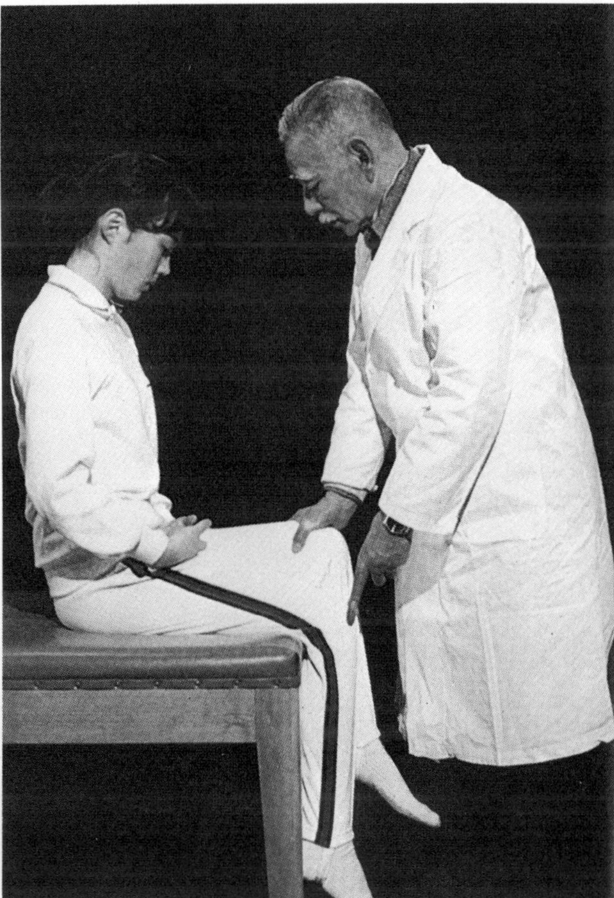

Fig. 22 Seated A

Seated A

Dōshin: Sitting with her legs over the edge of the table, the patient alternately lifts the left and the right leg (Fig. 21). The difference in the sensation of comfort and discomfort produced by these movements is noted.

Sōtai: When this mobility examination indicates that lifting of the right leg produces the greater sensation of discomfort, the patient lifts her left leg as the therapist gently applies resistance against this movement (Fig. 22). (Refer to page 90 for detailed instructions.)

Mobility Examination and Sōtai Technique for Rotation of Trunk
—*Eliminating pain and fatigue in the back and lumbar areas*

Seated D-1

In this technique, the rotational mobility of the trunk and the difference in sensation of comfort or discomfort produced by these bilateral movements of the trunk are examined (Fig. 23).

The patient must rotate her trunk without shifting the center of gravity. Movements which displace the body's center of gravity greatly reduce the effectiveness of the technique. The therapist must be sure the patient understands this point before proceeding with the movements. (Refer to page 100 for detailed instructions.)

Mobility Examination and Sōtai Technique for Lateral Trunk Flexion
—*Eliminating pain and fatigue in the back and lumbar areas*

Seated D-2

The difference in sensations produced by the alternate flexion of the trunk to the left and right are examined in this technique (Fig. 24). As in D-1, it is important that careful attention is paid to maintain the body's center of gravity. (Refer to page 102 for detailed instructions.)

Fig. 23 Seated D-1

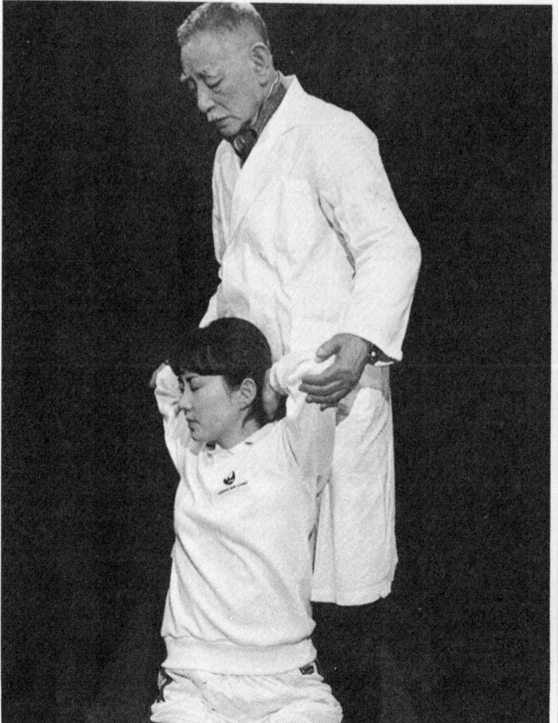

Fig. 24 Seated D-2

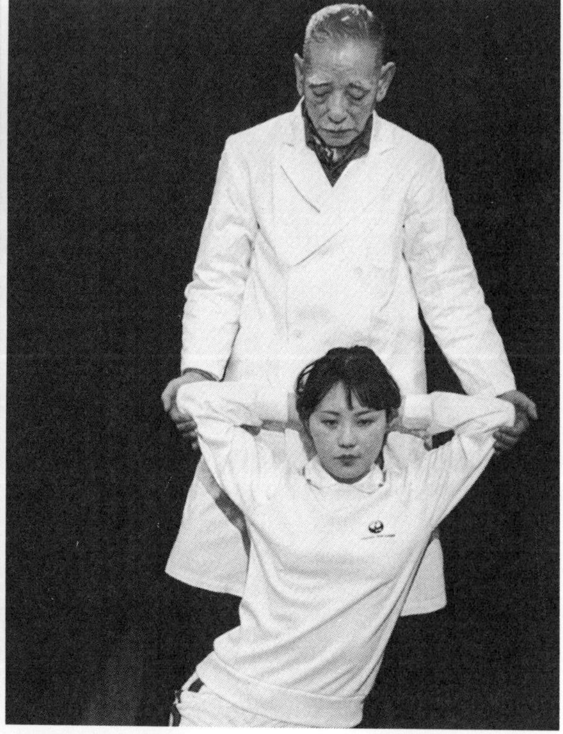

Sōtai Technique for Anterior Flexion of Trunk
—Eliminating pain and fatigue in the back and lumbar areas; alleviation of hypotension and digestive problems; increasing mobility at the waist

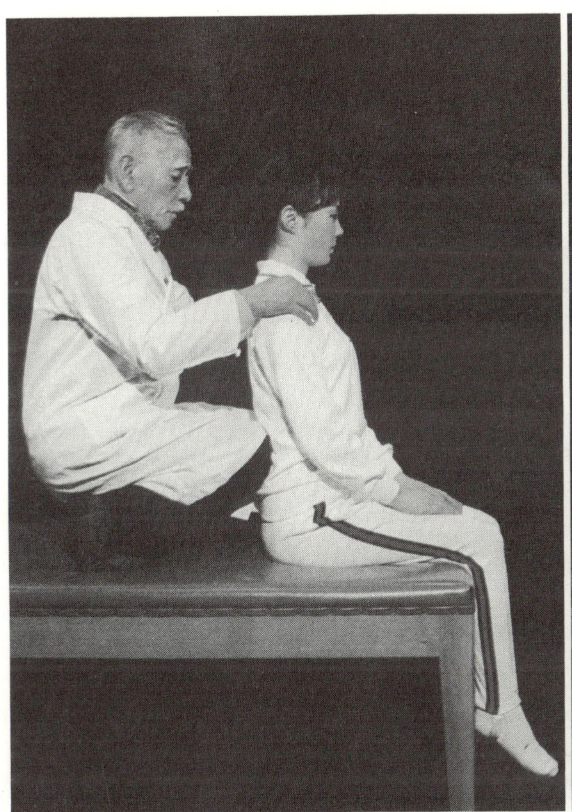

Fig. 25 Seated I

Fig. 26 Seated I

Seated I
The therapist provides support to limit the mobility of the patient by placing his knees against the patient's back at the point where the discomfort is felt. The therapist then places his hands on the patient's shoulders and applies resistance as the patient flexes her trunk forward in the Sōtai movement (Figs. 25 and 26).

By the therapist using his knees to provide points of support which limit the mobility of the spine, it becomes possible to effect anteflexion of the spine from the fifth thoracic vertebra up. This technique is used for restoring the normal spinal curvature. (Refer to page 118 for detailed instructions.)

Sōtai Technique for Extension of Trunk
—*Eliminating pain and fatigue in the back and lumbar areas; relief from tension in cervical and cranial areas; increasing mobility at the waist*

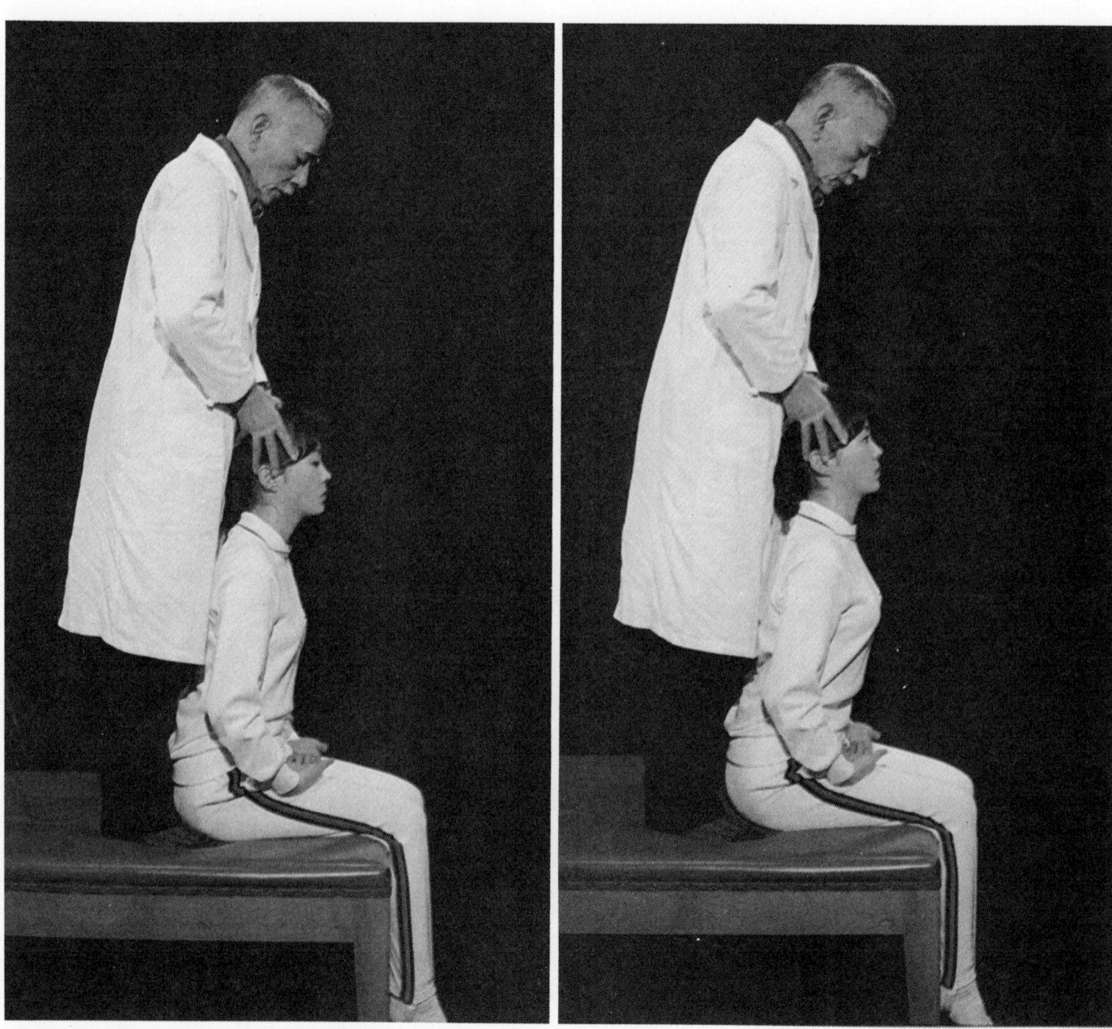

Fig. 27 Seated I *Fig. 28 Seated I*

Seated I
As the patient extends her torso in an upward direction, the therapist applies resistance either at the top of her head, or at the first thoracic vertebra (Figs. 27 and 28). The patient relaxes this movement of extension all at once after three to five seconds. This technique is also used to restore the normal spinal curvature.

Mobility Examination and Sōtai Technique for Rotation of Trunk
—*Relief from fatigue, tension, and pain in the back and lumbar areas*

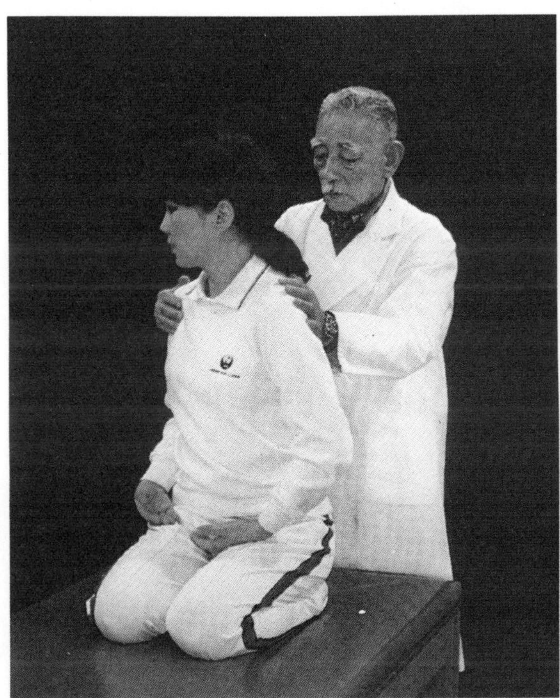

Fig. 29 Seiza D

Fig. 30 Seiza D

Seiza D

This is the same technique as the Seated D-1 Sōtai technique, shown in Figure 23, except that it is executed in the Seiza posture; the movements are exactly the same (Figs. 29 and 30). Since the freedom in the joints of the legs differes between the Seiza and seated positions (lower legs hang over the edge of the table free of the floor in the seated position), the effect of the same Sōtai technique also differs.

2. MOBILITY EXAMINATION AND SŌTAI TECHNIQUES

In Japanese, the characters used in the word *Sōtai* are the same but in the reverse order as those used in the word *Taisō*, which means exercise. The character *Sō* (操) means to work or manipulate as one would manipulate a puppet, and the character *Tai* (体) means body. The meaning of Sōtai therefore, is manipulation or movement of the body for the purpose of restoring or maintaining health. The important features of Sōtai Therapy are as follows:

1. *Tiring and painful movements are avoided,* unlike many exercise programs on television and elsewhere.
2. *No set rhythm is followed,* differing from the feats of gymnasts.
3. *Power and speed are not required.* Gentle movements are made in the most comfortable direction which is judged subjectively by the patient.
4. *Movements are made in the most relaxed manner possible while exhaling.* Natural principles of motion are applied. What exactly is the direction of most comfortable movement? In order to find this direction, the part of the body in question is moved in all possible directions by alternately flexing and extending as well as rotating it to the right and left. The patient's sensations accompanying these movements are noted.
5. *Mobility examination (Dōshin)* refers to this examination of mobility in which the direction of comfort and discomfort in movement are determined.
6. *Comfort* refers to movements made with ease.
7. *Discomfort* refers to movements made with difficulty. When the direction of most comfortable movement is determined, the body should be—
8. *Relaxed* as completely as possible, and while—
9. *Exhaling* the breath, the movement is executed—
10. *Slowly.* This movement is made against—
11. *Light resistance* applied by the therapist. When the—
12. *Comfortabe extent of mobility* has been reached, the body is—
13. *Held* motionless for three to five seconds, after which all tension is—
14. *Released* at once, whereupon a therapeutic effect is obtained. The nature of this effect is such that—
15. *Reduction or elimination of pain and discomfort* experienced while motionless, as well as during movement is obtained. (This includes pain resulting from organic disorders.) At times, the effect extends to elimination of mental and physical symptoms, as well as reducing restrictions in mobility stemming from various causes. In Sōtai Therapy, with the exception of special patients, the patients make the movements themselves, using their own strength. This is hereafter referred to as—
16. *Active movement.* A similar effect can be obtained by producing these movements with another person providing the necessary motive force, so long as the movement is in the direction of greatest comfort. This movement made with assistance from a therapist is hereafter referred to as—
17. *Passive movement.* It can be said that our bodies possess a propensity toward comfort through motion. This principle is utilized in the techniques introduced in this book.

Definition of Terms

Although only the fundamental techniques of Sōtai Therapy are covered in this book, some specialized terms are used in referring to parts of the body and their movements. The special terms used often in Sōtai Therapy are defined below.

Therapist—The person who performs the mobility examination and Sōtai techniques

Patient—The person who receives the Sōtai treatment

Intrinsic force—The force exerted by the patient to effect active movement

Extrinsic force—The force applied by the therapist to produce passive movement of the patient; movement not dependent upon the patient's own strength

Comfort—Ease in movement or in being moved; a state in which movement does not create in sensations of pain or discomfort

Discomfort—Difficulty in movement or in being moved; movement is not smooth and easy, and causes pain in some cases.

Difference in sensation—The difference between the sensations felt by the patient when making a movement in one direction, compared to that felt during movement in the opposite direction: The phrase "ease in movement" and "difficulty in movement" refer only to ease and difficulty in relation to movement in the opposite direction, or with the opposing limb. This is a comparison of subjective sensations reported by the patient during two movements in the opposite direction or with opposing limbs.

Mobility examination (Dōshin)—A technique by which a part of the body is moved in order to determine whether that movement is easy or difficult: The movements of this examination are performed slowly and gently. Refer to Supine L-1-1 and -2 (see p. 67 and p. 68), where the patient's head is rotated to the left and the right. When the direction in which the movement is more comfortable is judged by the patient while making Sōtai movements, this is called an active mobility examination. When the therapist uses his hands to rotate the patient's head for this purpose, as in the figures, this is called a passive mobility examination.

Pressure sensitive point—A point or area on the body where tenderness or pain is felt when pressed by the fingers or palm.

Tension (stiffness)—On a healthy body, any area that is relaxed feels soft to the touch when lightly pressed with the fingers or palm. Tension is the condition in which due to various causes, hardness develops in the muscular and connective tissues over a broad area.

Induration (knot)—Similar to tension, but affecting a smaller area (from that barely palpable to the fingertips, to hard areas the size of a large marble).

Special patient—A patient incapable of initiating Sōtai movements with own strength (i.e., incapable of active movement).

Distortion—An abnormal morphological condition in which a part or the whole of the body is structurally unsound.

Tortility—An abnormal morphological condition in which a certain part of the body is chronically twisted or turned

Curvature—An abnormal morphological condition in which a part of the body is curved or "warped."

Protrusion—An abnormal morphological condition in which a part of the body projects out, or is slightly elevated compared to normal.

Inclination—An abnormal morphological condition in which the body or a particular part of it leans toward a certain direction.

Sensation of weight—When the therapist lifts both the patient's feet by holding the same toe on either foot (refer to page 35 for this Dōshin technique), in some cases the therapist can feel a distinct difference between the sensations of weight produced when lifting with the fifth toes as compared to lifting with the third toes.

Bilateral movement—In movement of a single segment, this term refers to two identical movements performed in opposite directions, such as the rotation of the head to the left and right. In movement of paired segments (limbs) it refers to identical movements performed on the left and right, such as extension of the right and left legs.

Seiza (say-za)—This is the traditional Japanese sitting posture where one sits with the legs folded underneath. This posture is becoming less common with the increasing trend toward westernization in Japan today. Nevertheless, it is the formal sitting posture, especially in rooms with *tatami* floors (rice straw matting), where simple sitting cushions are provided for this purpose. This posture with its straight back is traditionally held in Japan to be the most proper posture. Hence, its name "Seiza," which literally means "right sitting." (Refer to page 25 and 140 for illustrations.)

Guidlines for Using This Manual

Much consideration has been given to arrange the figures in this book in a simple and easy to use format. Therefore they should be studied in the numerical order which they are presented. Refer to the captions under the figures or look for that particular figure number to find the explanation for each procedure.

1. The symbols: "Supine G-1" signifies the first procedure (movement) of technique G with the patient lying in the supine position. Accordingly, "Seated I-5" is the fifth procedure (movement) of technique I executed with the patient in the seated position.

2. Morphological observation (figures with black background): See chapter 4 "Checkpoints for Morphological Observation."

3. Palpation examination (figures with black background): In this examination, the therapist looks for indurations or abnormal tension in specific areas of the patient's body. The therapist probes for pressure sensitive points with his hands, and the painful or pleasant sensations produced when applying pressure are noted.

4. Dōshin (mobility examination) (figures with black background): This always indicates bilateral movement of the right and left sides, or that in opposite directions, for the purpose of comparison.

5. Sōtai technique (figures with white background): This indicates movement in one direction only. In the actual Sōtai treatment, the therapist first examines the mobility and the accompanying sensations produced in the patient by performing a mobility examination. The Sōtai technique is performed immediately following this, based on the initial observations.

6. Hand placement and applying resistance: Care must be taken when the therapist uses his hands in moving or resisting movement made by the patient; no more force than is absolutely necessary must be used. The resistance applied against the patient's movements should be as light and steady as possible so as to enable a balanced and steady movement. (Refer to Chapter 3.)

7. Performing the Sōtai techniques

A. Hardness of the working surface—Sōtai can be performed on any surface including the floor, a bed, a long desk, or a table, provided that it is covered with an appropriate amount of padding. (*Tatami* floors are commonly used in Japan.) If the surface which the body comes in contact with is too soft, this could cause the patient to make the Sōtai movement in a less than ideal manner. Sinking down on a soft surface is quite undesirable. The appropriate firmness for the working surface is that of a sheet of plywood covered with a blanket.

B. Slipping—A little slipping or sliding of the patient on the working surface while performing the Sōtai movements is no cause for concern. There are actually cases where a certain amount of slipping increases the effectiveness of a Sōtai movement.

C. Relaxing the body as completely as possible—In our daily lives forceful movement are usually made to accomplish specific objectives. The movements described in this book are for the purpose of transforming difficulty of movement (discomfort) into ease of movement (comfort). Since forceful movements make it difficult to ascertain the subtle differences in sensation, the use of force in making these movements is absolutely unacceptable

D. Exhaling with each movement—When exhalation accompanies the movement of the body, the movement becomes controlled and stable and allows for increased sensitivity. In illustration of this fact, when striking another person, one usually holds his breath while striking. Inhaling while striking is extremely difficult. Taking this analogy a step further, the effect is much more pronounced if one strikes while exhaling.

E. Slow movement—The proper speed for these movements may be likened to the speed for moving one's hand immersed just below the surface of water without creating ripples. The proper speed differs between children and adults, and even between adults in many cases. Slow movement is essential when examining for physical sensations produced by Sōtai movements.

F. Appropriate resistance—Refer to the Supine L–1–1 and –2 on pages 67 and 68 in which the patient's head is rotated bilaterally. When it is found that rotation to the left causes discomfort (more difficulty in turning the head to the left), the patient uses her own strength to turn her head in the opposite direction (toward the right). The therapist applies gentle resistance against this movement which should be relaxed and slow.

G. Suitable position—The proper range of movements in performing Sōtai is between the farthest points on either extreme of the comfortable range of mobility for the patient. The suitable position is reached at the farthest extent of the particular motion, at which the patient is still comfortable. The Sōtai movement is brought to a stop at this point.

H. Holding—In holding, the therapist and the patient continue to apply approximately the same amount of force used during the movement portion of the Sōtai technique. Only the movement is brought to a stop while the therapist maintains the same steady resistance.

I. Releasing tension—The force applied during the motionless period while holding is released all at once. The tension held by the therapist and patient must be released completely and instantaneously rather than partially or gradually*.

When the mobility examination is performed gently and slowly according to the above instructions, sensations of comfort and discomfort in movement can be readily discerned by the patient. Using these initial movements and the sensations they produce as a guide, the Sōtai movement is performed slowly in unison with exhaling of the patient's breath.

---

*The patient is first to relax all effort (release) so that the resistance provided by the therapist causes a brief movement in the opposite direction. The controlled force applied by the therapist is maintained just an instant longer to move the patient back to the original position, and is released before the movement goes beyond the starting point. For all practical purposes the releasing action on the part of the patient and therapist are simultaneous, so it is described as such.

Supine Position

Supine A-1

Dōshin: The therapist places a hand on the patient's side and alternately applies pressure on the left and then on the right hip from above (Figs. 1 and 2). Next the therapist alternately lifts the left and right hips from bleow (Figs. 3 and 4), and checks for sensations of comfort or discomfort

Objective of procedure:

a. In cases where there is no abdominal pain or discomfort, to determine whether pain or discomfort is sensed when the patient's hip is pressed from above or lifted from below to a height of 5 to 10 centimeters.
b. In cases where abdominal pain is present, to determine whether discomfort increases or pain becomes worse when the patient's hip is pressed from above or lifted from below.
c. In cases where the patient does not feel anything in the supine position, to determine whether application of pressure or lifting produces sensations of heaviness discomfort, or pain in other parts of the body.

Fig. 1 Supine A-1–1

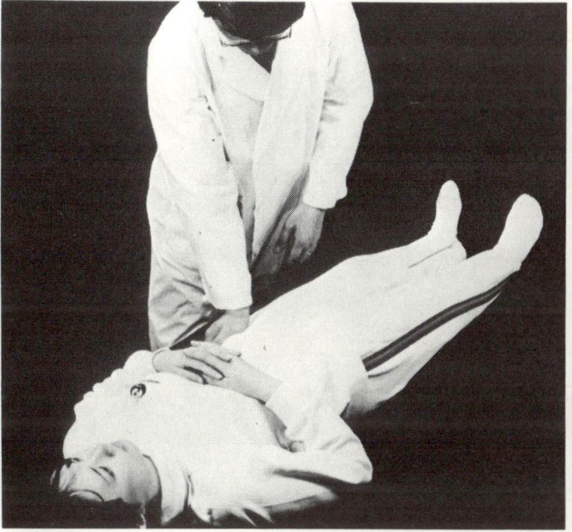

Fig. 2 Supine A-1–2

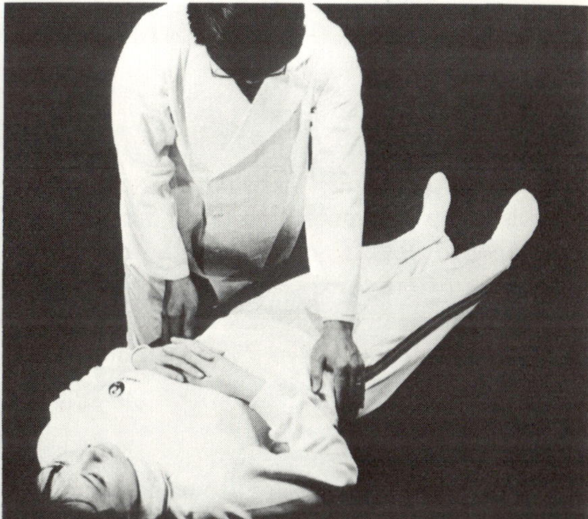

Fig. 3 Supine A-1–3

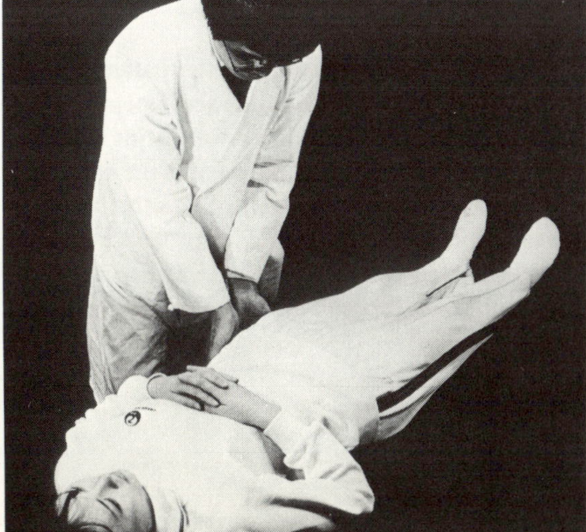

Fig. 4 Supine A-1–4

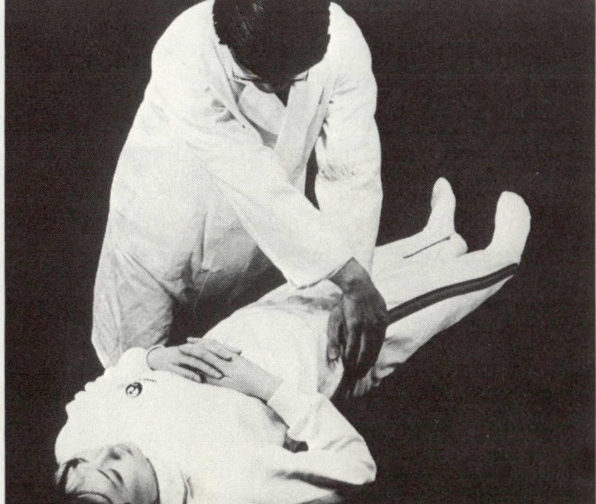

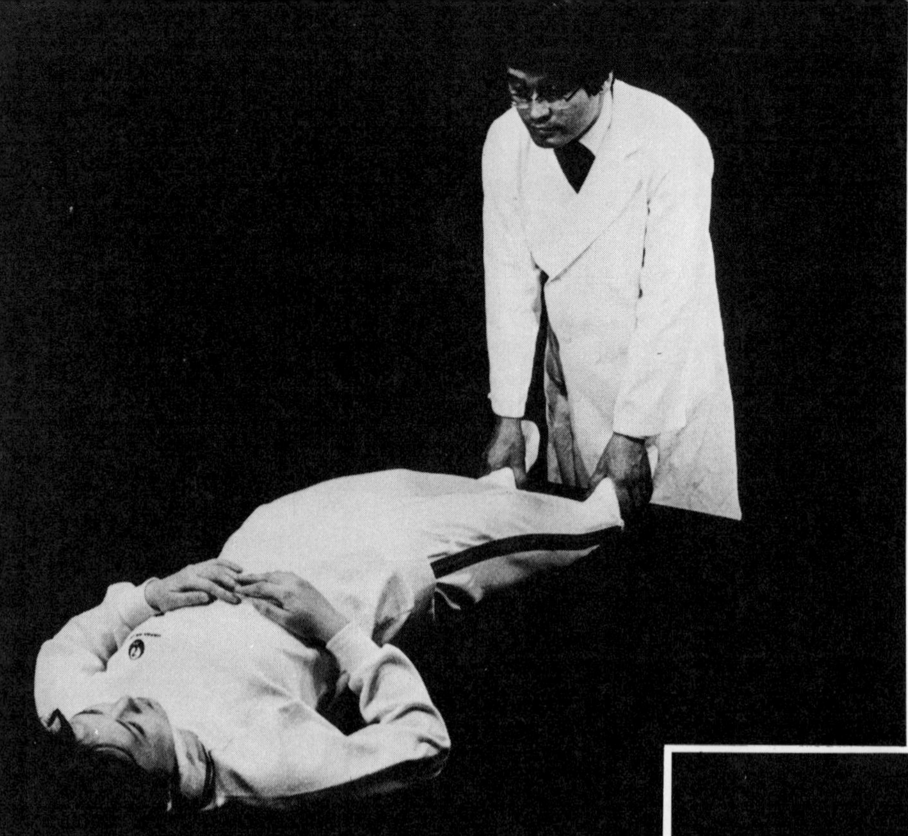

Fig. 5 Supine A-2–1

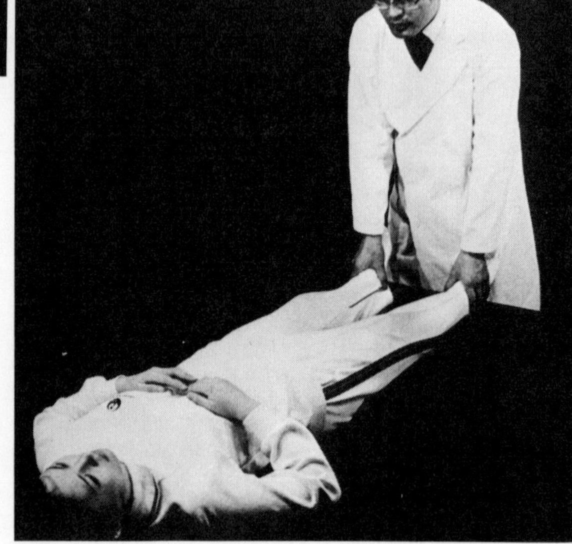

Fig. 6 Supine A-2–2

Supine A-2

Sōtai: The patient uses her shoulders and heels as points of support and raises her buttocks upward (Figs. 5 and 6). After holding this posture for two to three seconds, the patient releases the tension of her body all at once and lets her hips fall back down. This procedure is repeated two or three times.

Objective of procedure:

a. To release excess tension from the patient's body.
b. To help the patient, as far as possible, to assume a natural and straight posture.
c. In cases where there is no complaint of pain, to examine the extent to which pain is produced and the manner in which pain radiates from the hips to other parts of the body when the hips are dropped suddenly.
d. To give patients self confidence in knowing that they are capable of performing such movements.

Supine B-1

Dōshin: The therapist holds the patient's feet (Figs. 7 and 8), and turns the feet laterally and medially (eversion and inversion) using the line through the center of the heel and the third toe as the axis. The amount of comfort or discomfort is determined. This procedure is performed by holding the ankle at the most natural angle vertically, for the patient.

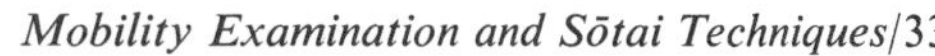

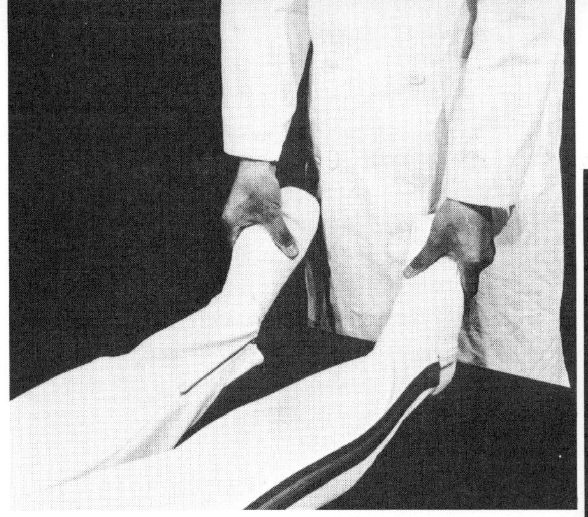

Fig. 7 Supine B-1–1

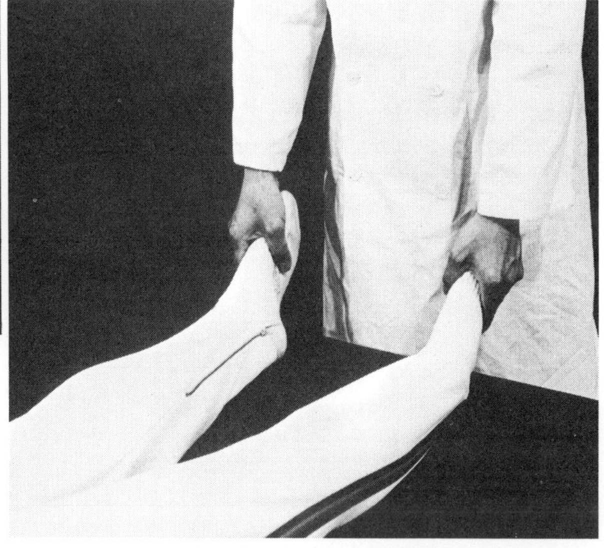

Fig. 8 Supine B-1–2

Supine B-2

Dōshin: The therapist grasps the patient's toes (Figs. 9 and 10), and rotates the feet to the left and then to the right using the heels as pivot points. Sensations of comfort and discomfort are noted. As an alternative procedure, both feet may be turned outward to the open position, and inward to the closed position by pivoting the movement on the heels (Figs. 11 and 12); any sensation of discomfort at this time is noted.

Fig. 9 Supine B-2–1

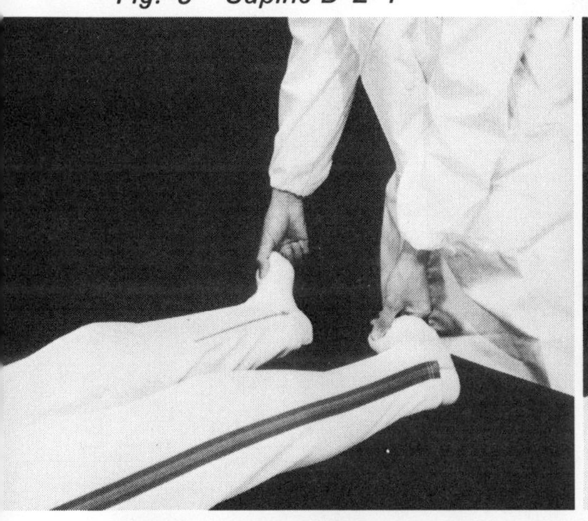

Fig. 10 Supine B-2–2

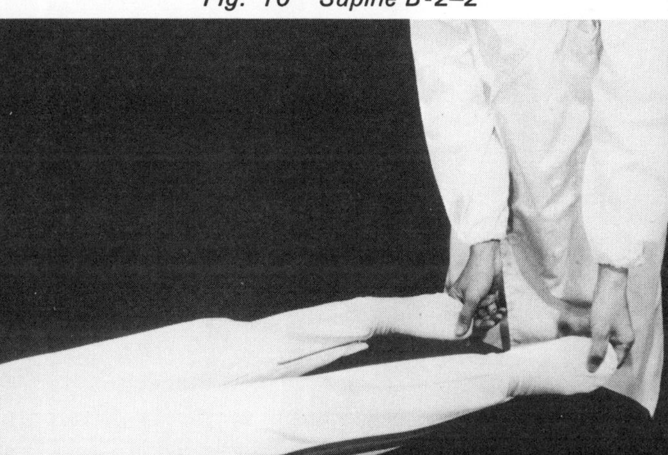

Fig. 11 Supine B-2–3

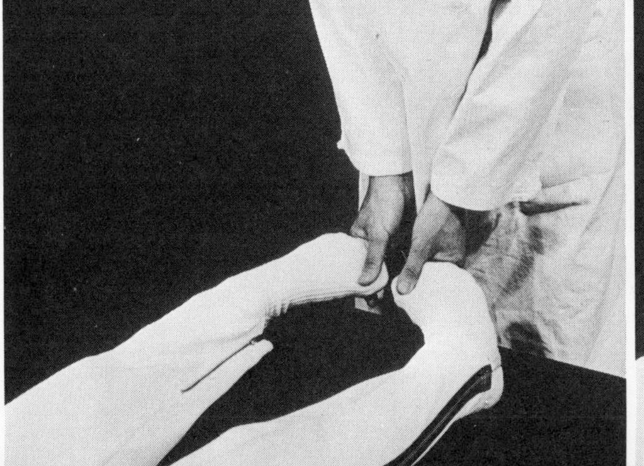

Fig. 12 Supine B-2–4

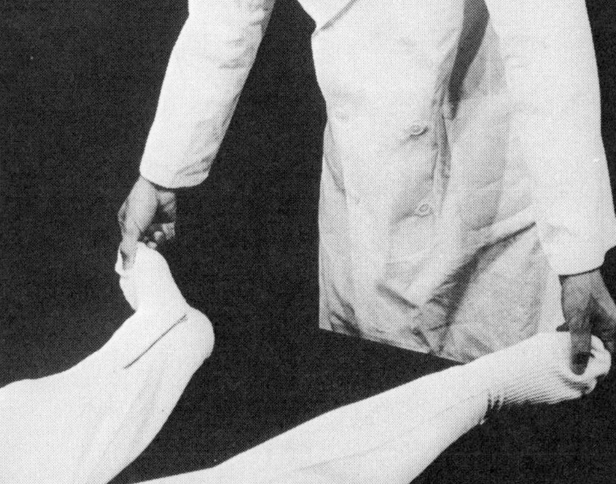

Supine B-3

Dōshin: The therapist places his hands on both the patient's feet (Fig. 13), and stretches the ankles by pressing the toes downward. Then, placing his hands on the toes (Fig. 14), the ankles are flexed by pressing the toes back toward the shins. Comfort and discomfort as well as the difference in the amount of mobility between the right and the left feet are examined.

Although the therapist is shown performing the mobility examination on both feet at once in the pictures for Supine B-1, B-2, and B-3, it is also possible to perform the examination separately for each foot to account for impediments in either foot. Figures 15 and 16 of Supine B-3 show this examination being performed separately on each foot.

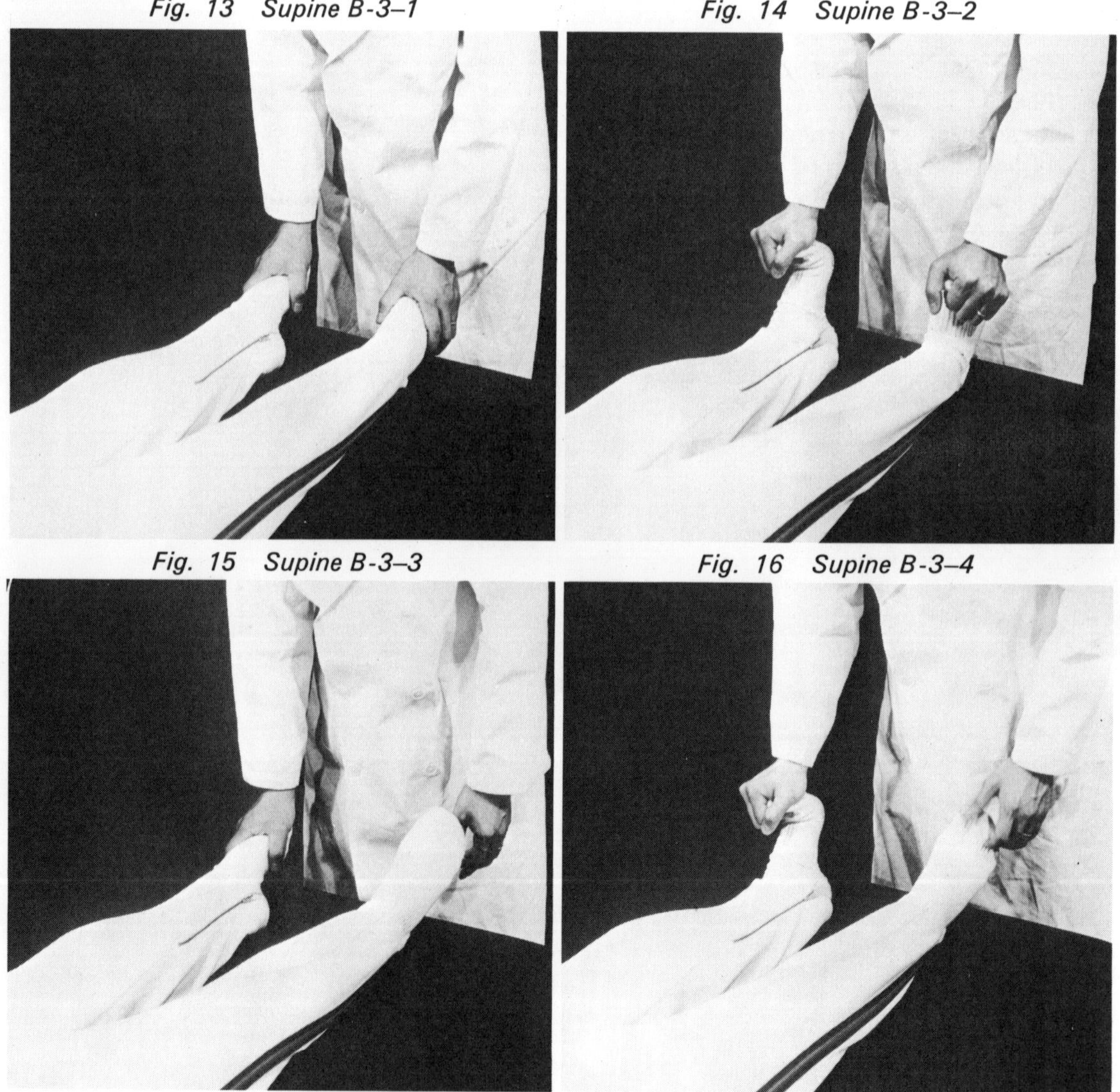

Fig. 13 Supine B-3–1

Fig. 14 Supine B-3–2

Fig. 15 Supine B-3–3

Fig. 16 Supine B-3–4

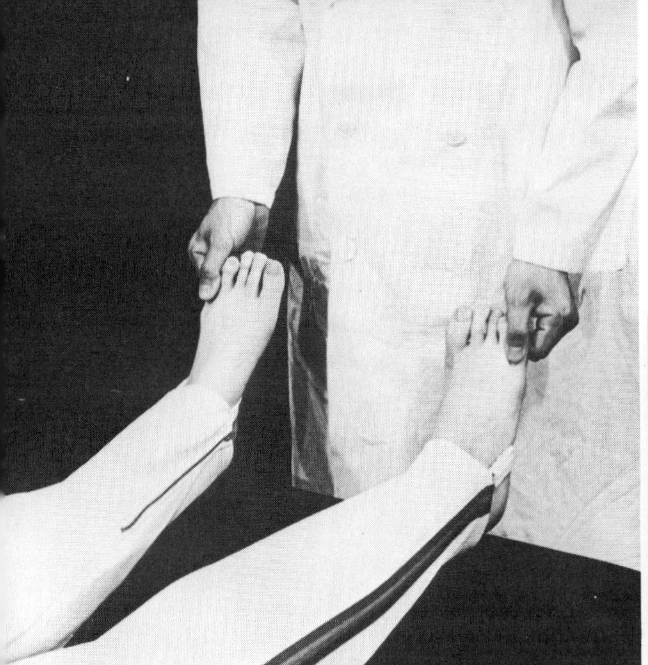

Fig. 17 Supine B-4–1

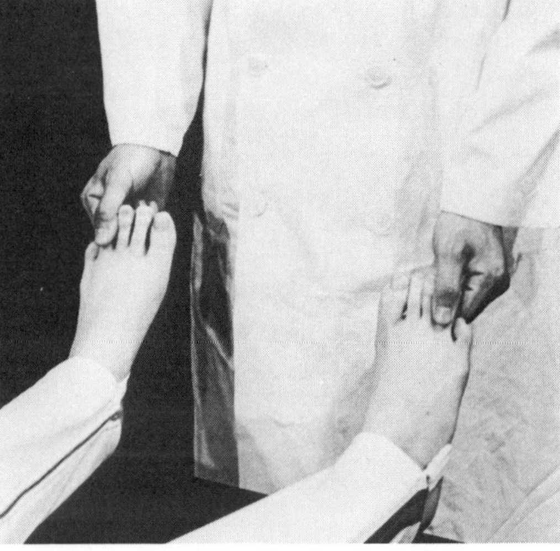

Fig. 18 Supine B-4–2

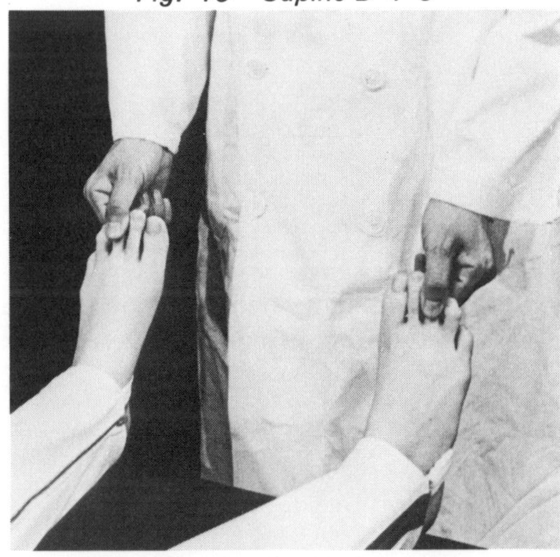

Fig. 19 Supine B-4–3

Supine B-4

a) The therapist grasps a pair of toes successively from the first toes through the fifth, and the patient's legs are lifted each time by the pair of toes to see if any difference can be felt in their weight (Figs. 17 to 19). When the therapist feels a greater weight when lifting the legs with a certain pair of toes, this indicates that there is resistance in the movement of the patient's feet or toes.

b) Sensations of comfort or discomfort as well as the hardness of the joints are examined by flexing, rotating, and twisting each toe (Figs. 20 and 21).

c) The toes are palpated to examine their hardness, softness, stiffness, induration, and abnormal tension of their surface and muscles.

Fig. 20 Supine B-4–4

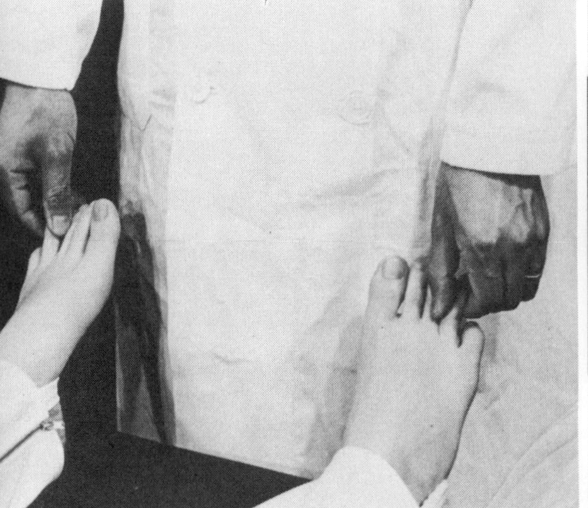

Fig. 21 Supine B-4–5

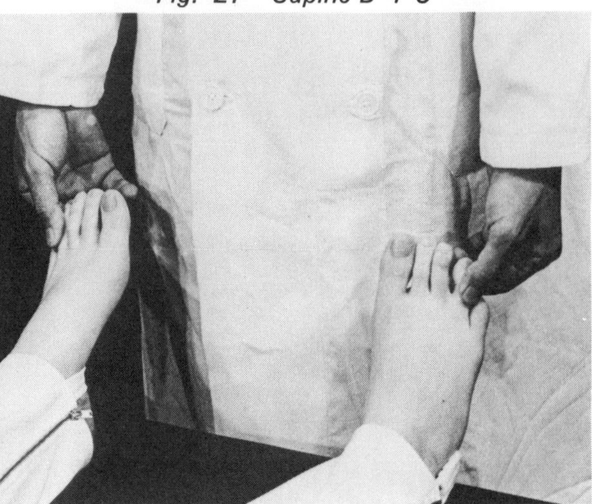

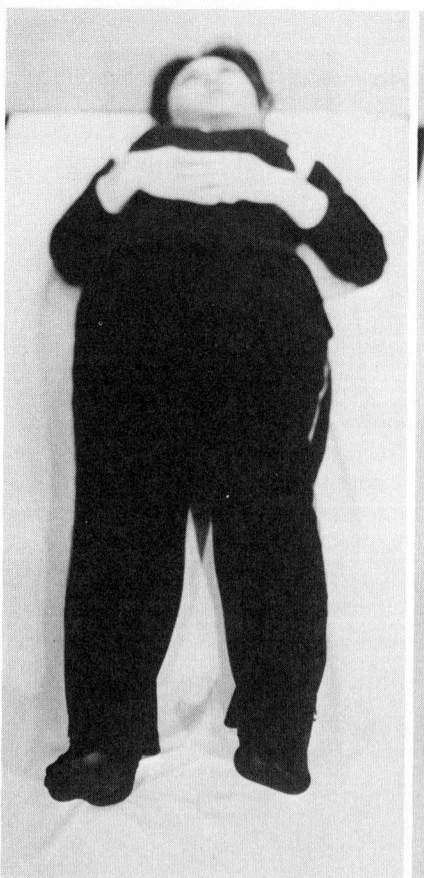

Fig. 22 Supine C-1–1

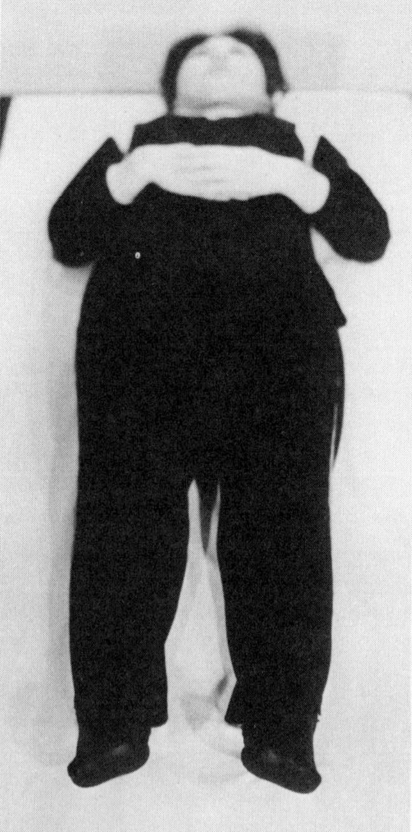

Fig. 23 Supine C-1–2

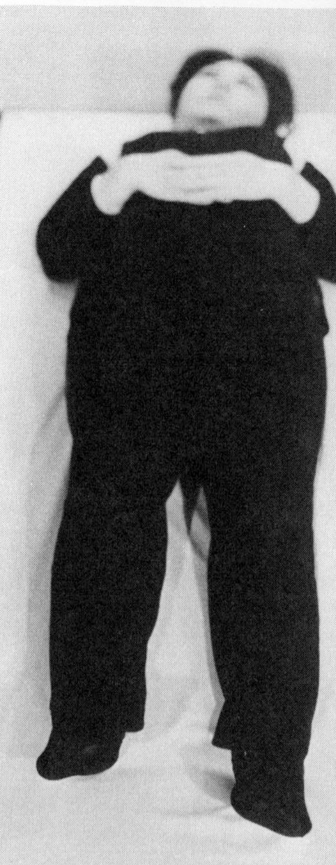

Fig. 24 Supine C-1–3

Supine C-1

Dōshin: In the supine position, the patient slowly extends and then retracts (shortens) one leg at a time, paying attention to any sensation of comfort or discomfort (Figs. 22 to 24). If the patient's movements are observed closely at this time, it can be seen that the extension of one leg corresponds with the retraction of the other.

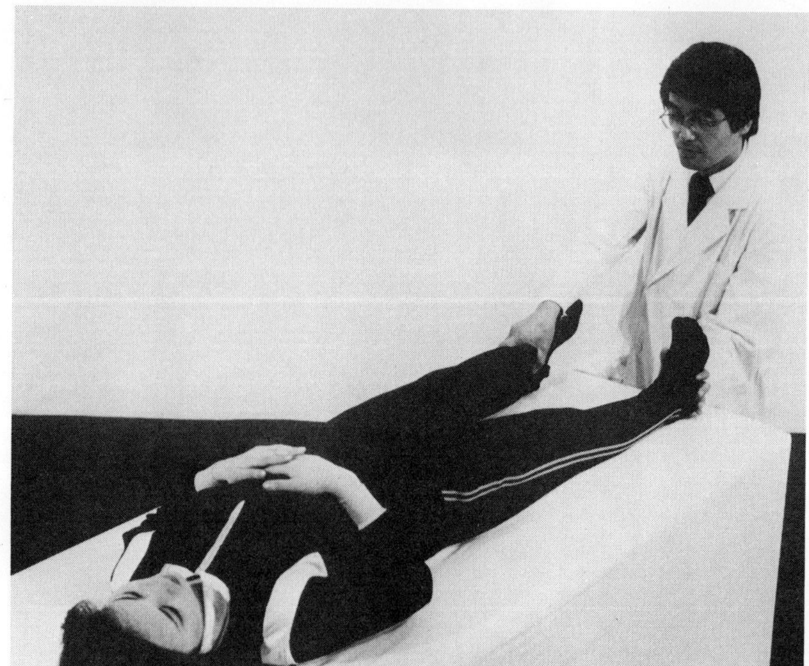

Fig. 25 Supine C-1–4

Sōtai: The patient extends her right leg and retracts her left leg at the same time. The therapist applies resistance to these movements by pushing the bottom of the foot (specially the heel) on the extending foot, and by holding the ankle of the retracting leg (Fig. 25). When the full extent of mobility is reached, they both hold the tension for three to five seconds; after which, the patient and therapist release this tension simultaneously. This procedure is repeated two or three times.

Supine C-2

Dōshin: With the patient in a supine position, the therapist lifts first the right leg, and then the left leg to a height of 10 centimeters from the working surface. The therapist extends and then pushes the lifted leg inward, inquiring about the presence of any discomfort (Figs. 26 through 29).

Sōtai: The therapist lifts the patient's left leg about 10 centimeters up from the floor or treatment table (Fig. 30). While the patient retracts her lifted leg, the therapist applies resistance against this movement (Fig. 31). When the full extent of retraction is reached, both persons hold the tension for three to five seconds, and then relax their efforts simultaneously. This is repeated two or three times.

Fig. 26 Supine C-2–1

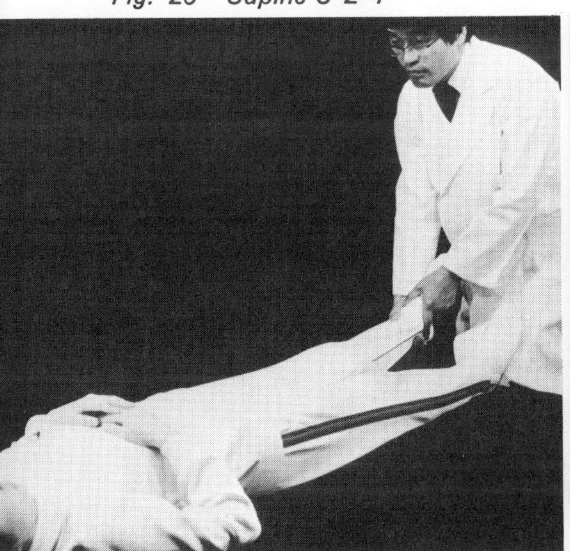

Fig. 27 Supine C-2–2

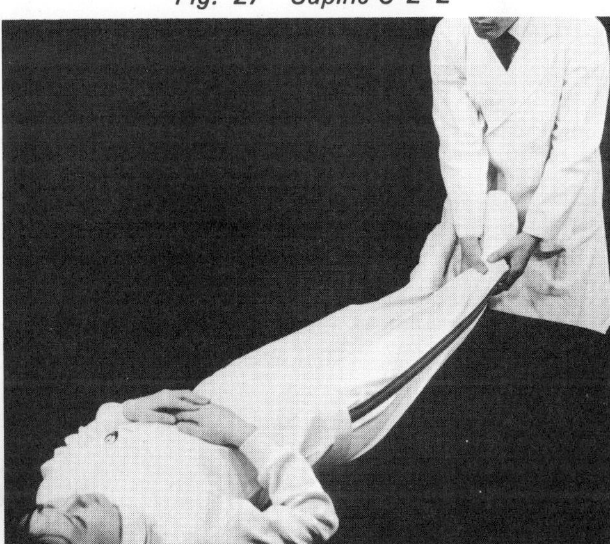

Fig. 28 Supine C-2–3

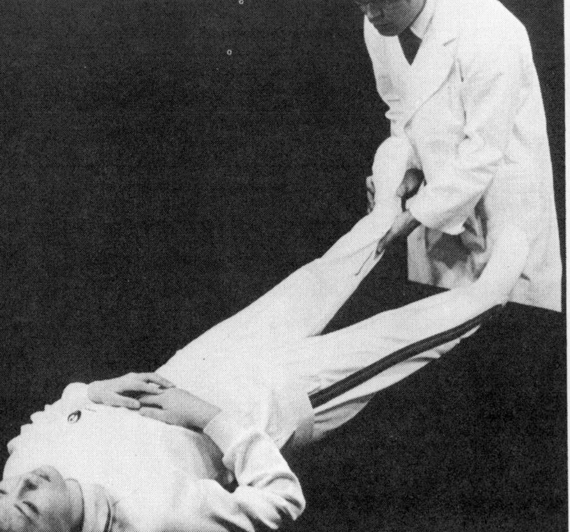

Fig. 29 Supine C-2–4

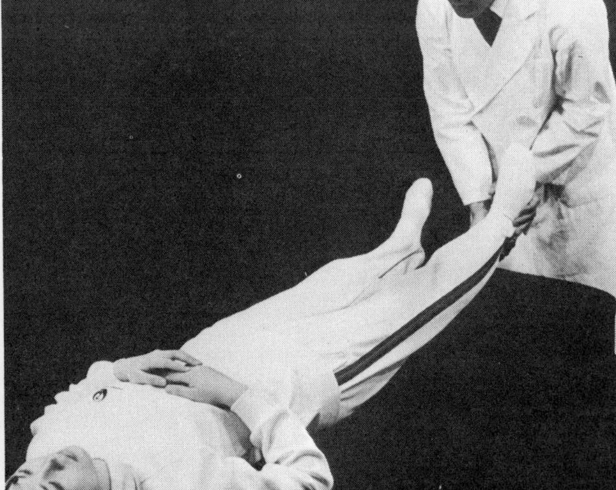

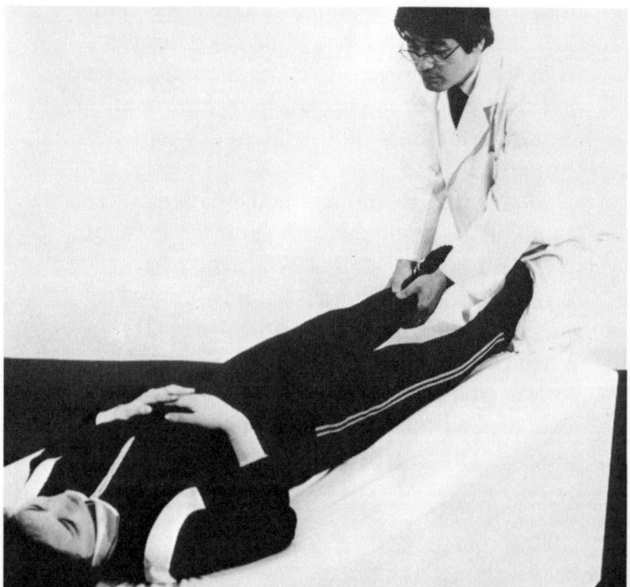

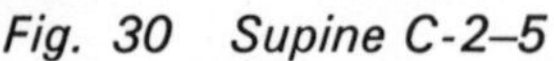

Fig. 30 Supine C-2–5

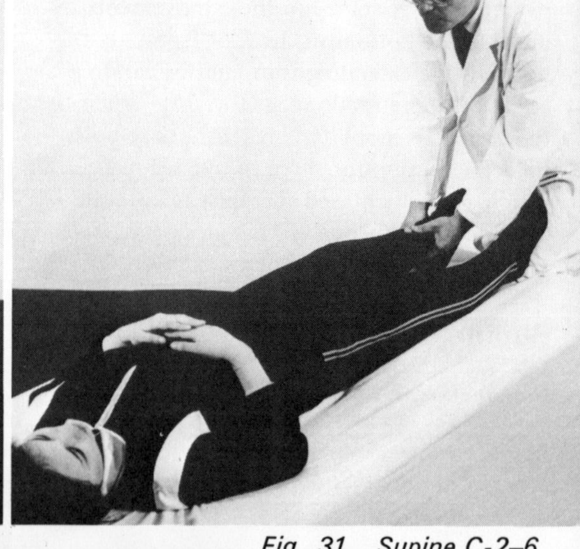

Fig. 31 Supine C-2–6

Supine D-1

Dōshin: The therapist places one hand on the patient's right or left heel and lifts the leg to a height of about 10 centimeters. With his other hand, the therapist grips the toes of the lifted foot and rotates the foot medially and laterally (to the inside and outside) pivoting the movement on the heel. Any sensation of comfort or discomfort are noted.

Fig. 32 Supine D-1–1

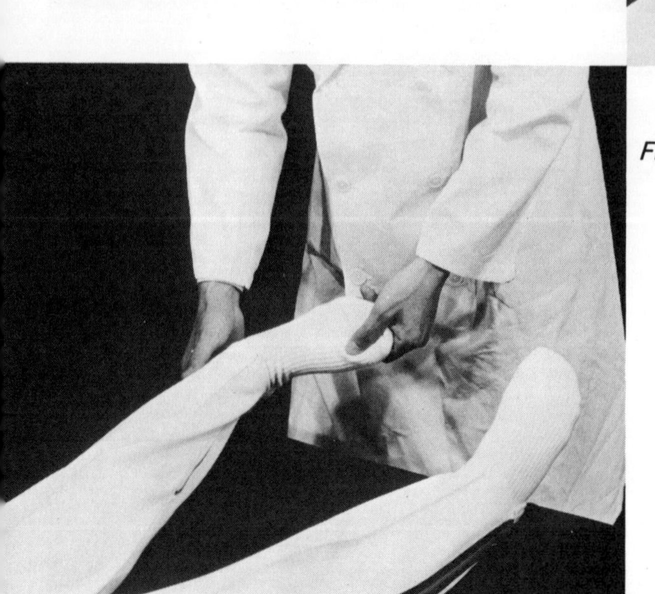

Fig. 33 Supine D-1–2

In Figure 32, the toes of the left foot are rotated laterally. Figure 33 shows medial rotation of the left foot. Figure 34 shows lateral rotation of the right foot, while Figure 35 shows medial rotation of the right foot.

Fig. 34 Supine D-1–3

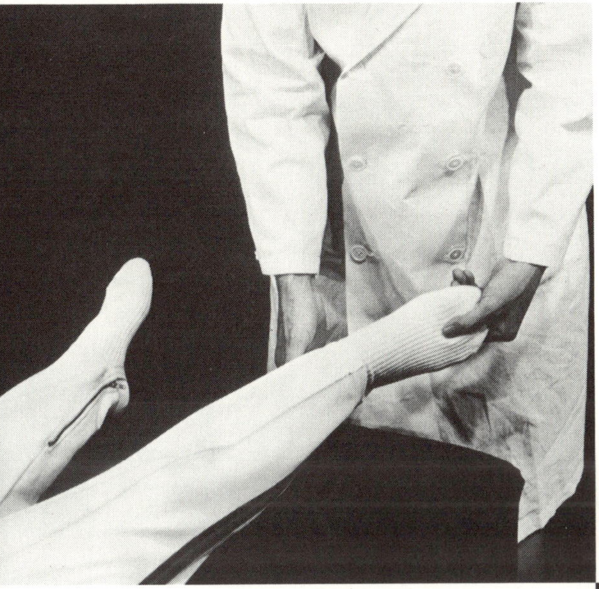

Sōtai I: Placing one hand under the patient's right heel, the therapist lifts the leg about 10 centimeters (Fig. 36). The patient rotates the toes of her right foot medially, pivoting this movement on the heel. The therapist applies resistance against this movement by gently holding the patient's toes with his other hand (Fig. 37). After holding tension for three to five seconds at a suitable position, both persons simultaneously release the tension. This is repeated two or three times.

Fig. 35 Supine D-1–4

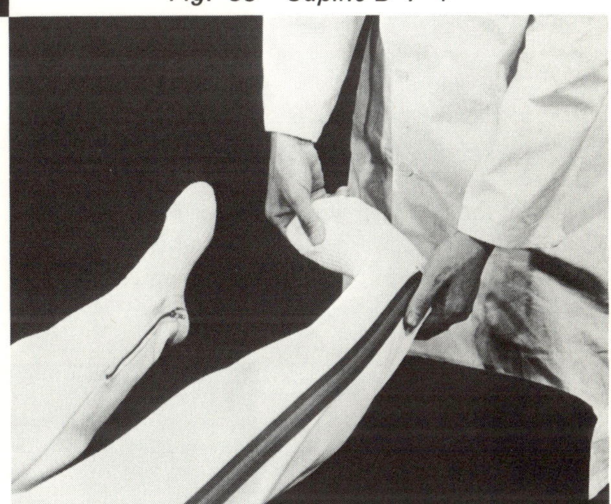

Sōtai II: The therapist raises the leg of the patient slightly (about 10 centimeters) by lifting with one hand under the heel (Fig. 38). The patient rotates her foot laterally, pivoting the movement on the right heel. The therapist applies resistance to this movement with his other hand by holding the toes of the patient's right foot (Fig. 39). After a suitable position has been reached, they both maintain tension for three to five seconds, and then relases in unison. This procedure is repeated two or three times.

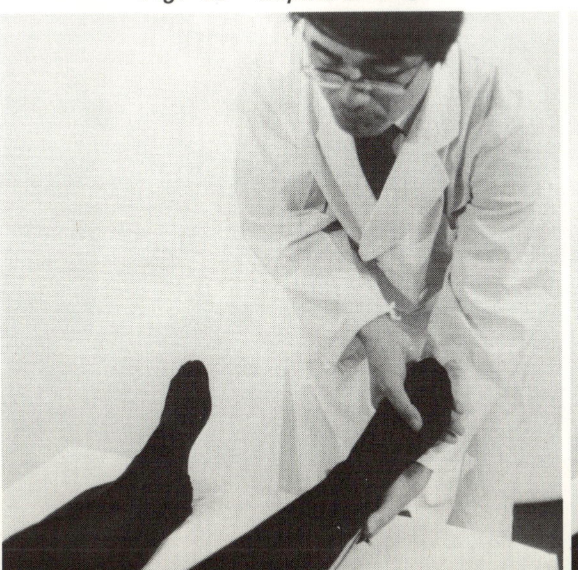

Fig. 36 Supine D-1–5

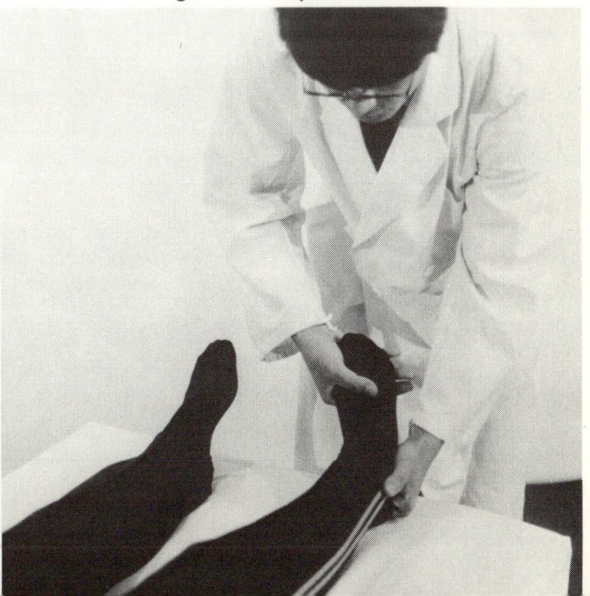

Fig. 37 Supine D-1–6

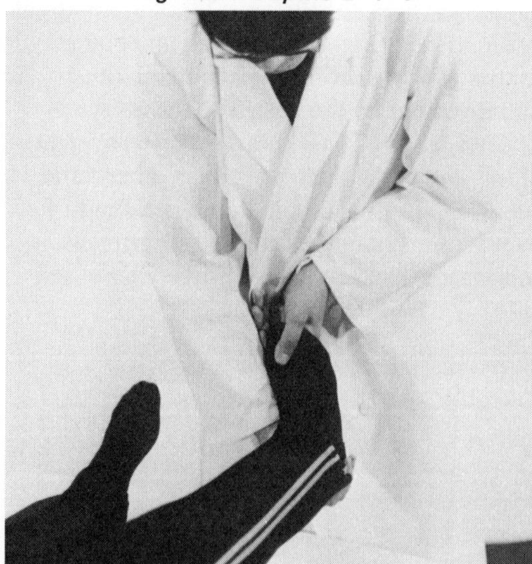

Fig. 38 Supine D-1–7

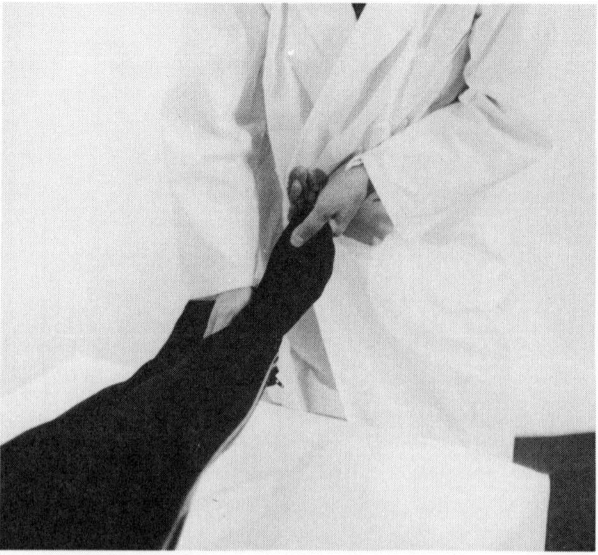

Fig. 39 Supine D-1–8

Supine D-2

Dōshin: Grasping the toes of the right or left foot with one hand, the therapist lifts the patient's leg about 10 centimeters. Holding the heel of the lifted leg with the other hand, the heel is rotated toward the right, and then toward the left, using the toes as the pivoting point. Any sensation of comfort or discomfort are noted.

The heel of the left foot is rotated medially in Figure 40, and laterally in Figure 41. In Figure 42, the heel of the right foot is rotated medially, while Figure 43 shows the right heel rotated laterally.

Fig. 40 Supine D-2–1

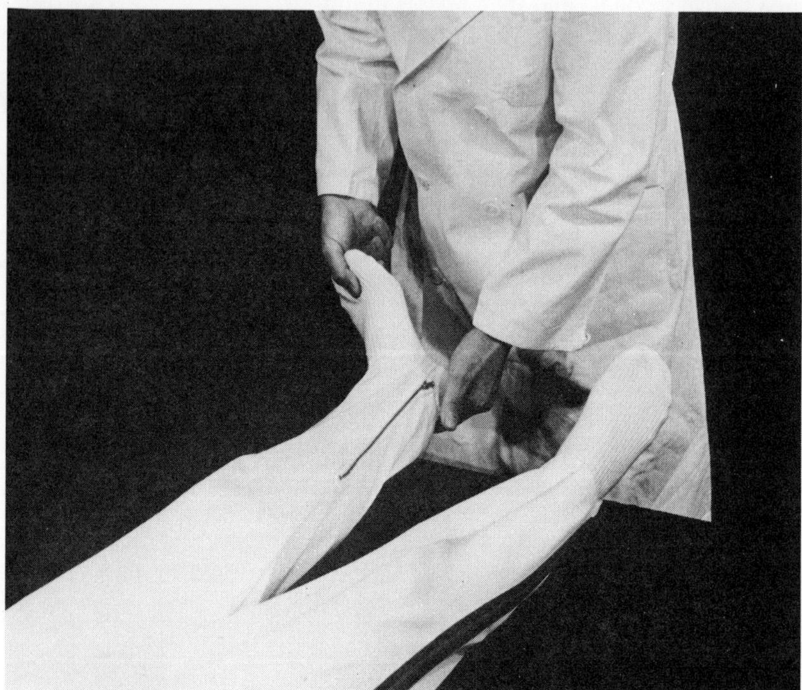

Sōtai I: Grasping the toes of the patient's left foot with one hand, the therapist slightly lifts the leg about 10 centimeters (Fig. 44). The patient rotates her heel laterally, pivoting the movement on the toes of her left foot. The therapist applies resistance against this movement by placing his other hand against the outside of the left heel (Fig. 45). After holding tension for three to five seconds at a suitable position, they release the tension together. This procedure is repeated two or three times.

Fig. 41 Supine D-2-2

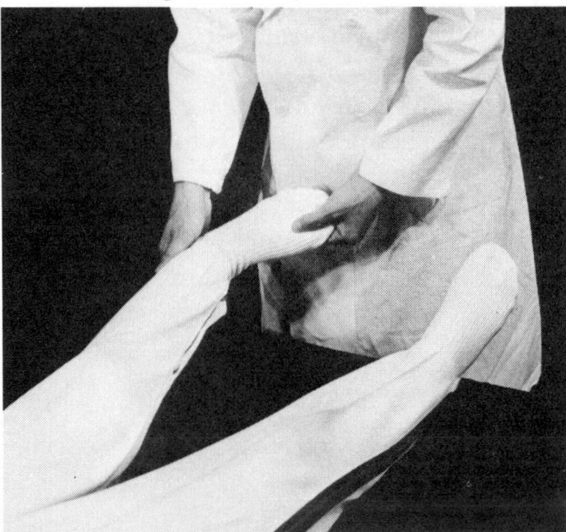

Fig. 42 Supine D-2-3

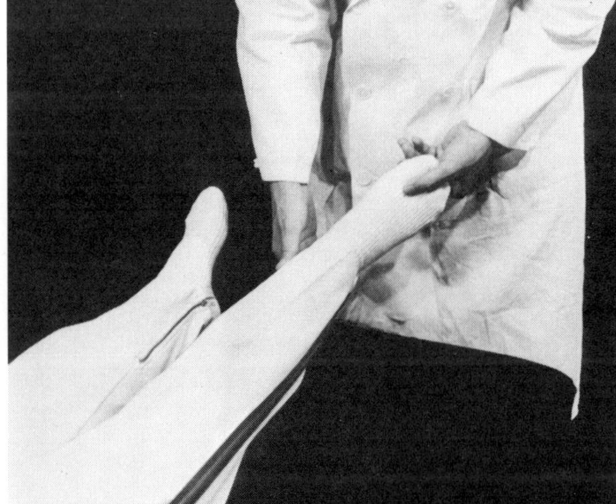

Fig. 43 Supine D-2-4

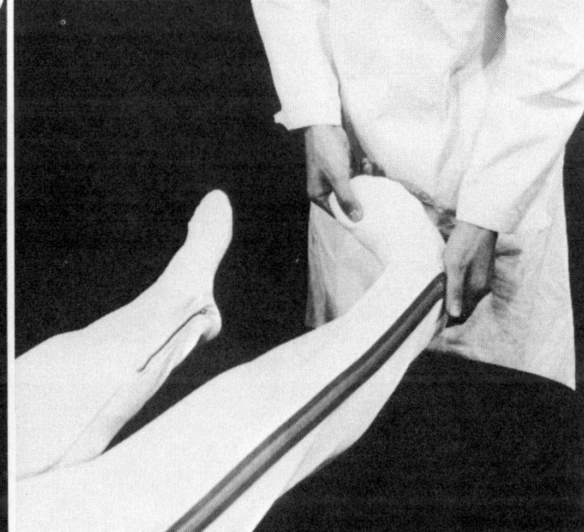

Fig. 44 Supine D-2-5

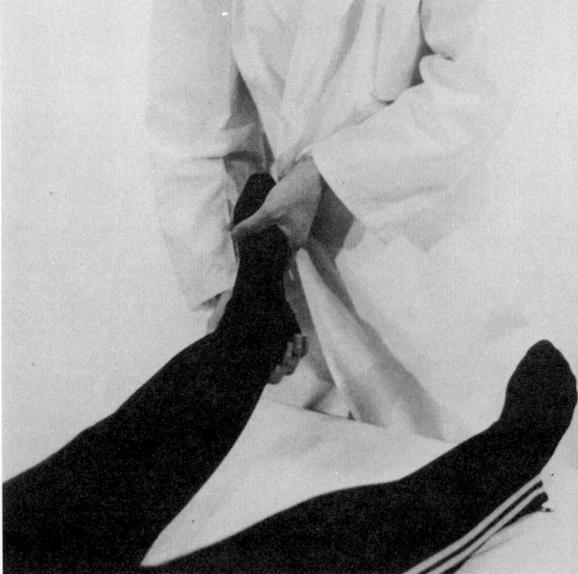

Fig. 45 Supine D-2-6

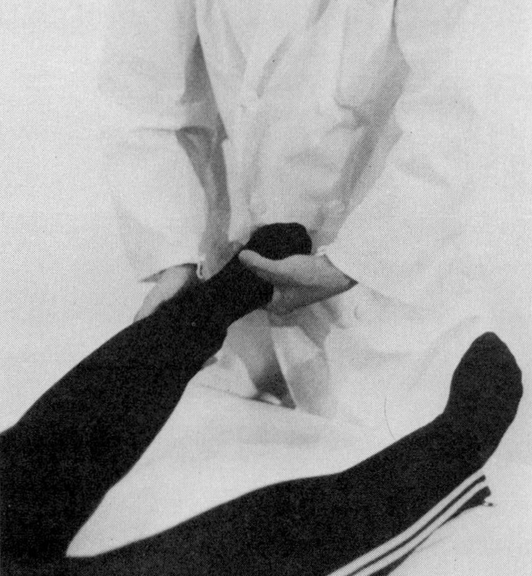

Sōtai II: Grasping the toes of the patient's left foot with one hand, the therapist lifts that leg slightly (about 10 centimeters) from the working surface (Fig. 46). The patient rotates her heel medially, pivoting at the toes. The therapist applies resistance against this movement by holding his other hand against the inside of her heel (Fig. 47). After holding tension for three to five seconds at a suitable position, they both release the tension. This procedure is repeated two or three times.

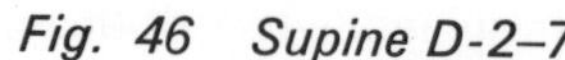
Fig. 46 Supine D-2–7

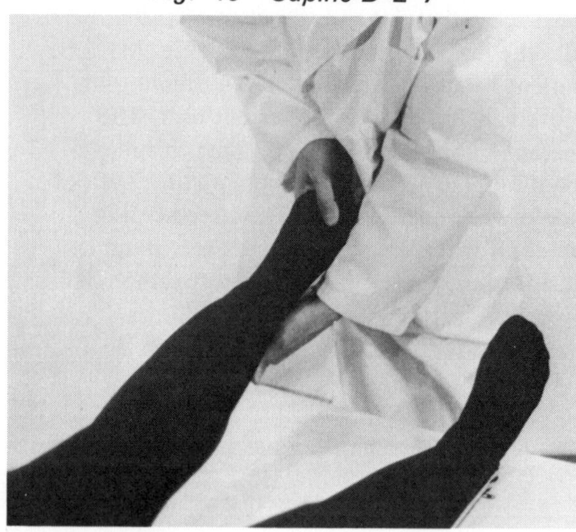

Fig. 47 Supine D-2–8

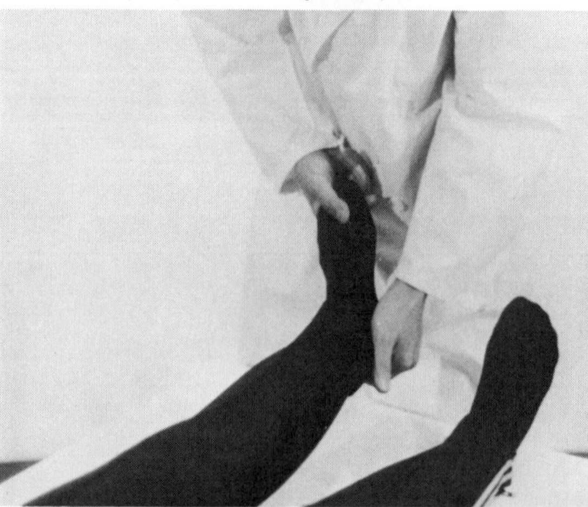

Supine E-1

Dōshin: In the supine posture, the patient alternately raises her right and left legs, keeping the knees extended. The patient checks for any sensations of comfort or discomfort produced, and for differences between the left and right legs (Figs. 48 and 49).

Fig. 48 Supine E-1–1

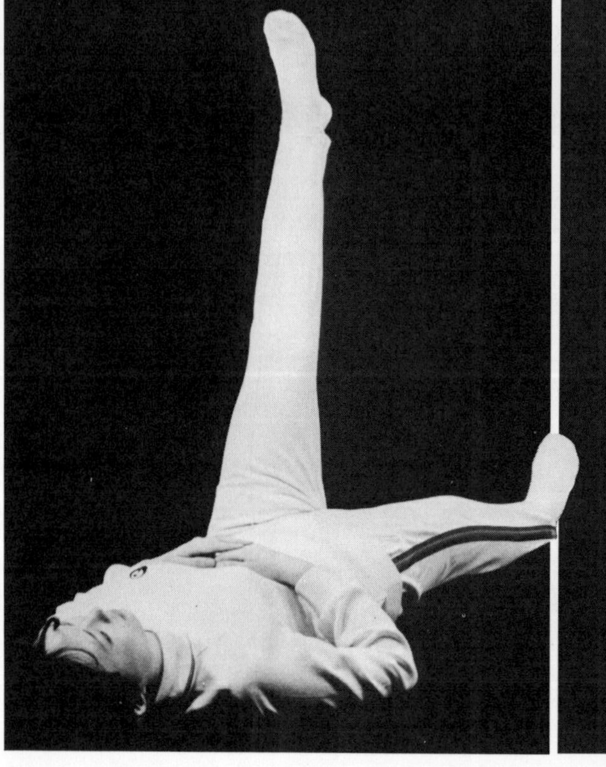

Fig. 49 Supine E-1–2

Note: For examination by passive movement, the comparison between the heaviness of the left and right legs which is judged in technique Supine B-4 may be used. That is to say, the leg which was found to be the heavier one in technique Supine B-4 is normally found to be also the leg with the most discomfort during movements of technique Supine E.

Sōtai: The patient raises her right leg, and then begins to lower it back down. The therapist applies resistance against this lowering movement by holding the heel of the right foot.

Fig. 50 Supine E-1–3

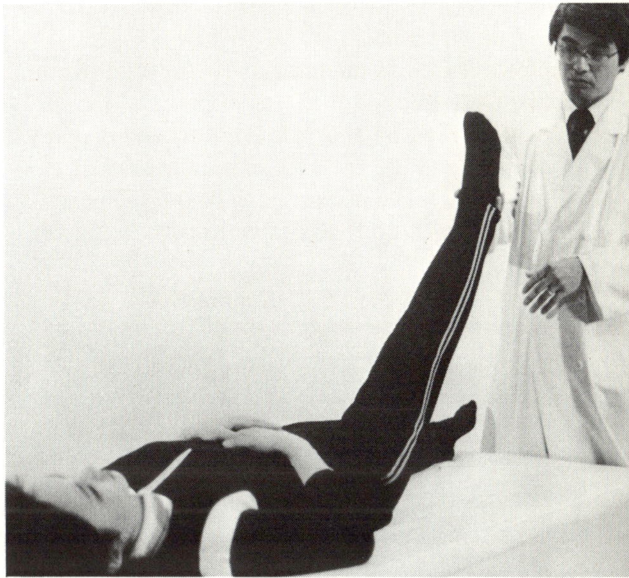

Fig. 51 Supine E-1–4

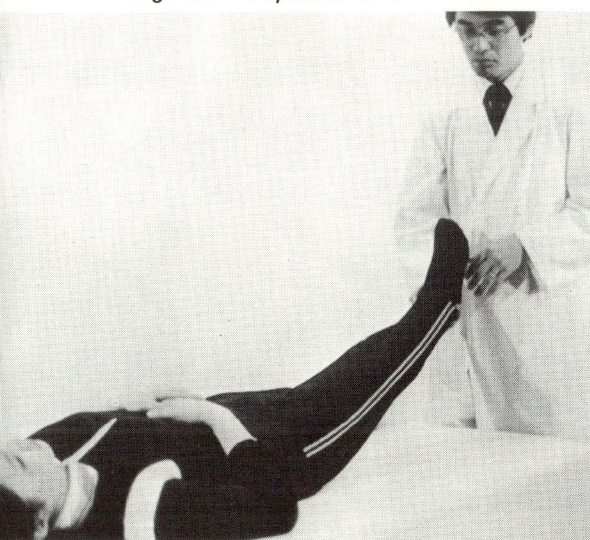

After holding tension in a suitable position for three to five seconds, the therapist instructs the patient to release tension. This procedure is repeated two or three times (Figs. 50 to 52). When executing this movement, the height to which the leg is first raised can be varied. For instance, in cases where raising the leg past a certain height causes pain, it is more effective to raise the leg to a point just below that height, and then to begin lowering it.

Fig. 52 Supine E-1–5

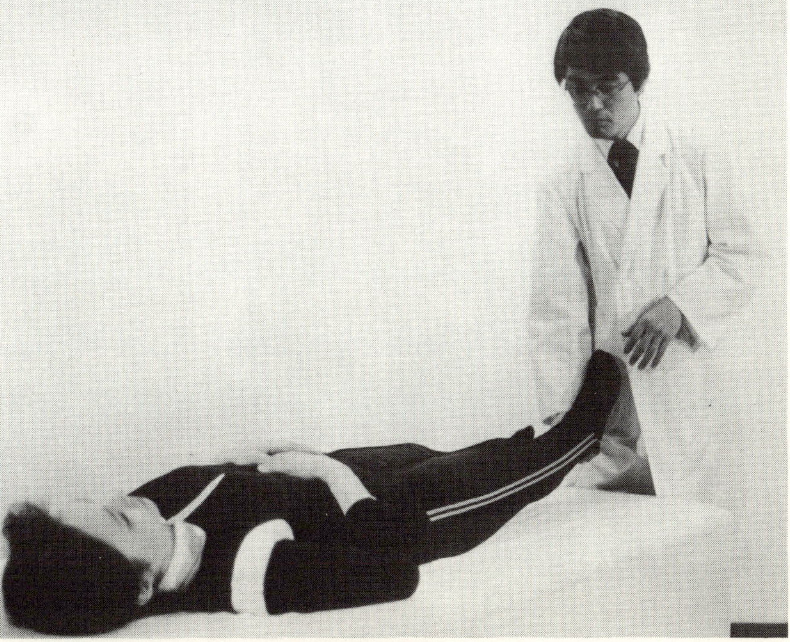

Supine F-1

Palpation examination: The therapist gently places his hands on and slowly presses down on first the right, and then the left knee of the patient (Figs. 53 and 54). Comfort and discomfort and the presence of pain are noted.

Sōtai I: The patient lying in the supine position with both legs extended, flexes (raises) her right knee. The therapist places one hand upon the patient's right knee and the other hand upon her right ankle. He applies resistance against her movement (Figs. 55 and 56). They both hold tension for three to five seconds at a suitable position, and then release this simultaneously. This procedure is repeated two or three times.

Fig. 53 Supine F-1–1

Fig. 54 Supine F-1–2

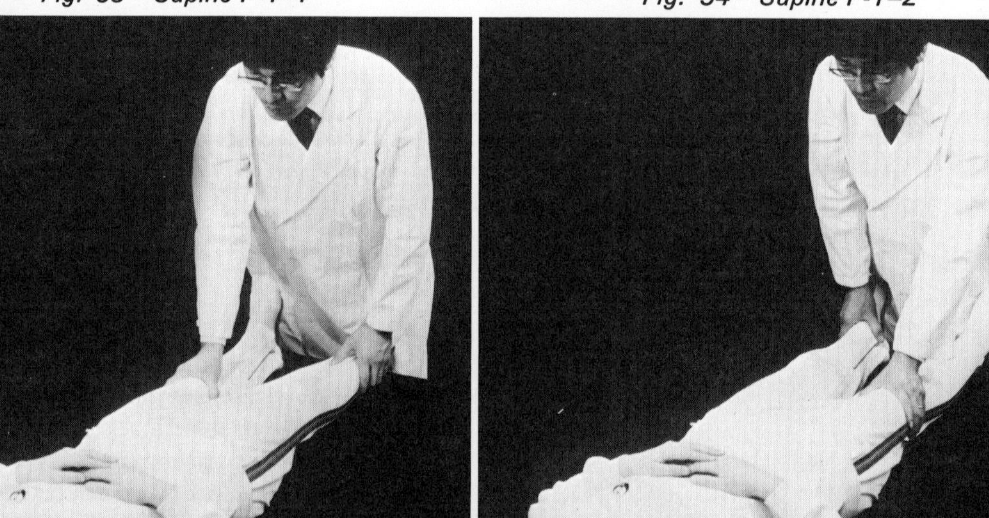

Fig. 55 Supine F-1–3

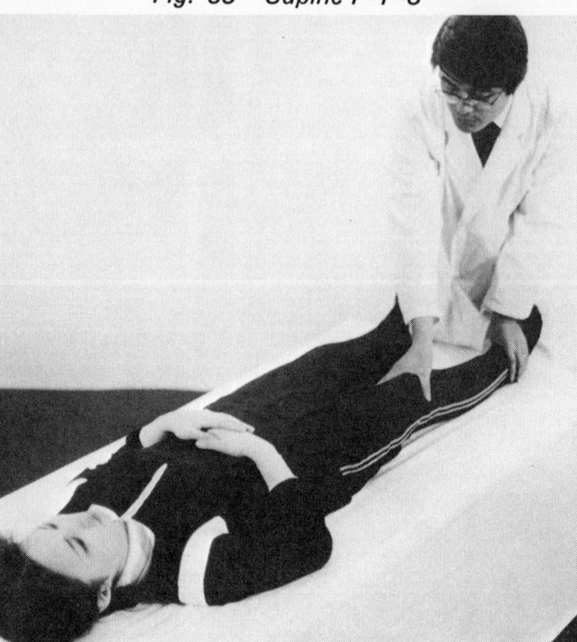

Fig. 56 Supine F-1–4

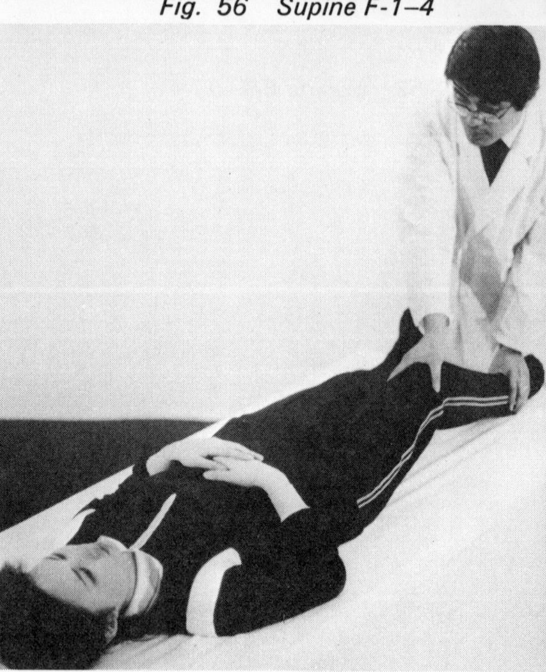

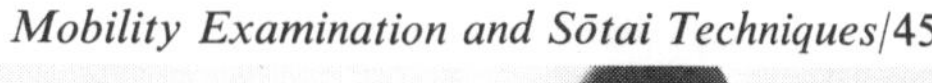

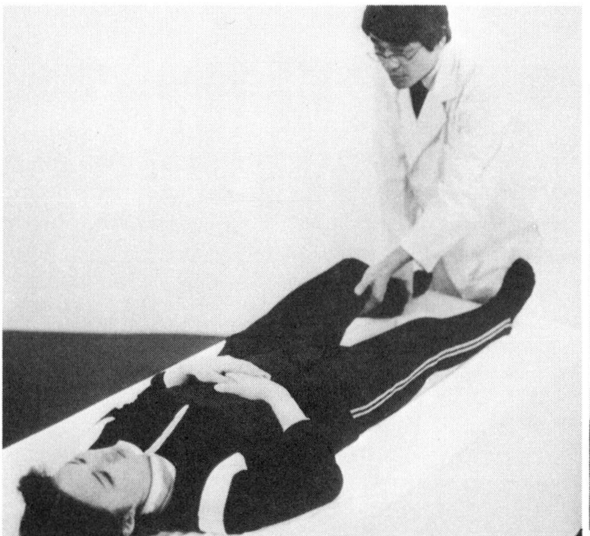

Fig. 57 Supine F-1–5

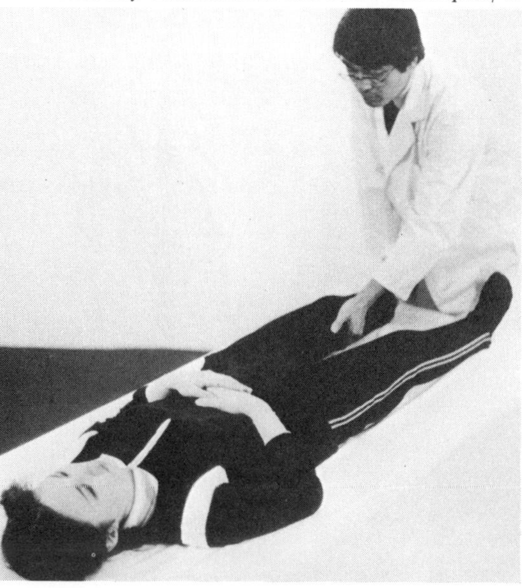

Fig. 58 Supine F-1–6

Sōtai II: The patient first raises her left knee several inches (Fig. 57). Then, while keeping her foot on the table or floor surface, she lowers her knee by extending her leg. The therapist applies resistance to this movement by placing one hand under the knee and the other hand on the ankle of the left leg (Fig. 58). They both hold tension for three to five seconds, and then release simultaneously. This procedure is repeated two or three times.

Supine G-1

Palpation examination: From the supine position, the patient lightly flexes her knees to an angle of 90° to 100°. Keeping the knees together, the feet are positioned apart about the width of the patient's waist (Fig. 59). The therapist probes for pressure sensitive points accompanying muscle tension (stiffness and indurations) at the back of the knee inside the bend (upper extreme of calf: popliteal fossa). These abnormally tense and sensitive points may be regarded as a product of distortion and imbalance in the body as a whole, or otherwise, as abnormal pressure from the inside manifested in a concentrated form in the muscles of this area.

This area where muscular tension and pressure sensitivity can be most often found is marked in Figure 60. Figure 61 is an anatomical diagram of the lower leg.

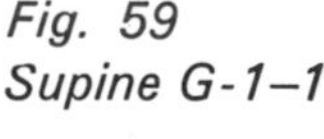

Fig. 59
Supine G-1–1

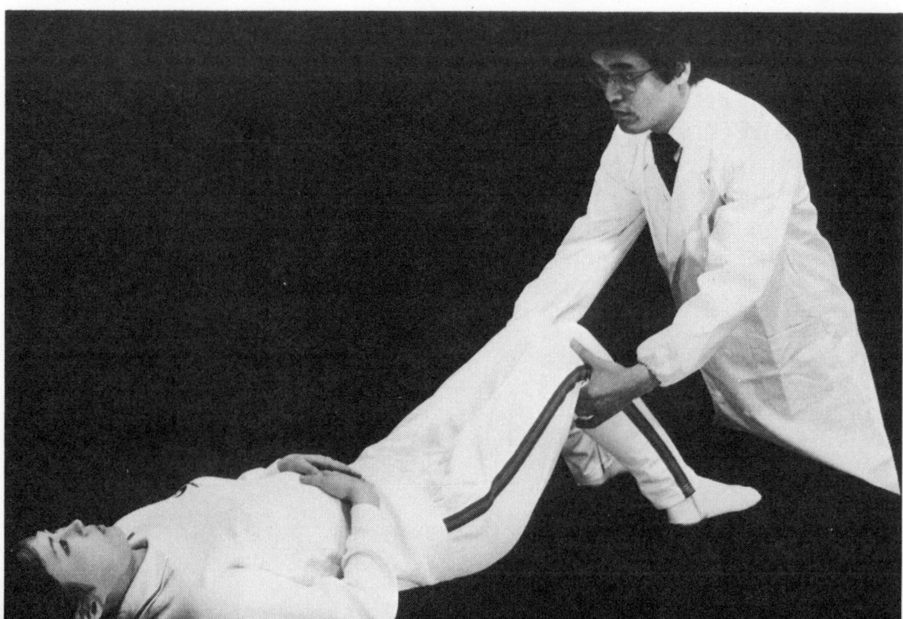

Fig. 60 Anatomical Diagram of Leg

Fig. 61

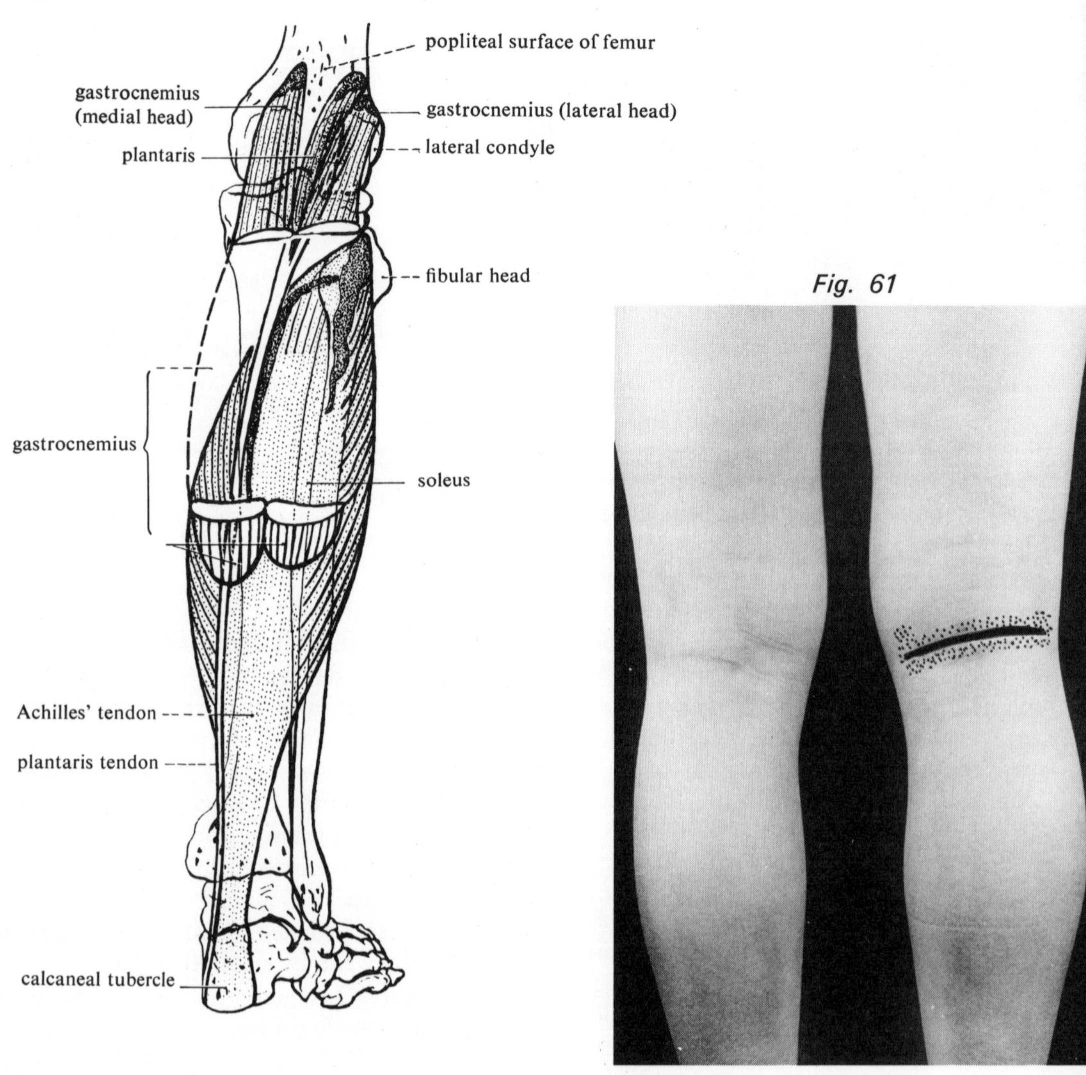

Note: Although procedures (a) through (d) are given for Sōtai technique Supine G-1, it is not necessary to perform all of these in every case. When the palpation examination and subsequent performance of procedure (a) does not produce any improvement in the original sensation of discomfort, only then proceed with one or more of the other procedures of (b), (c), and (d).

Supine G-1-a

Sōtai I: The patient assumes the same posture as during the palpation examination. The therapist instructs the patient to lift the distal ends of her feet using the heels as a fulcrum (base support point) and to bend the ankles into dorsiflexion as far as they will go. Next, the therapist instructs the patient to hold her ankles at this maximum angle of flexion as he applies gentle downward pressure on the dorsal

Fig. 62 Supine G-1-a-2

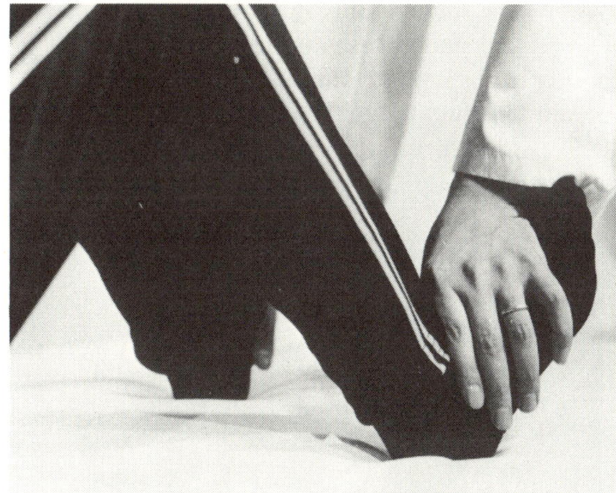

Fig. 63 Supine G-1-a-3

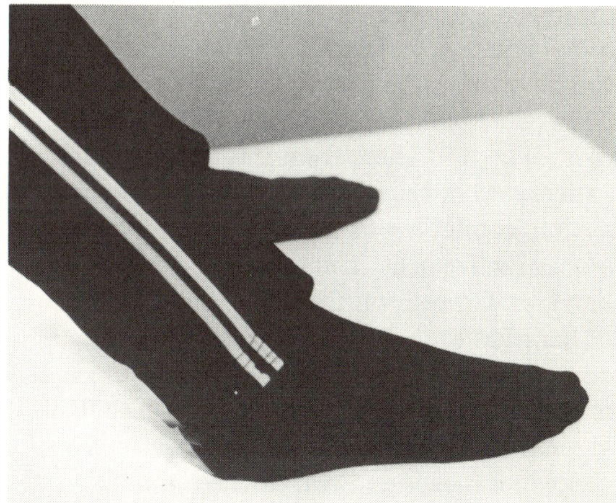

surface of the feet from above (Fig. 62). In this manner, they both maintain opposing tension for three to five seconds, and then release the tension simultaneously. When the patient releases tension, the soles of both feet should drop back to the surface.

Sōtai II: The patient assumes the same posture as during the palpation examination. This time, it is essential that the entire sole of the patient's foot contact the working surface completely (Fig. 63). The therapist applies light pressure upon the dorsal surface of the feet with both hands (Fig. 64). Next, using the heels of both feet as the fulcrum, the patient slowly raises her feet into dorsiflexion (Fig. 65). Pressing the dorsal surface of her feet downward, the therapist applies resistance to the patient's dorsiflexion (Fig. 66). They both maintain tension in a suitable position for three to five seconds, and then release the tension simultaneously. This procedure is repeated two or three times.

Fig. 64 Supine G-1-a-4

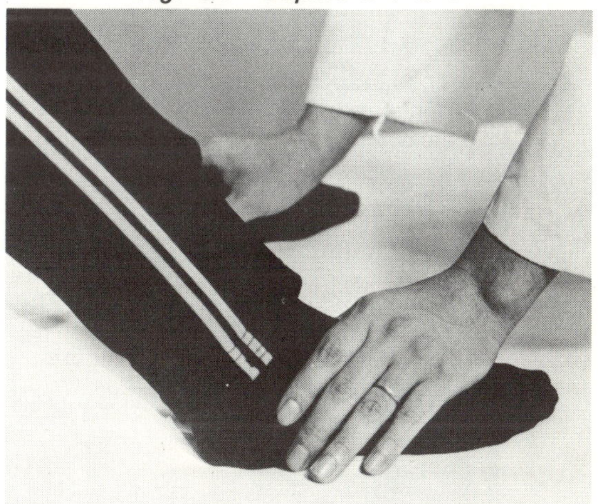

Fig. 65 Supine G-1-a-5

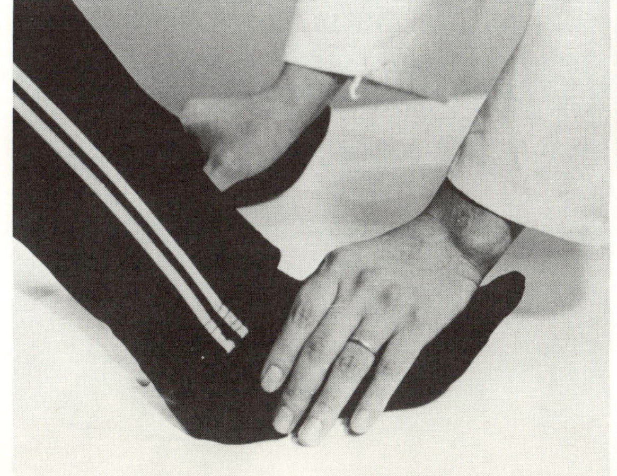

Fig. 66 Supine G-1-a-6

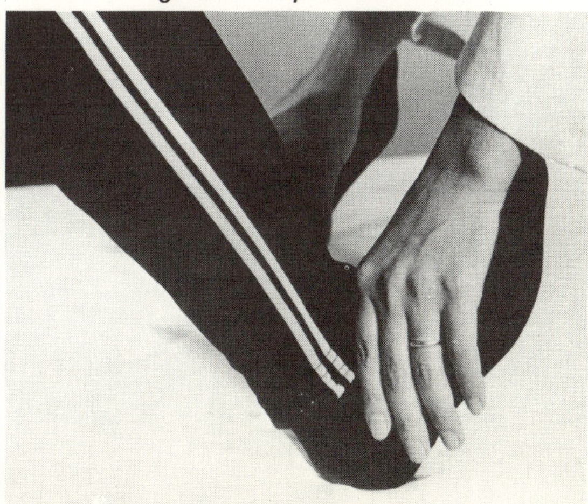

Supine G-1-b

Sōtai: In a posture with both knees comfortably flexed, the patient first raises the distal end of her right foot using the heel as the fulcrum (Fig. 67). Then, from this position, the patient lowers her foot back down into plantar flexion, continuing to use the heel as the fulcrum of movement. The therapist places his hands underneath on the distal end of the sole of her right foot and applies resistance to her downward movement (Fig. 68). They hold the tension at a suitable position for three to five seconds and then release simultaneously. This procedure is repeated two or three times.

Supine G-1-c

Sōtai: Assuming a posture in which both knees are comfortably flexed, the patient raises the heel of her right foot using the toes (phalanges) as fulcrums. The therapist grips her ankle, and resists her movement as she moves her soles upward in dorsiflexion (Figs. 69 and 70). At a suitable position, they maintain opposing tension for three to five seconds and then release it simultaneously. This procedure is repeated two or three times.

Supine G-1-d

Sōtai: Assuming a posture in which both knees are comfortably flexed, the patient first raises the heels of her right foot using the toes (phalanges) as fulcrums (Fig. 71). Next, from that position she lowers the heel toward the working surface while keeping the toes stationary. The therapist provides resistance by placing his hand underneath and holding the heel as it is being lowered (Fig. 72). They both maintain tension at a suitable position for three to five seconds and then release this simultaneously This procedure is repeated two or three times.

Fig. 67 Supine G-1-b-7

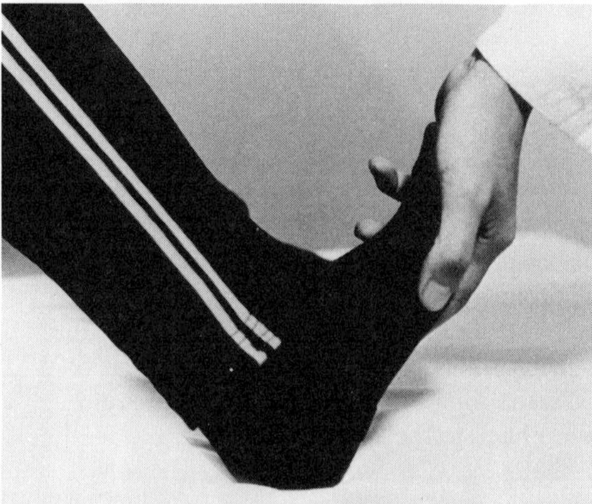

Fig. 68 Supine G-1-b-8

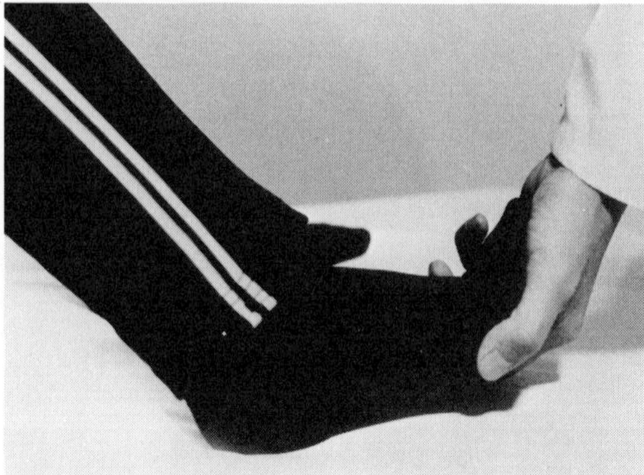

Fig. 69 Supine G-1-c-9

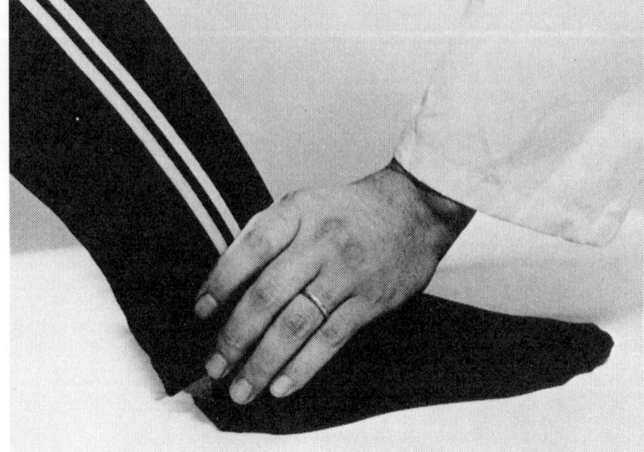

Fig. 70 Supine G-1-c-10

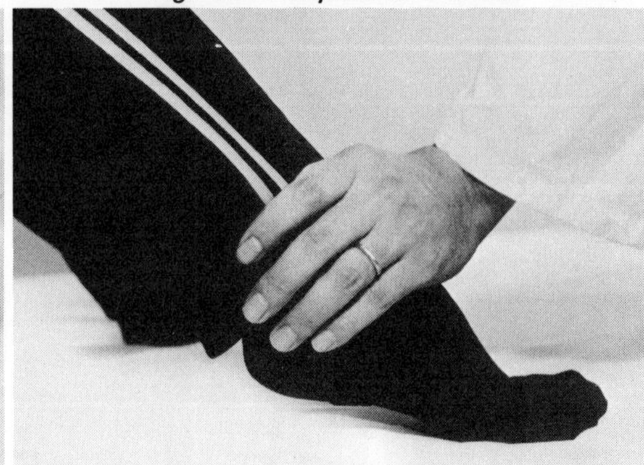

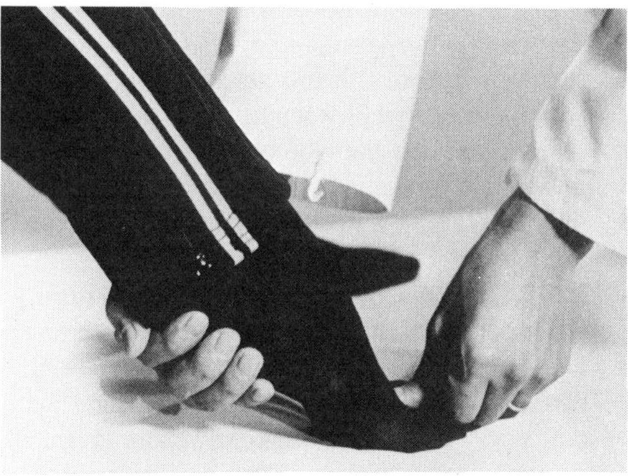
Fig. 71 Supine G-1-d-11

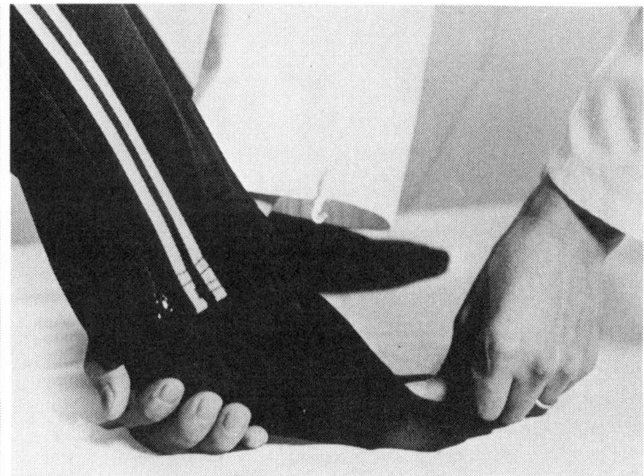
Fig. 72 Supine G-1-d-12

Supine G-2

Sōtai: These are the same Sōtai procedures as Supine G-1, but are performed with slight variation in the patient's posture. That is to say, the angles of the hip and knee joints are varied by changing the position of the feet as illustrated in Figures 73 through 76.

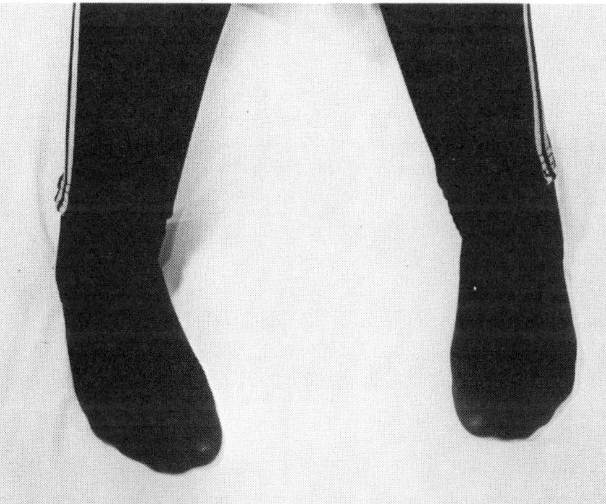
Fig. 73 Supine G-2–1

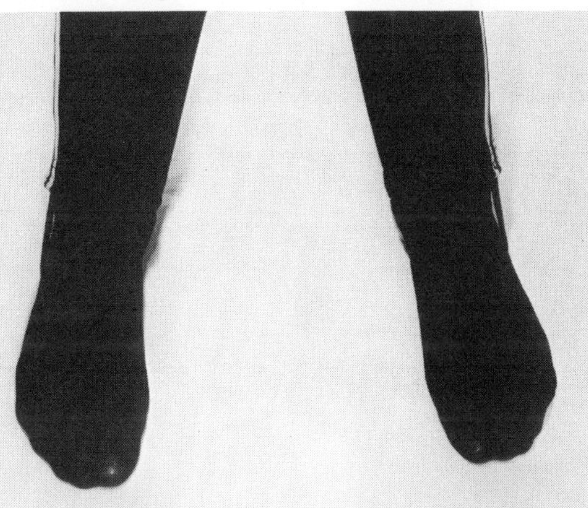
Fig. 74 Supine G-2–2

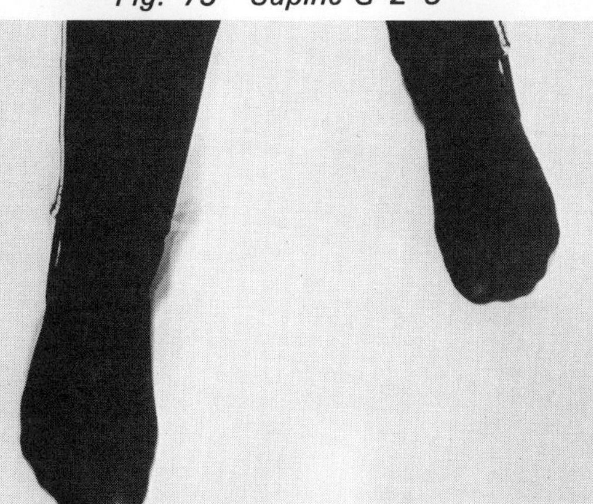
Fig. 75 Supine G-2–3

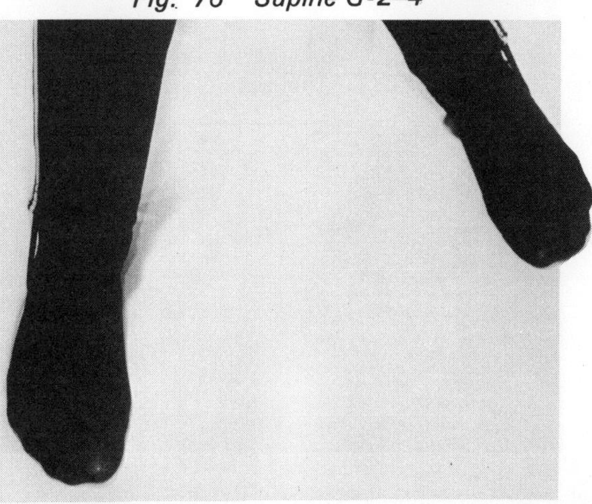
Fig. 76 Supine G-2–4

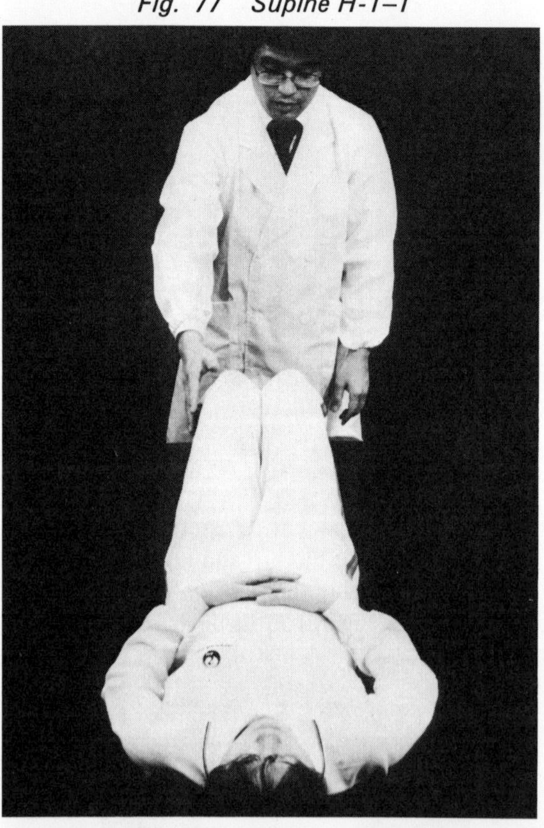
Fig. 77 Supine H-1–1

Supine H-1

Dōshin: After assuming a supine position, the patient raises (flexes) her knees to a comfortable angle while keeping them together. The therapist moves the patient's knees laterally and downward to the left, and then to the right, inquiring about any comfort or discomfort in the movement (Figs. 77 to 79).

Sōtai I: Assuming the posture used during the mobility examination, the patient keeping her knees together, swings her knees laterally from left to right. Placing his hands, the therapist gives resistance to this movement (Figs. 80 through 83). Tension of these opposing movements is maintained at a suitable position for three to five seconds, after which they are relaxed simultaneously. This procedure is repeated two or three times.

Sōtai II: Active movement by the patient is a part of each Sōtai technique and is always made in a manner and direction which is "away from discomfort and toward greater ease." The

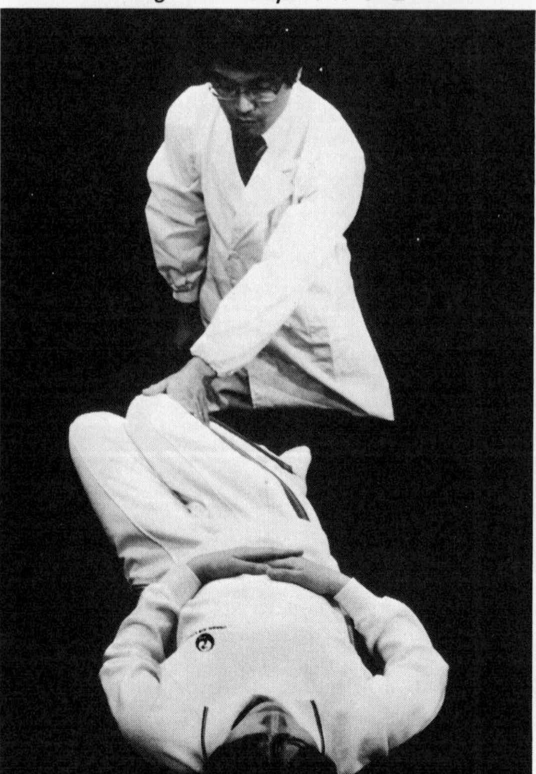
Fig. 78 Supine H-1–2

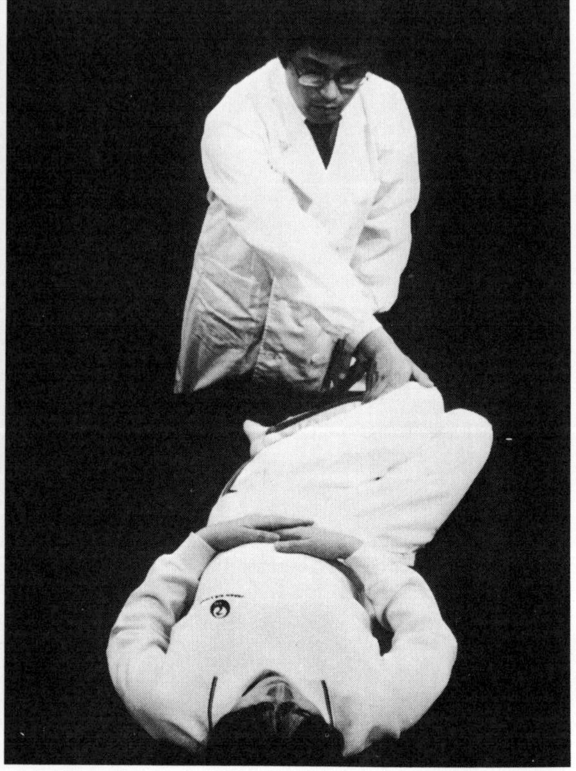
Fig. 79 Supine H-1–3

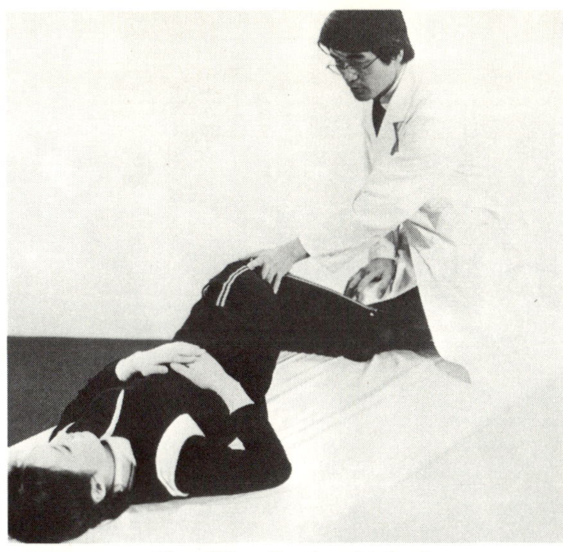
Fig. 80 Supine H-1–4

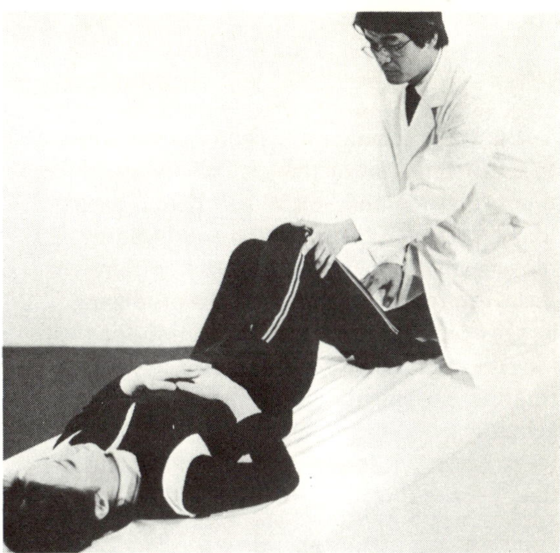
Fig. 81 Supine H-1–5

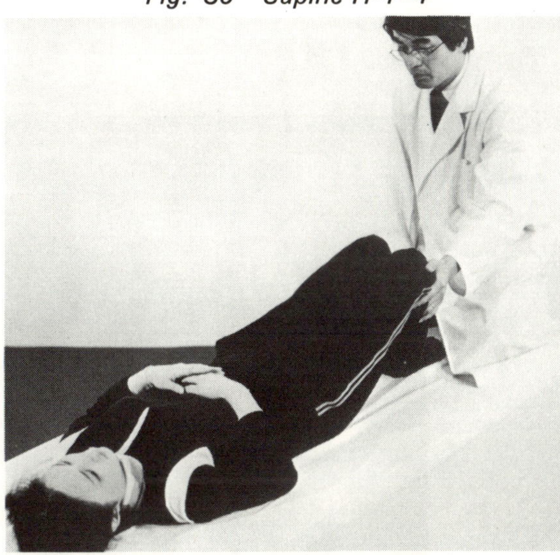
Fig. 82 Supine H-1–6

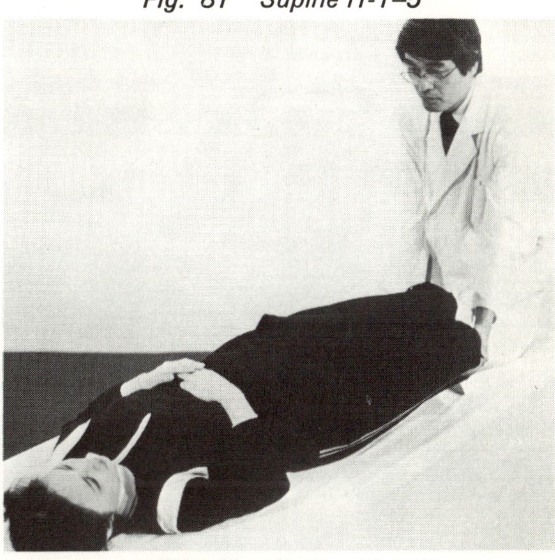
Fig. 83 Supine H-1–7

patient therefore, can also perform these techniques alone without the aid of the therapist.

The knees are raised in a half flexed position lightly in contact with each other. The heels should be placed apart approximately the width of the hips. The toes, in this case, should point slightly inward (Fig. 84).

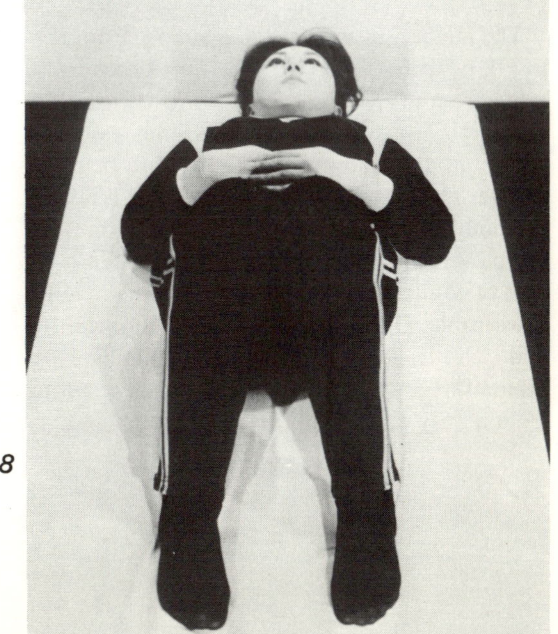
Fig. 84 Supine H-1–8

The knees together are swung down laterally to either the right or the left side two or three times (Figs. 85 and 86). When there is a difference between the sensation produced by movements to the right and left sides, the knees are moved in the direction producing less discomfort. The correct direction for the movement is therefore determined by which rotation movement with the knees flexed together is less difficult or strained, and less painful or "heavy," as compared to movement in the opposite direction.

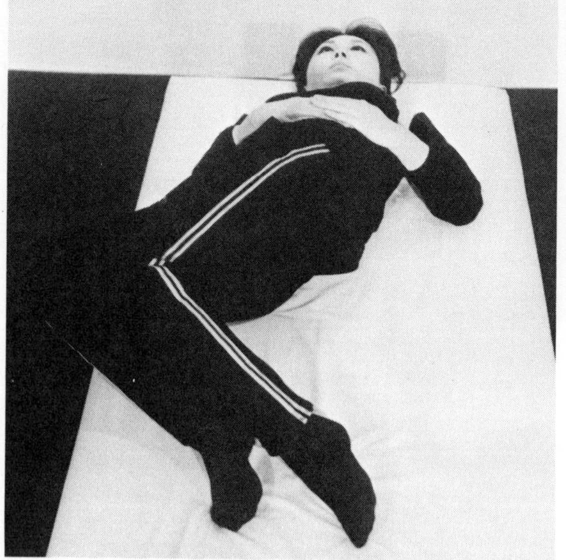

Fig. 85 Supine H-1–9

Fig. 86 Supine H-1–10

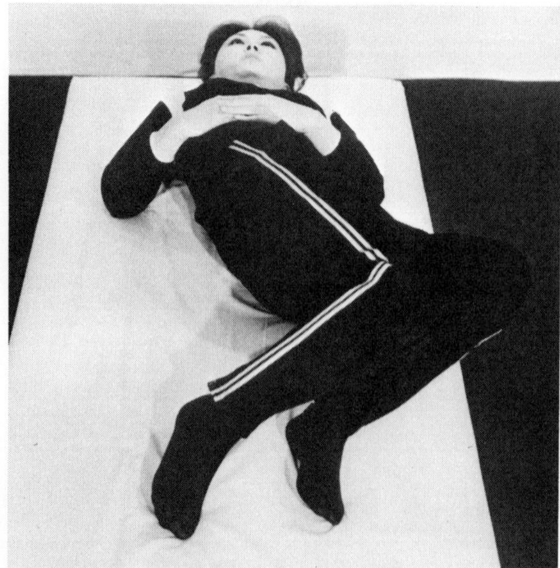

The method of movement is simply from (8) to (9), or from (8) to (10). The time taken to move from (8) to (9) or from (8) to (10) should be at least five seconds since anything less would produce movement too rapid to be effective. The secret of effectiveness is to relax the body as much as possible before beginning the movement. When this is practiced, sensation of comfort and discomfort become readily discernable. One good way to maintain health and well-being is to systematically eliminate discomfort and to dispel fatigue which resulting from a busy day, using these techniques.

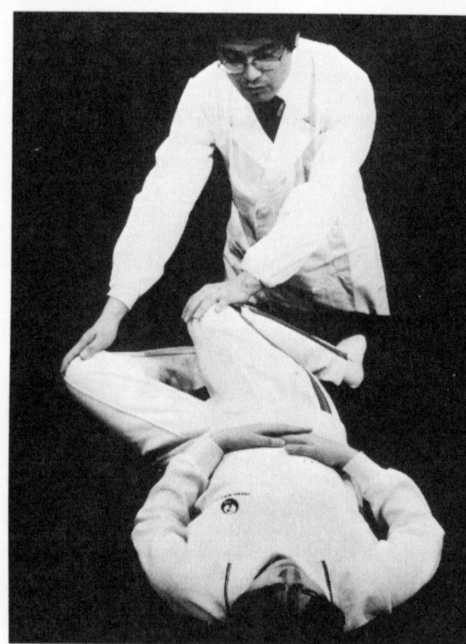

Fig. 87 Supine H-2–1

Supine H-2

Dōshin: Keeping her knees apart, the patient lightly flexes both knees upward. The therapist pushes the knees down laterally to the right, keeping the knees the same distance apart and then reverses the motion to the left to check which direction produces more discomfort (Figs. 87 and 88).

Fig. 89 Supine H-2–3

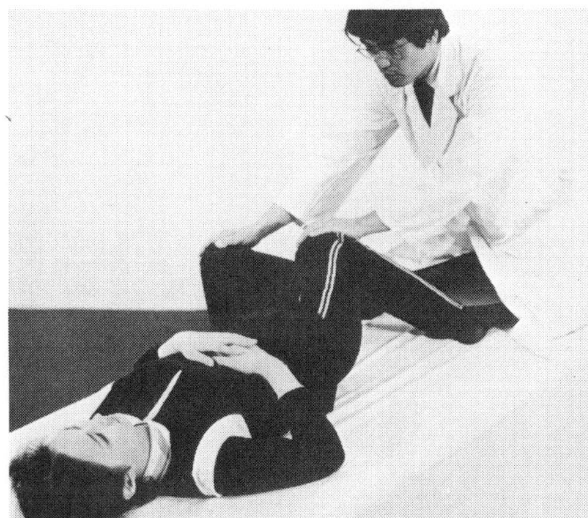

Fig. 90 Supine H-2–4

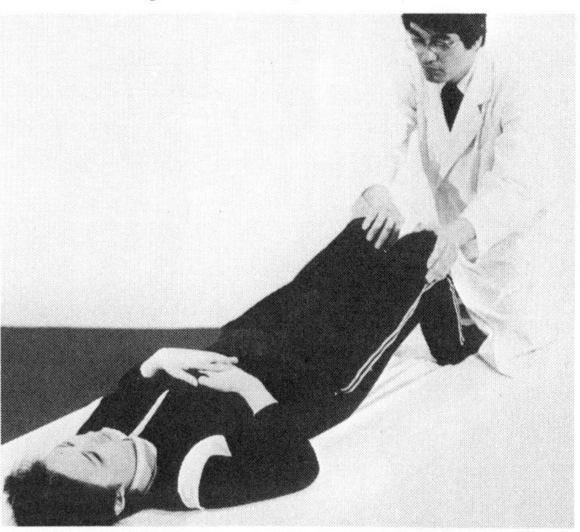

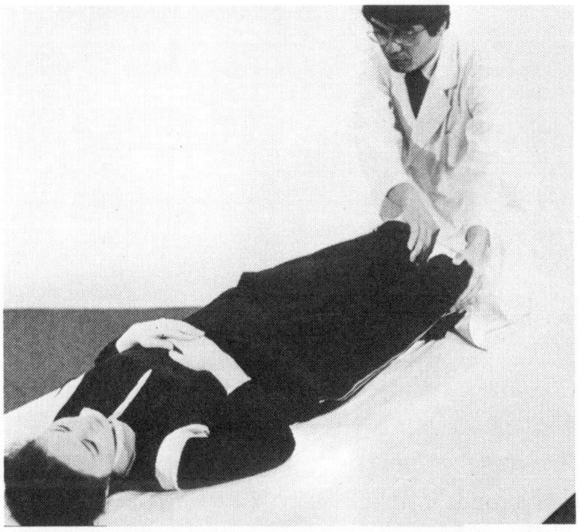

Sōtai: Keeping her knees slightly apart, the patient moves her knees from left to right. The therapist places his hands on the patient's knees in order to provide resistance to her movement (Figs. 89 through 92). At a suitable position, they maintain opposing pressure for three to five seconds, and then release this simultaneously. This procedure is repeated two or three times.

Fig. 91 Supine H-2–5

Fig. 88 Supine H-2–2

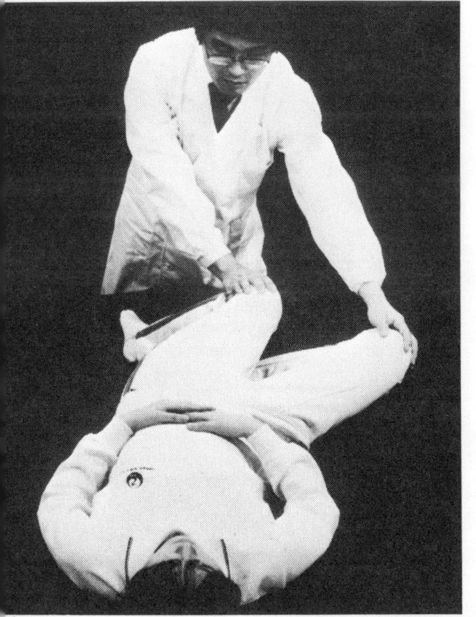

Fig. 92 Supine H-2–6

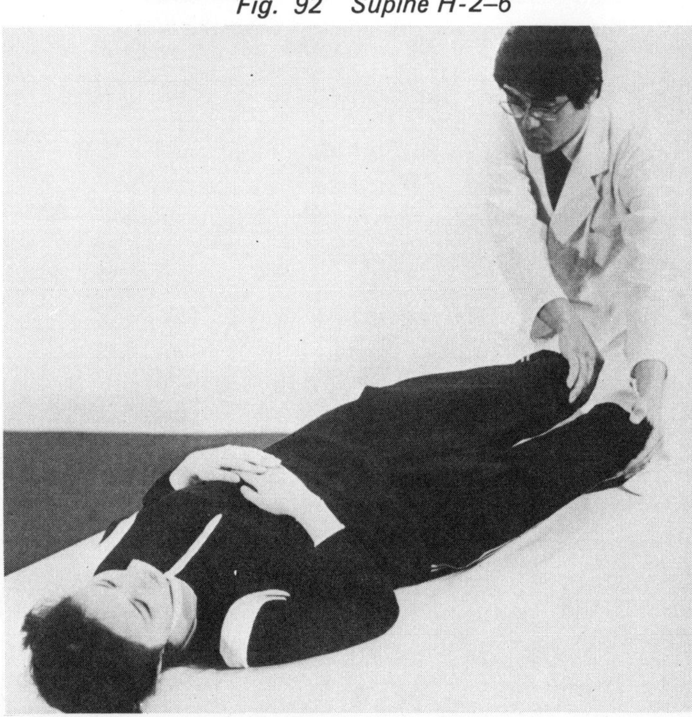

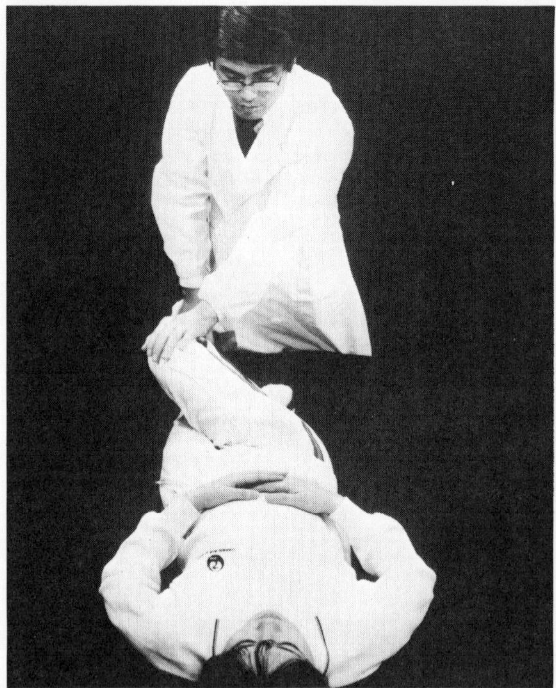

Fig. 93 Supine H-3–1

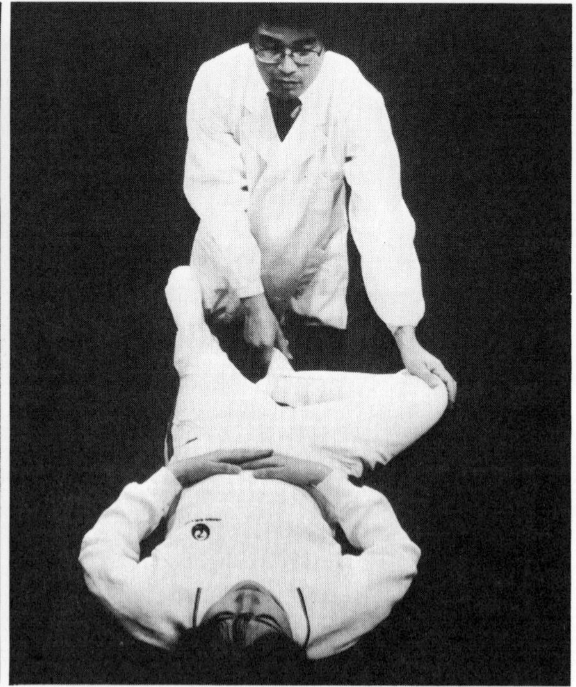

Fig. 94 Supine H-3–2

Supine H-3

Dōshin: From the supine position, the patient flexes her right or left knee upward into a comfortable position. The therapist rotates the patient's flexed knee downward first medially and then laterally, and determines the direction of greater discomfort (Figs. 93 and 94).

Note: If when preforming the procedures Supine H-1 and H-2, it is found that one leg is especially sore, or that there is an impediment present in one leg, this Sōtai procedure should be performed.

Sōtai I: The patient first flexes her left knee upward and rotates the leg laterally. Next, from this opened position, she lifts the knee still flexed, back up to the upright position and continues the movement rotating the leg medially. The therapist places his hand on the knee provides resistance to the patient's movement (Figs. 95 and 96). At a suitable position

Fig. 95 Supine H-3–3

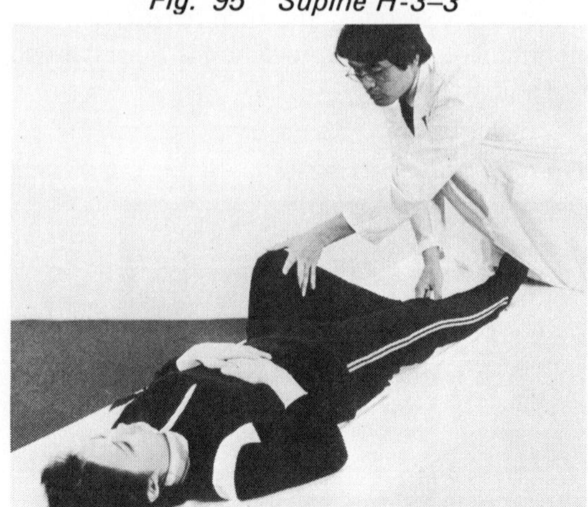

Fig. 96 Supine H-3–4

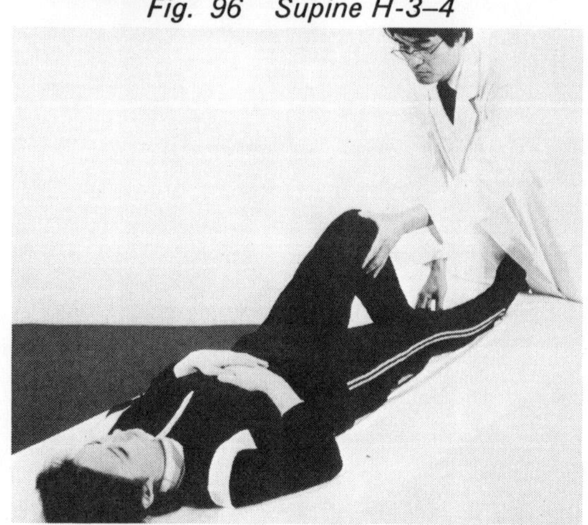

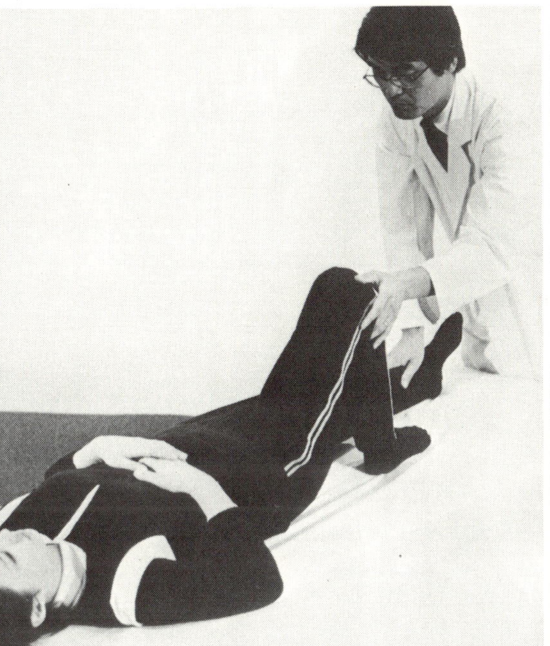

Fig. 97 Supine H-3–5

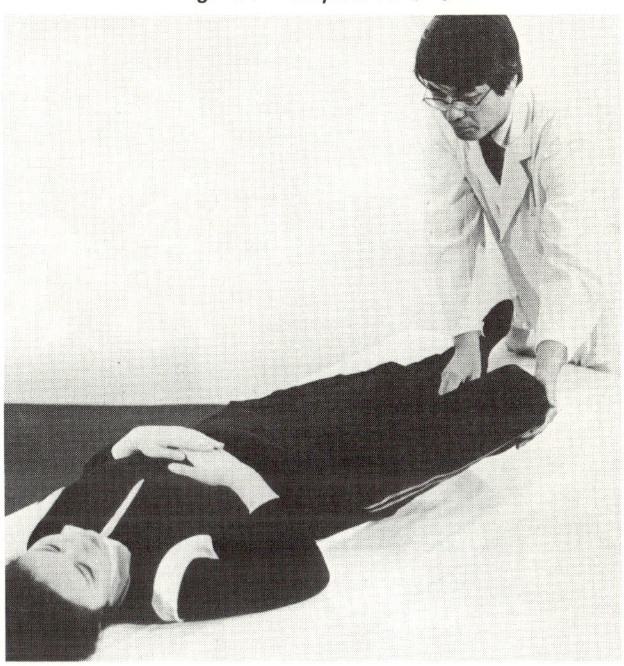

Fig. 98 Supine H-3–6

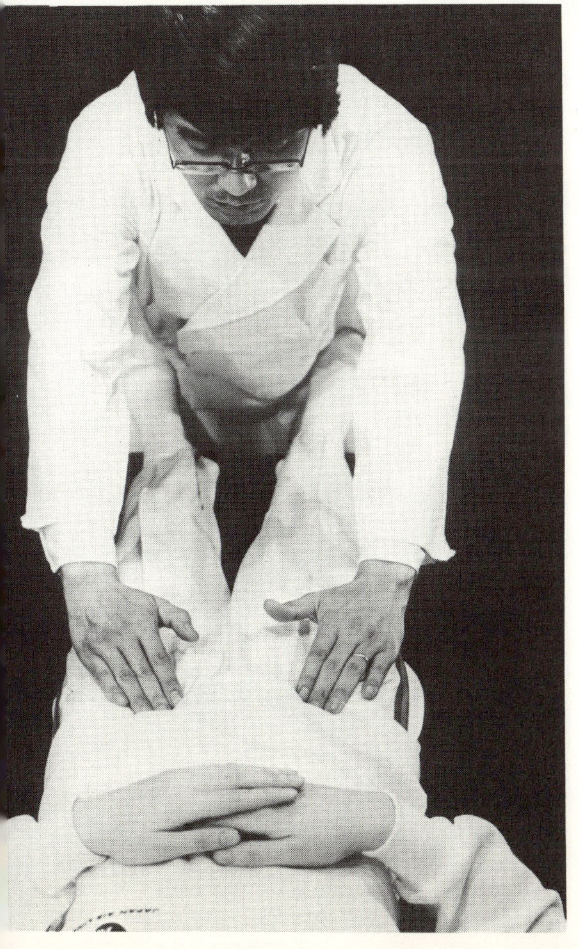

Fig. 99 Supine I-1–1

they maintain opposing pressure for three to five seconds, and then relax their efforts simultaneously. This is repeated two or three times

Sōtai II: The patient flexes her right knee upward to a comfortable position. Then this raised knee is rotated laterally to the open position. The therapist places his hand on her knee and provides resistance to the rotation of the leg (Figs. 97 and 98).

Supine I-1

Palpation examination I: In the supine position, the patient either extends both legs keeping them spread slightly apart, or lightly flexes her knees while keeping them even. The therapist palpates the inguinal region as shown in Figure 99. He checks for the presence of pressure sensitive areas which often accompany abnormal tension in muscles. Figure 100 is the anatomical diagram of anterior abdominal musculature.

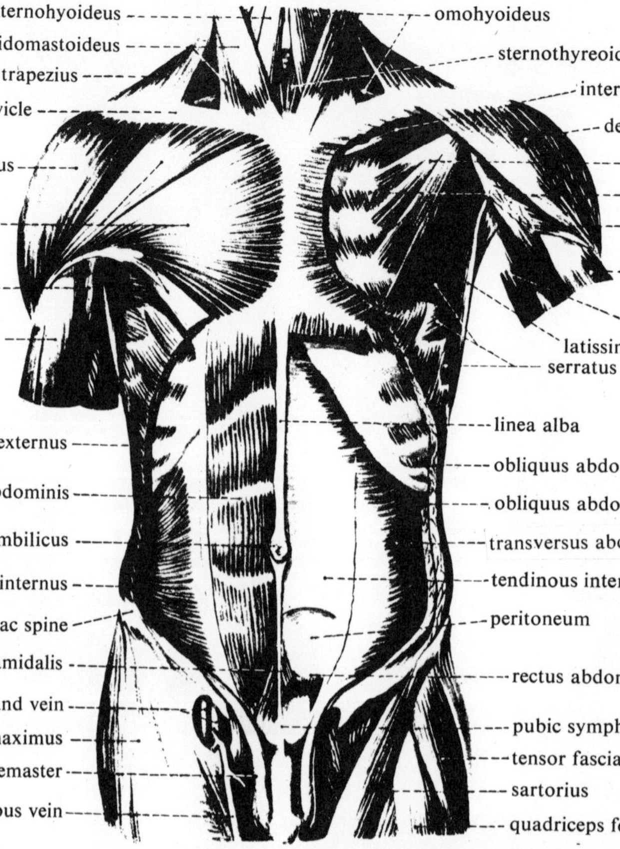

sternohyoideus
sternocleidomastoideus
trapezius
clavicle
deltoideus
pectoralis major
coracobrachialis
biceps brachii
obliquus abdominis externus
rectus abdominis
umbilicus
obliquus abdominis internus
anterior superior iliac spine
pyramidalis
femoral artery and vein
gluteus maximus
cremaster
long saphenous vein
omohyoideus
sternothyreoideus
intercostales interni
deltoideus
pectoralis minor
intercostales interni
pectoralis major
biceps brachii
triceps brachii
latissimus dorsi
serratus anterior
linea alba
obliquus abdominis externus
obliquus abdominis internus
transversus abdominis
tendinous intersections of rectus abdominis
peritoneum
rectus abdominis
pubic symphysis
tensor fasciae latae
sartorius
quadriceps femoris

Fig. 100 Anatomical Diagram of Chest and Abdomen

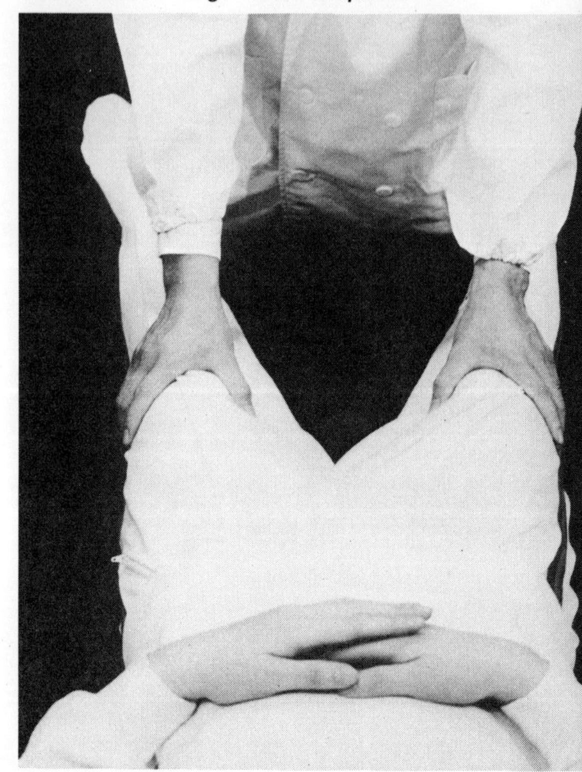

Fig. 101 Supine I-1–2

Palpation examination II: As in Supine I-1–1, the patient either extends or slightly flexes the knees. The therapist palpates the musculature around the adductor canal (canalis adductorius muscularis: on the anterior border of the medial aspect of the thighs, about a third of the way up from the patella) and checks for the presence of pressure sensitive areas (Fig. 101). Figure 102 is the anatomical diagram of musculature of the medial aspect of the thighs.

Sōtai: From the posture shown in Figure 103, the patient slowly rotates her knees apart laterally. The therapist places his hands on the lateral sides of her knees and provides resistance to this movement (Fig. 104). At a suitable position they both maintain opposing pressure for three to five seconds, and then release together. This procedure is repeated two or three times.

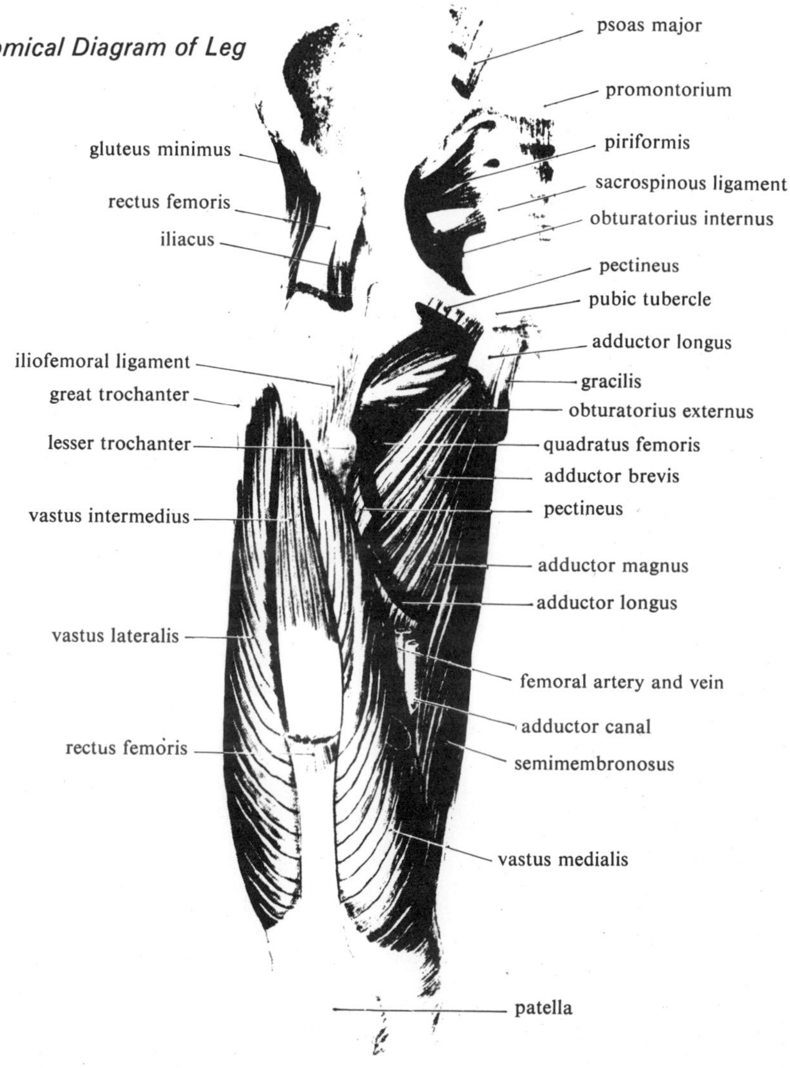

Fig. 102 Anatomical Diagram of Leg

psoas major
promontorium
gluteus minimus
piriformis
sacrospinous ligament
rectus femoris
obturatorius internus
iliacus
pectineus
pubic tubercle
adductor longus
iliofemoral ligament
gracilis
great trochanter
obturatorius externus
lesser trochanter
quadratus femoris
adductor brevis
vastus intermedius
pectineus
adductor magnus
adductor longus
vastus lateralis
femoral artery and vein
adductor canal
rectus femoris
semimembronosus
vastus medialis
patella

Fig. 103 Supine I-1–3

Fig. 104 Supine I-1–4

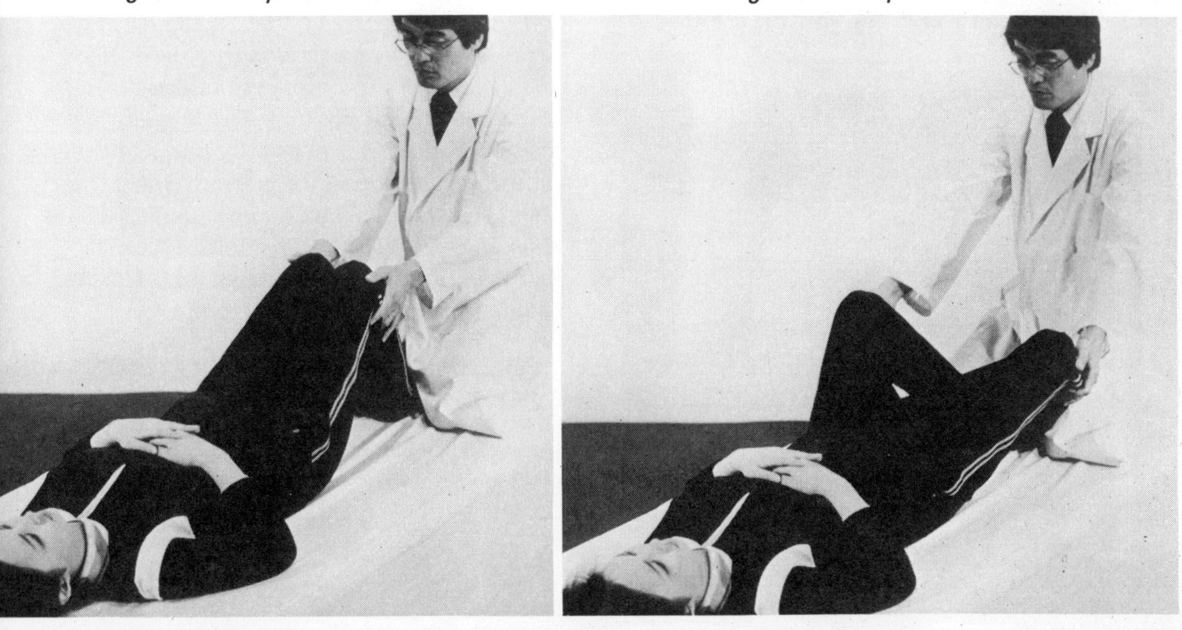

Relationship of the Adductor Muscle to Visual Function

The adductor muscles on the medial aspect of the thigh consist of a group of six muscles innervated by the femoral and obturator nerves, and are supplied by the femoral, external pudendal, and obturator arteries. The principle function of the adductors are the adduction of the thighs, though they do assist in hip flexion also. According to Dr. Hashimoto, when external stimulus is applied to these muscles (when tension is removed by Sōtai movement), visual function is clearly influenced. Dr. Hashimoto discovered a trigger point he termed Seigan (clear eyes) point which has the effect of clearing up blurred vision. Acupuncture stimulation here is also considered effective.

Sōtai techniques performed around this area have been shown to stimulate ocular function. However, the question remains to be answered as to whether this results from effects on the visual organs (e.g., ciliary body, macula lutea, retina, and light receptor organs), or from lowered excitation thresholds in the visual center of the cerebrum.

An attempt was made to study this question by examining the retinal blood vessels and pulse wave, as well as by giving eye tests and flicker tests to nine subjects before and after Sōtai treatments. Improved visual performance was recorded along with higher flicker fusion thresholds.* Also the focusing abilities of the subjects improved and a heightened level of cerebral excitation was evidenced. No change was observed in the blood vessels of the retina, however, so it was clear that there was no significant improvement in circulation to the visual organs.

Kawakami Laboratories
Miyagi University of Education

Supine I-2

Palpation examination: In the supine position the patient, keeping her knees together, flexes them up about halfway. The therapist palpates the mid-region of the lateral aspect of the thighs and looks for pressure sensitive points (Fig. 105). The specific area to be palpated is shown in Figure 106. This is the point where the tip of the fingers touch the thigh when the arms are held straight down at the sides in a standing position. Figure 107 is a diagram of the musculature of this region.

Fig. 105 Supine I-2–1

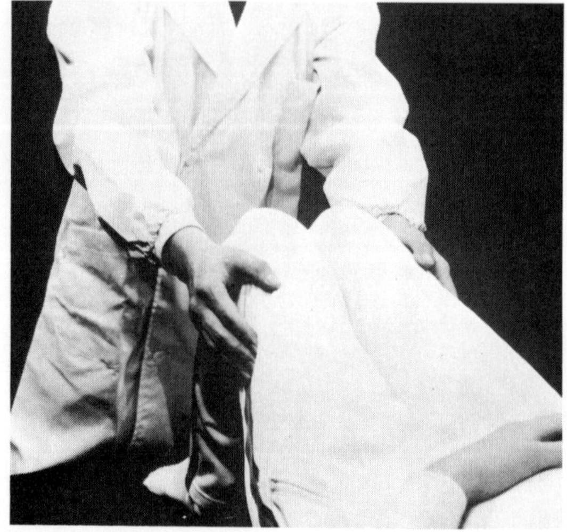

Dōshin: The patient first rotates her knees apart laterally as much as is comfortable (Fig. 108). Next she slowly rotates her legs medially toward the closed position. The therapist gives resistance to this movement by placing his hands on the medial side of the patient's knees (Fig. 109). They both maintain opposing pressure at a suitable position for three to five seconds, and then release this simultaneously. This procedure is repeated two or three times.

*The number of flashes per second at which a flickering light appears continuous. The flicker test is a determination of the flicker fusion threshold which lowers with fatigue.

Fig. 106 Area of Palpation

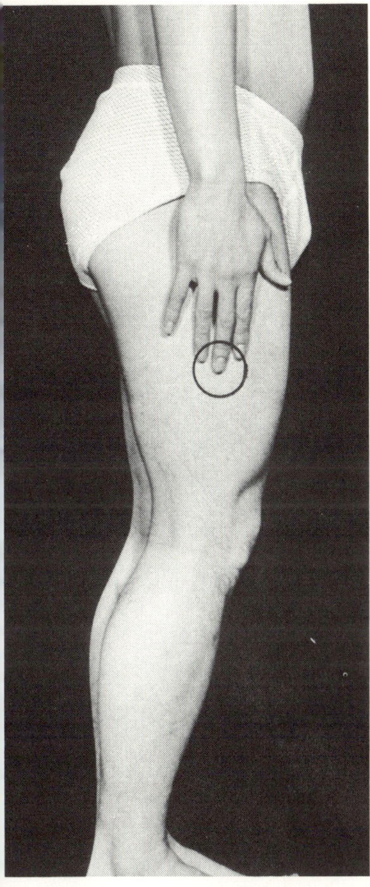

gluteus medius
iliac crest
anterior superior iliac spine
gluteus maximus
sartorius
great trochanter
tensor fasciae latae
rectus femoris
biceps femoris: long head
ilio-tibial tract
vastus lateralis
biceps femoris: short head
vastus intermedius
femur
patella
patellar tendon
head of fibula
tibial tuberosity
gastrocnemius (lateral head)
tibilalis anterior
extensor digitorum longus
soleus
peroneus longus
peroneus brevis
tendon of the peroneus tertius
Achilles' tendon
tendon of the extensoris hallucis longus
lateral malleolus
extensor digitorum brevis
calcaneus
abductor digiti minimi
cuboid bone
fifth metatarsal bone

Fig. 107 Anatomical Diagram of Leg

Fig. 108 Supine I-2–2

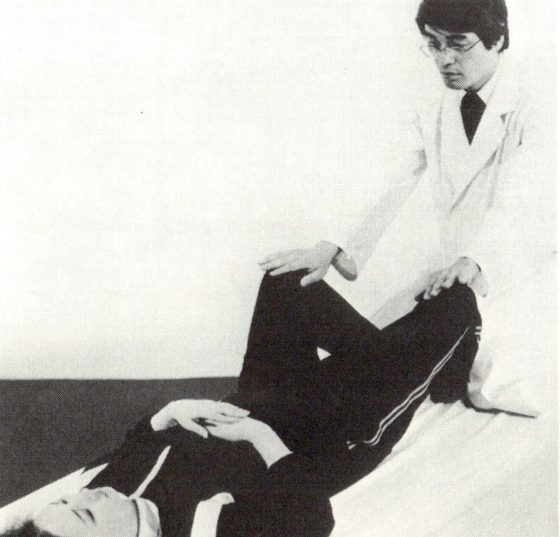

Fig. 109 Supine I-2–3

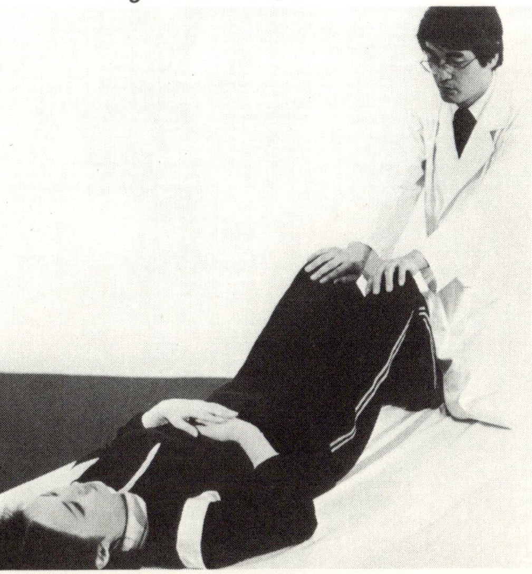

Fig. 110
Supine J-1–1

Supine J-1

Palpation examination: The patient assumes a supine position and while keeping her knees even, flexes them upward to a comfortable height. The therapist sits facing the patient's legs and places his fingers beneath the buttocks along the sacroiliac joint (Fig. 110). The therapist then palpates for the presence of pressure sensitive points alongside this joint. Figure 111 is the anatomical diagram illustrating the musculature in this region.

Fig. 111 Anatomical Diagram of Back

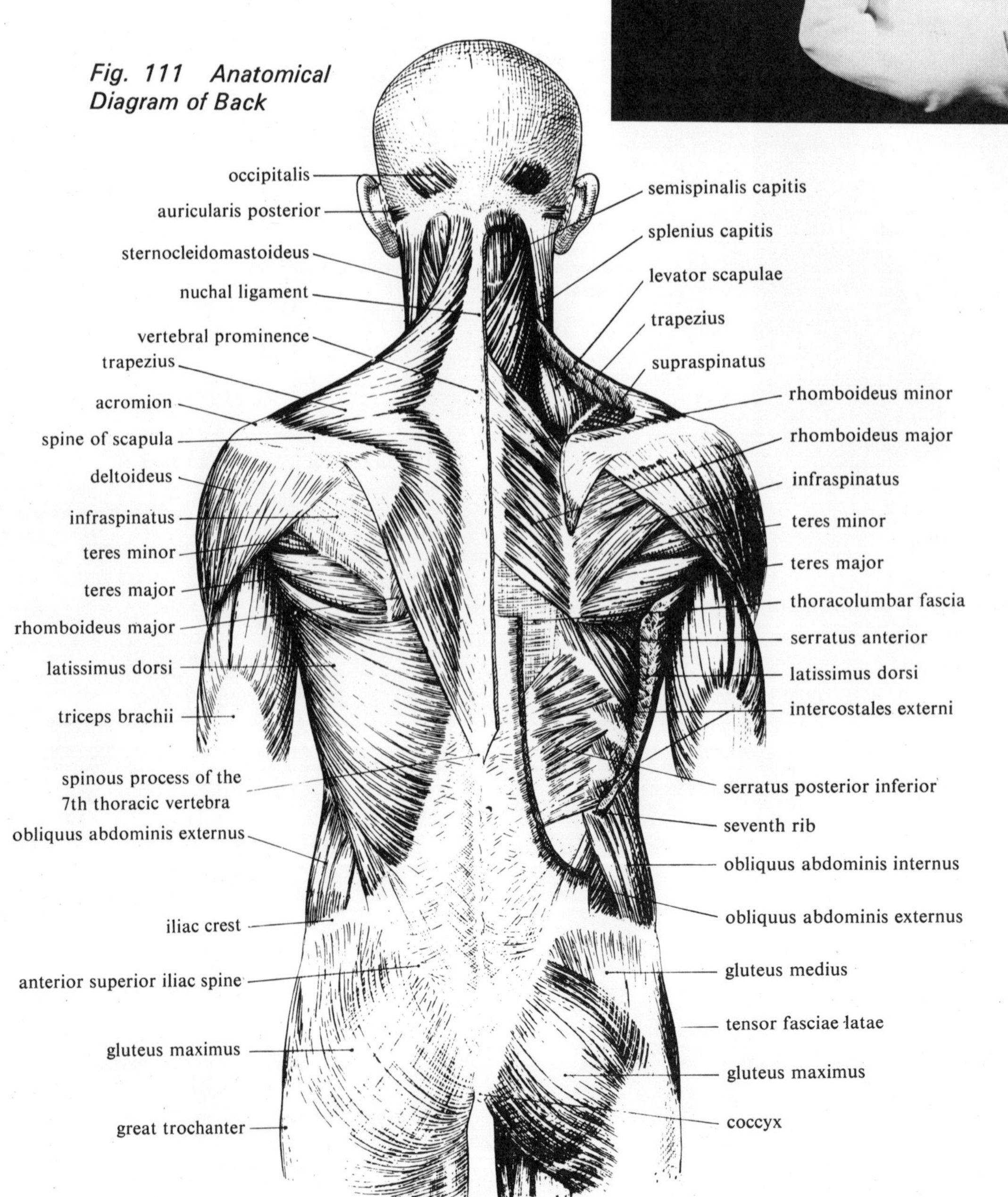

Dōshin: With the patient in a supine position, the therapist grasps the toes and lifts both feet (Figs. 112 and 113). Pushing and flexing the knees alternately so that the knees approach the abdomen, the therapist examines for comfort and discomfort as well as for any difference in the sensation caused in the right and left legs. (It is usual for the leg with pressure sensitive areas as determined by the previous palpation examination to experience greater discomfort during this passive mobility examination.)

Sōtai I: This Sōtai movement should be performed when pressure sensitive points are found in the palpation examination of Supine J-1–1, or when a difference in the sensation between the right and left legs is noticed during the mobility examination of Supine J-1–2 and J-1–3. The patient gently raises her knees to a flexed position, keeping them together. Then without moving her feet on the working surface, the patient attempts to simultaneously push the right knee down toward the tip of her feet and to draw her left knee up toward her abdomen (Fig. 114). Placing his hands on her knees as shown in Figure 115, the therapist applies resistance to the patient's movement. They both hold the tension at a suitable position for three to five seconds, and then release it. This procedure is repeated two or three times.

Fig. 112 Supine J-1–2

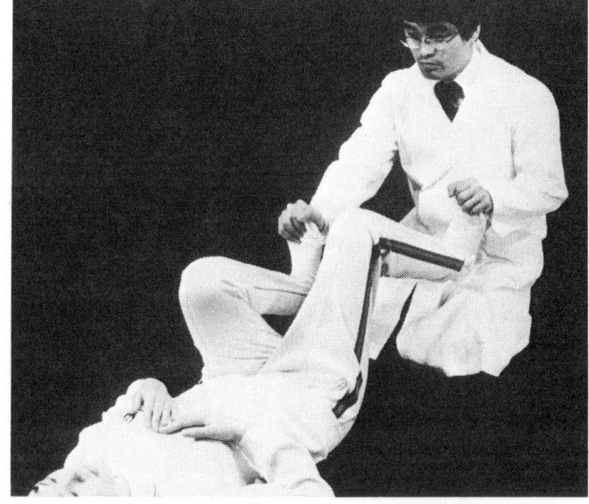

Fig. 113 Supine J-1–3

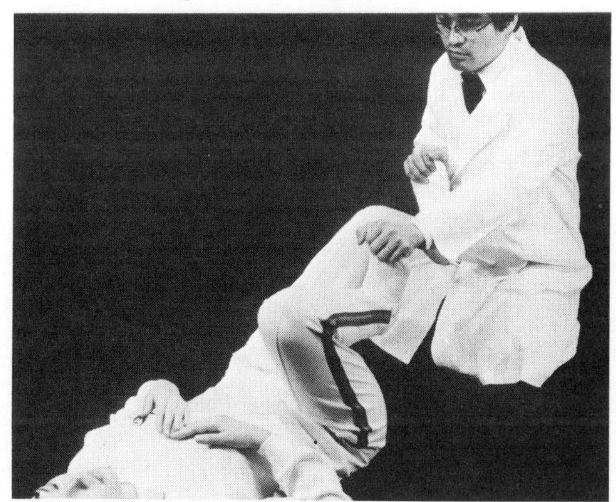

Fig. 114 Supine J-1–4

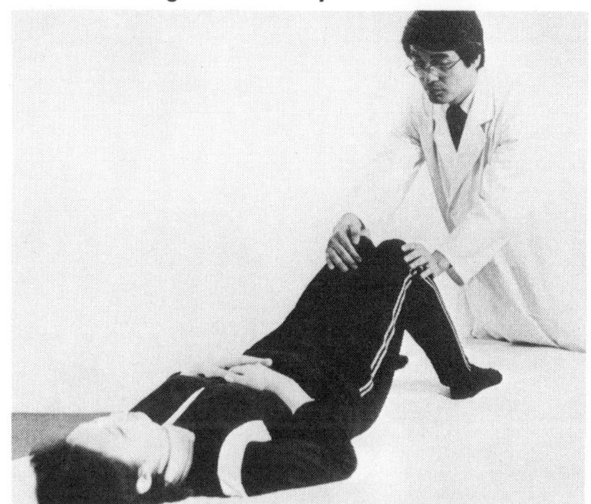

Fig. 115 Supine J-1–5

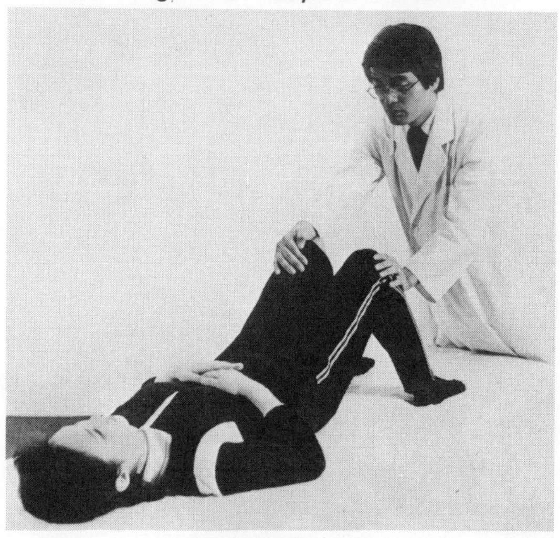

Sōtai II: In cases where pressure sensitive points were found on both sides in the palpation examination of Supine J-1–1, or when the mobility examination Supine J-1–2 and –3 caused discomfort in both legs, the patient should flex her knees upward, raising both feet a few inches off the working surface (Fig. 116). From this position, the patient lowers her feet toward the floor. The therapist gives resistance to this movement by applying counterpressure on the patient's legs below her knees (Fig. 117). They hold the tension for three to five seconds at a suitable position and then release it simultaneously. This procedure is repeated two or three times.

Fig. 116 Supine J-1–6

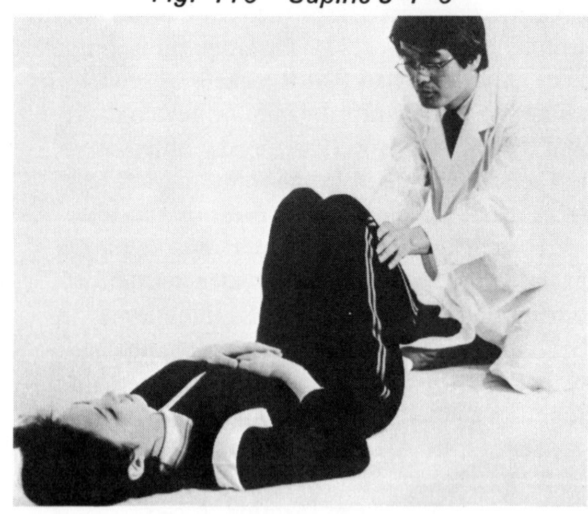

Fig. 117 Supine J-1–7

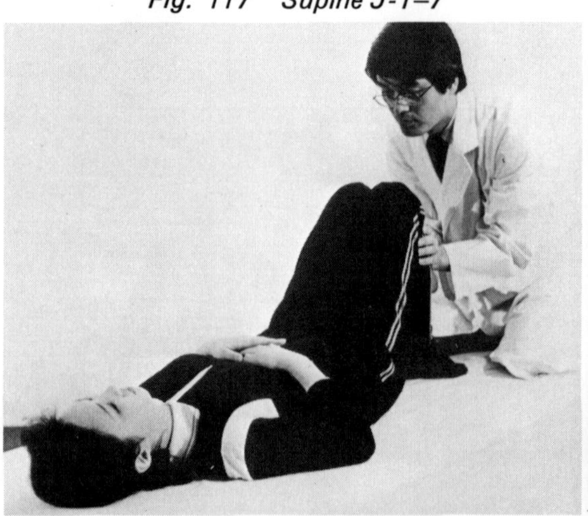

Fig. 118 Supine J-1–8

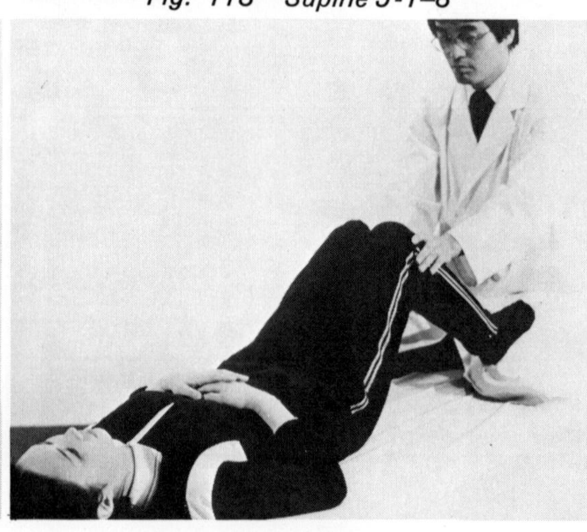

Fig. 119 Supine J-1–9

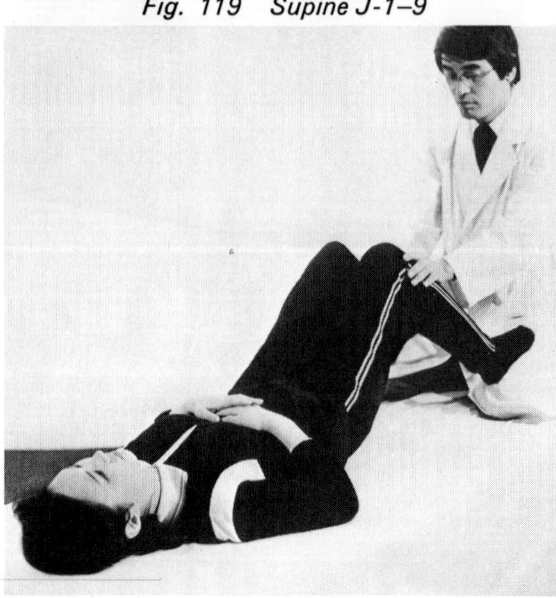

Sōtai III: This Sōtai movement should also be performed on the patients who have pressure sensitive points on both sides of the sacroiliac joint, or who experience discomfort in both legs during mobility examination. The therapist sits in the Seiza posture at the patient's feet. The patient in the supine position, flexes her knees upward and places her feet on the therapist's knees (Fig. 118). Then, with the soles of her feet securely planted on the therapist's legs, the patient pushes both of her knees in the direction of the therapist. Applying pressure to her knees, the therapist resists her movement (Fig. 119). They maintain opposing pressure at

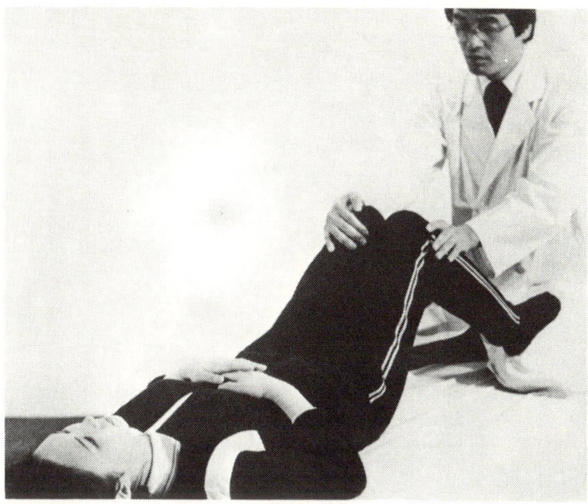

Fig. 120 Supine J-1–10

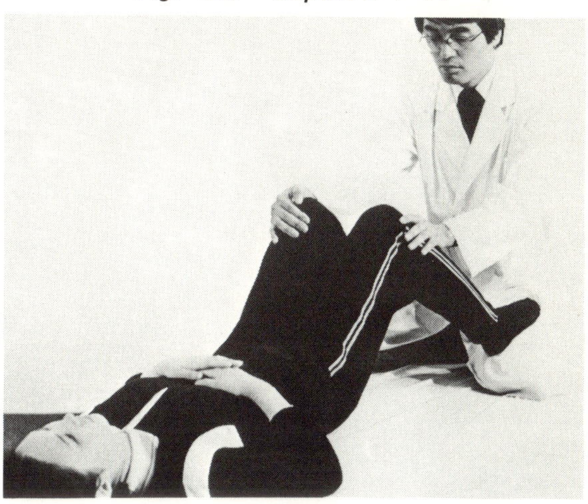

Fig. 121 Supine J-1–11

a suitable position for three to five seconds, and then release. This procedure is repeated two or three times.

Sōtai IV. The following are additional Sōtai movements which may be performed when discomfort or pressure sensitivity is experienced during the examinations of Supine J-1.

The therapist sits in the Seiza position at the patient's feet. The patient plants the soles of her feet on the therapist's legs just above his knees, and then attempts to push her right knee toward the therapist as she pulls her left knee back toward herself. Placing his hands as shown in Figures 120 and 121, the therapist gives resistance to these movements. They maintain opposing pressure for three to five seconds, and then release this simultaneously. This procedure is repeated two or three times.

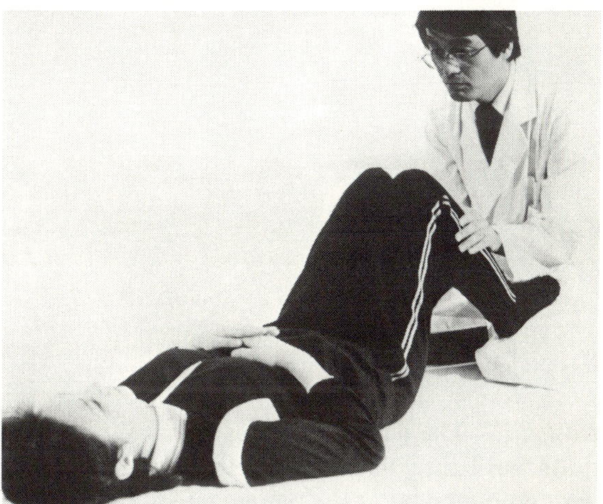

Fig. 122 Supine J-1–12

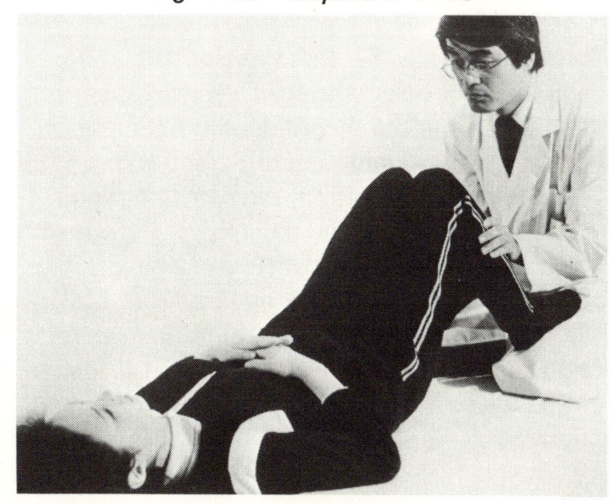

Fig. 123 Supine J-1–13

Sōtai V: In this movement also, the patient rests her feet on the knees of the therapist. She then tenses her leg muscles, pressing her feet down on to the therapist's legs. The therapist resists this movement by applying pressure against her legs below the knees (Figs. 122 and 123). At a suitable position they both hold opposing pressure for three to five seconds, and then release this simultaneously. This procedure is repeated two or three times.

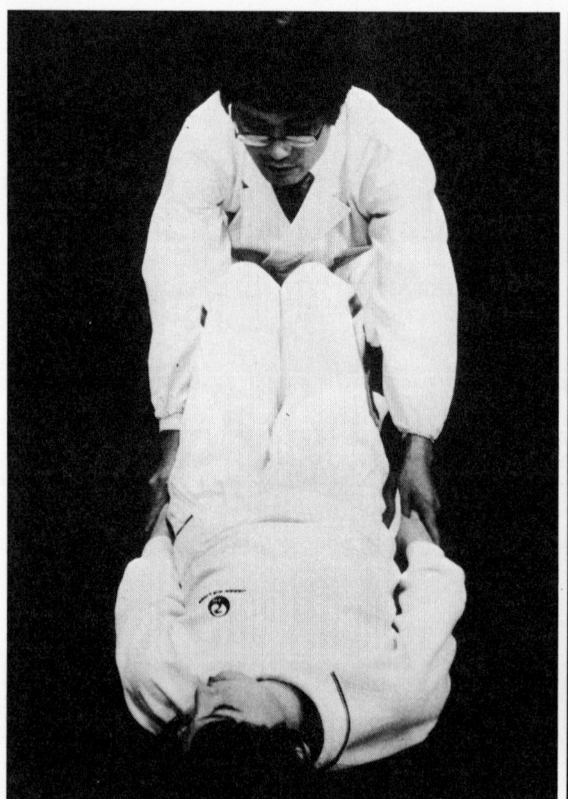

Fig. 124 Supine K-1–1

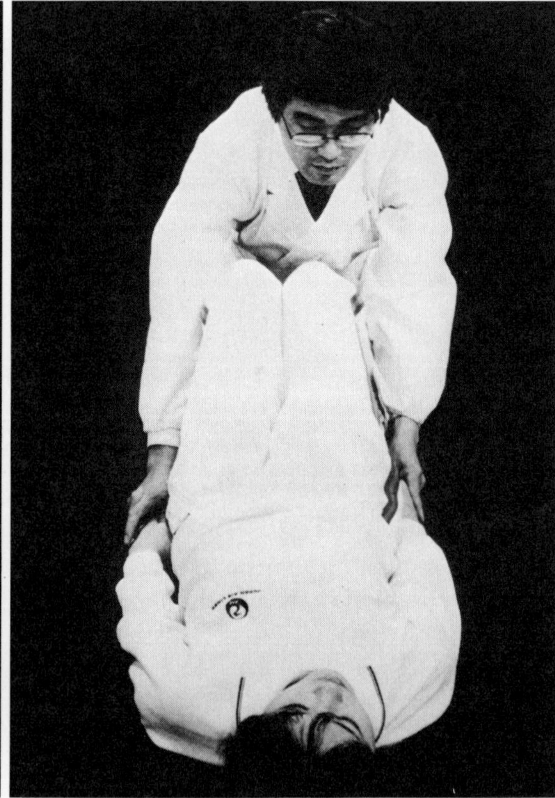

Fig. 125 Supine K-1–2

Supine K-1

Dōshin I; The patient assumes a supine position and lightly flexes her knees to a raised position. Standing at the patient's feet, the therapist grasps both of her hands and alternately pulls the left and right arms toward himself (Figs. 124 and 125). He inquires about the sensations of comfort and discomfort produced in these movements.

Dōshin II: After assuming a supine position, the patient extends her body. The therapist now stands at the patient's head and depresses her right and left shoulders alternately (Fig. 126 and 127). He again inquires about sensations of comfort and discomfort.

Note: During this examination, if the movement of the patient's entire body is observed carefully, it can be seen that both depressing the shoulders and pulling the arm produce physical movements of the same type. Consequently, it is usual for the sensations of comfort and discomfort, as well as their differences between the right and left sides to be just the same in both examinations.

Sōtai I: This Sōtai movement should be employed in cases where the greater discomfort was produced by pulling the right arm in the mobility examination of Supine K-1.

In the supine position, the patient elevates her right shoulder. The therapist at the patient's feet, holds her right wrist (Figs. 128 and 129). He gives resistance to the movement of her shoulder. They both hold tension in a suitable position for three to five seconds and then release. The procedure is repeated two or three times.

Fig. 126 Supine K-1–3

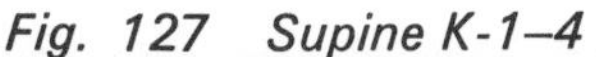

Fig. 127 Supine K-1–4

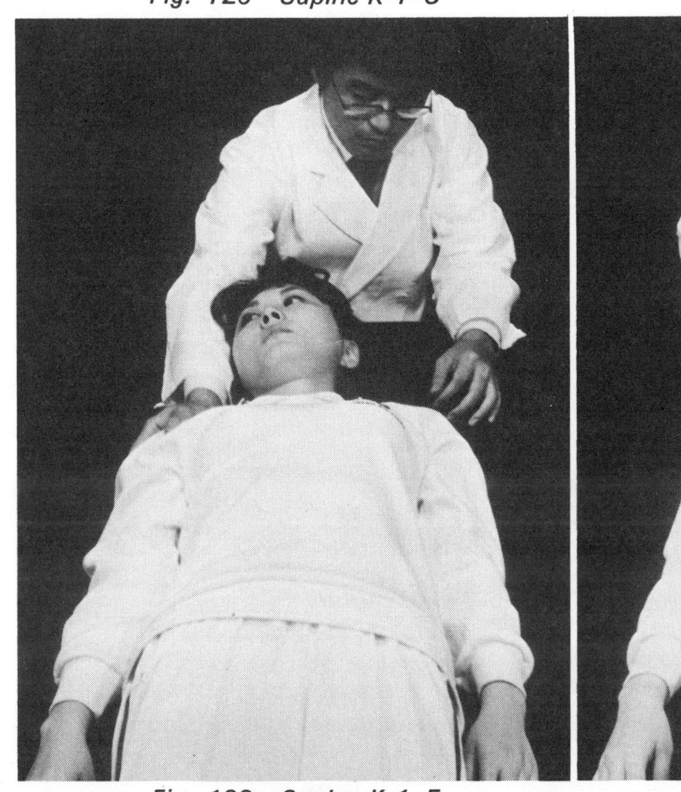

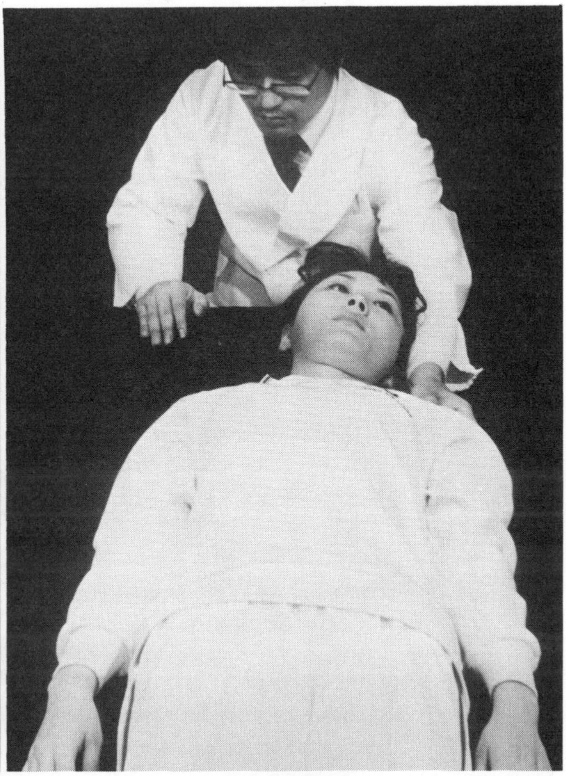

Fig. 128 Supine K-1–5

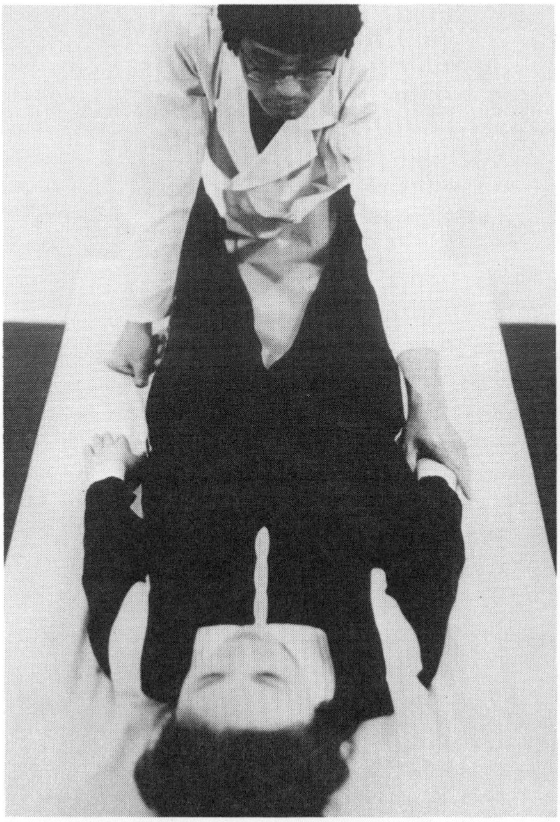

Fig. 129 Supine K-1–6

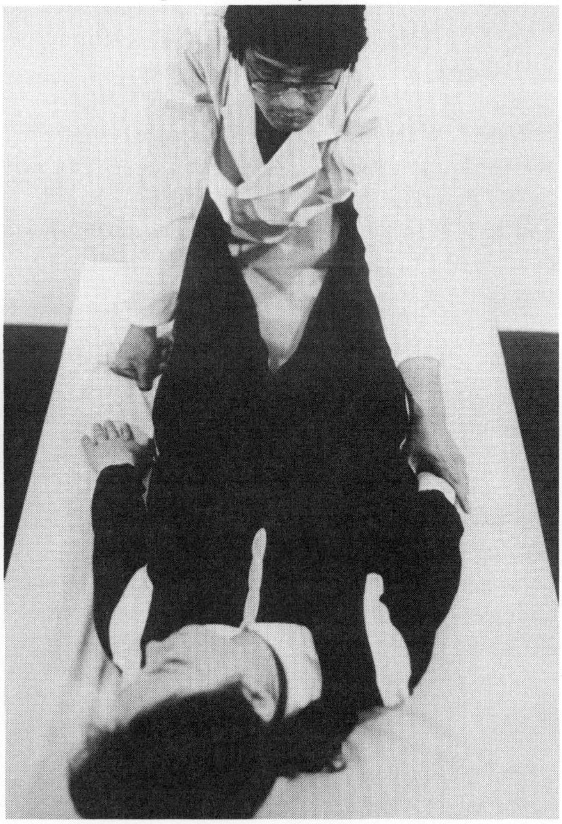

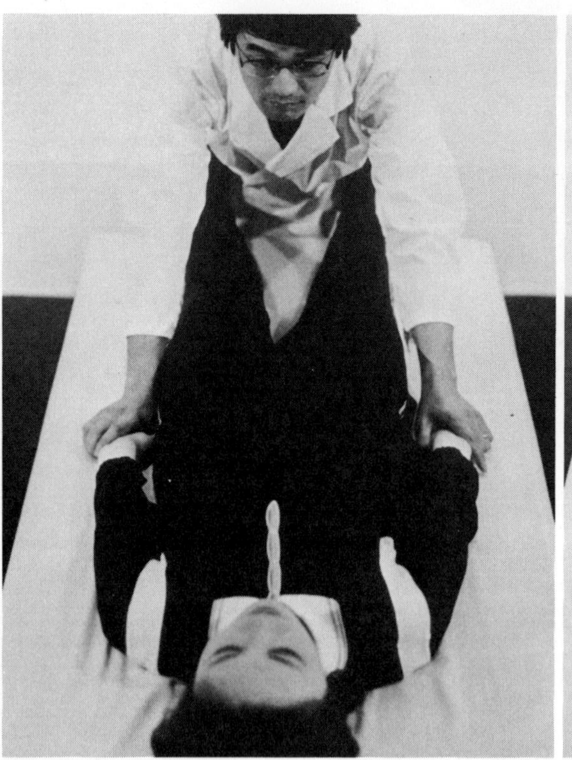

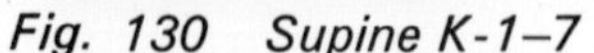
Fig. 130 Supine K-1–7

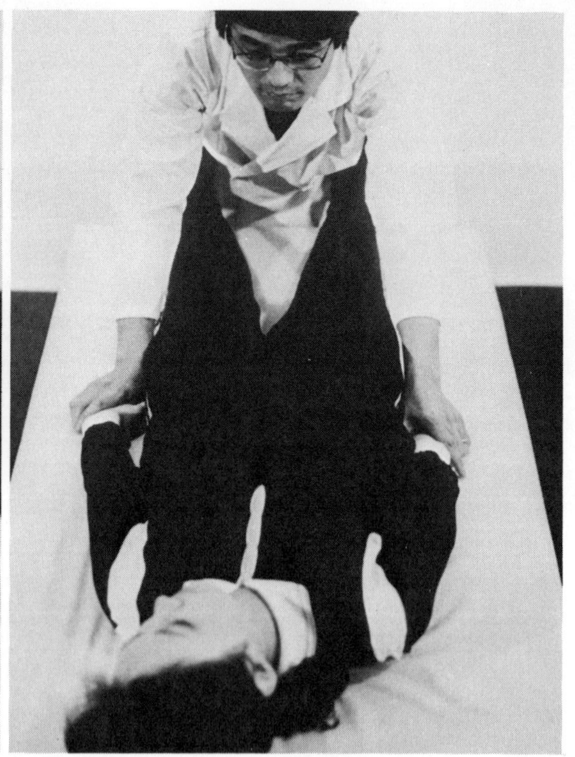

Fig. 131 Supine K-1–8

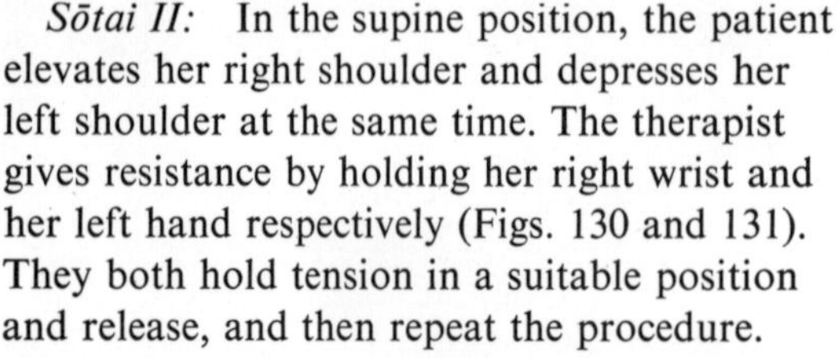
Sōtai II: In the supine position, the patient elevates her right shoulder and depresses her left shoulder at the same time. The therapist gives resistance by holding her right wrist and her left hand respectively (Figs. 130 and 131). They both hold tension in a suitable position and release, and then repeat the procedure.

Note: When performing Sōtai movements K-1–5 through K-1–8, the patient's knees can be lightly flexed as in mobility examination K-1–1 and K-1–2. In this variation, the therapist's chest can be used to stabilize the patient's knees, and this method could prove more effective.

Sōtai III: The patient again elevates her right shoulder. The therapist standing at the patient's head, applies resistance by placing his hand on her right shoulder (Figs. 132 and 133). They hold tension at a suitable position and release, and then repeat the procedure.

Sōtai IV: The patient simultaneously elevates her right shoulder and depresses her left shoulder. Placing his hands on her right shoulder and left axilla, the therapist provides resistance to her movement (Figs. 134 and 135). They maintain tension at a suitable position and release, and then repeat the procedure.

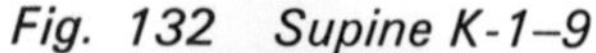
Fig. 132 Supine K-1–9

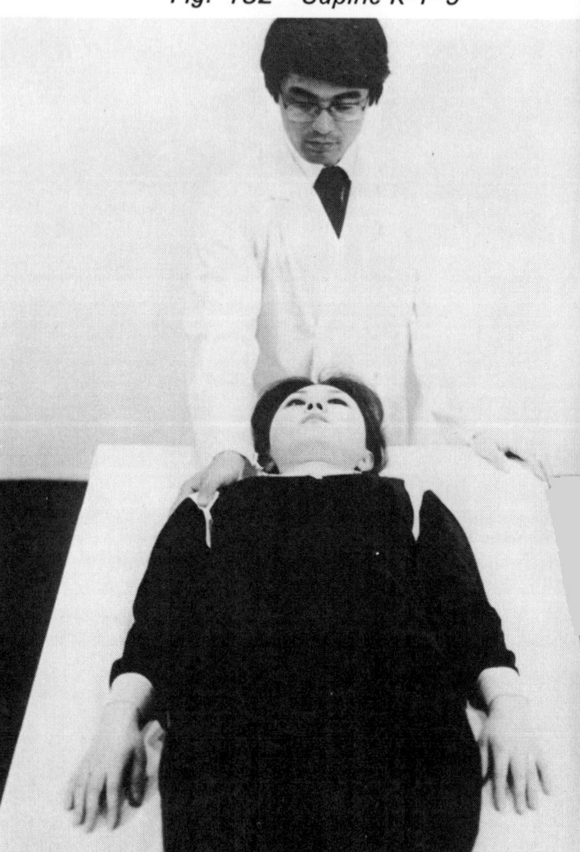

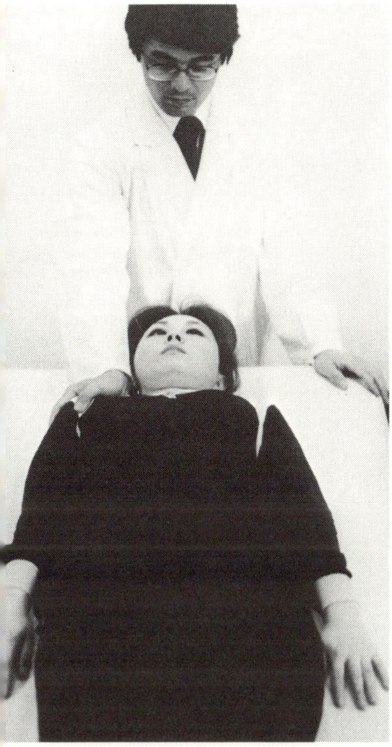

Fig. 133 Supine K-1–10 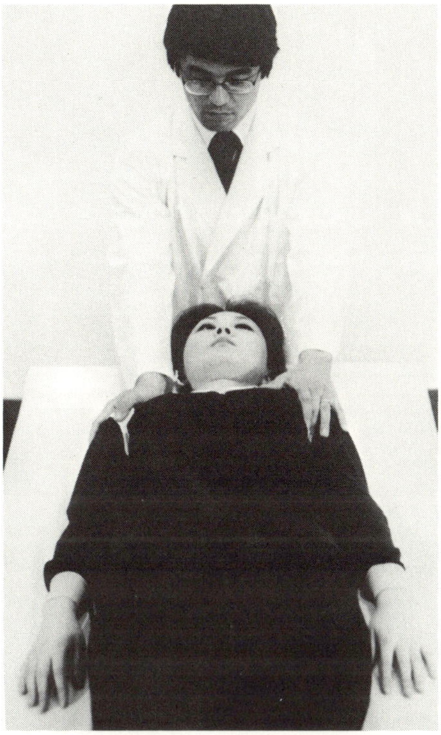 *Fig. 134 Supine K-1–11* 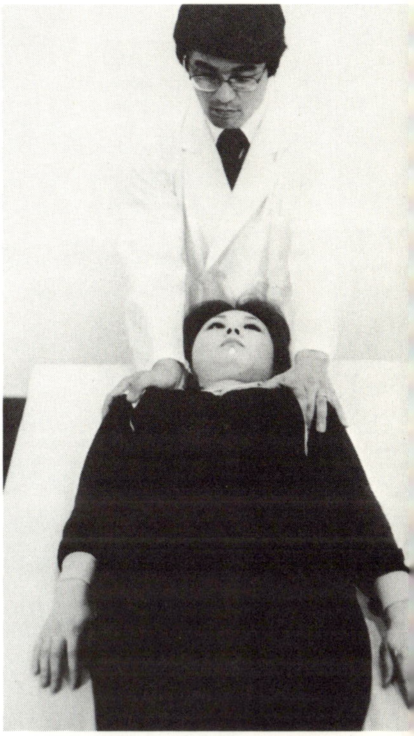 *Fig. 135 Supine K-1–12*

Supine L-1

Dōshin: The patient assumes a supine position and stretches her body, spreading her legs apart to shoulder width. Standing behind her head, the therapist rotates her head first to the right, and then to the left, inquiring about sensations of comfort and discomfort (Figs. 136 and 137). The patient compares the sensations of the rotation to the right and to the left.

Fig. 136 Supine L-1–1

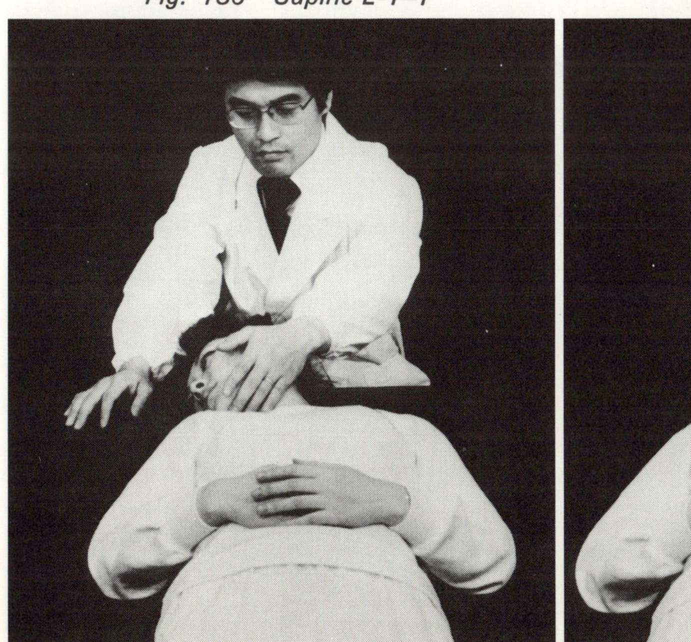

Fig. 137 Supine L-1–2

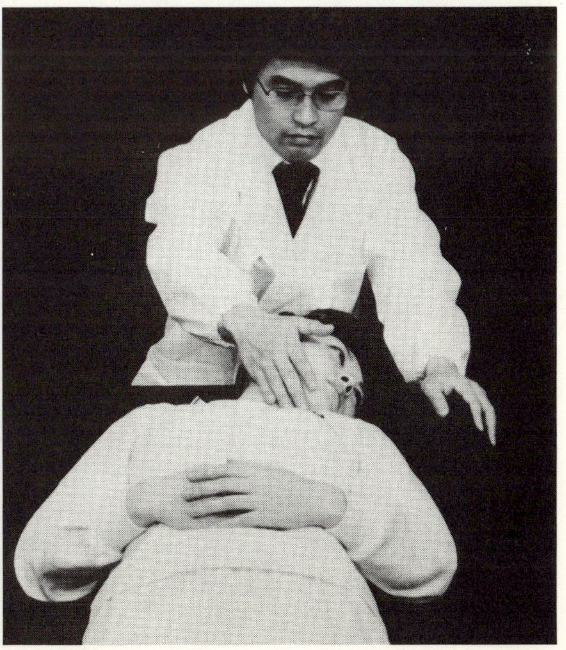

Fig. 138 · Supine L-1–3

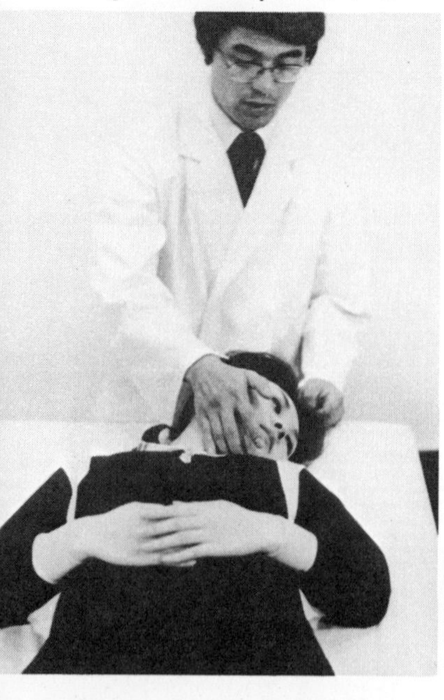

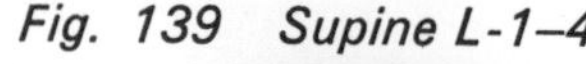

Fig. 139 Supine L-1–4

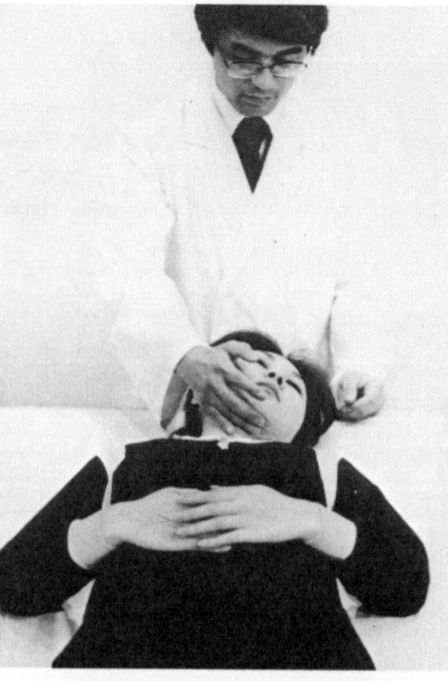

Fig. 140 Supine L-1–5

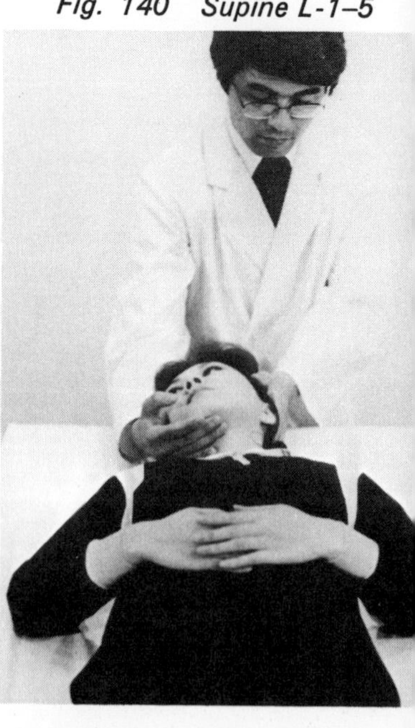

Sōtai: The patient rotates her head from left to right. The therapist applies resistance to her movement by pressing with his hands against her right zygomatic and maxillary area (Figs. 138 to 140). They hold tension at a suitable position and release, and then repeat the procedure.

Supine L-2

Dōshin: As in Supine L-1–1, the patient lies supine and stretches her body, spreading her feet apart shoulder width. Standing behind her head, the therapist flexes her head laterally, first to the right, and then to the left (Figs. 141 and

Fig. 141 Supine L-2–1

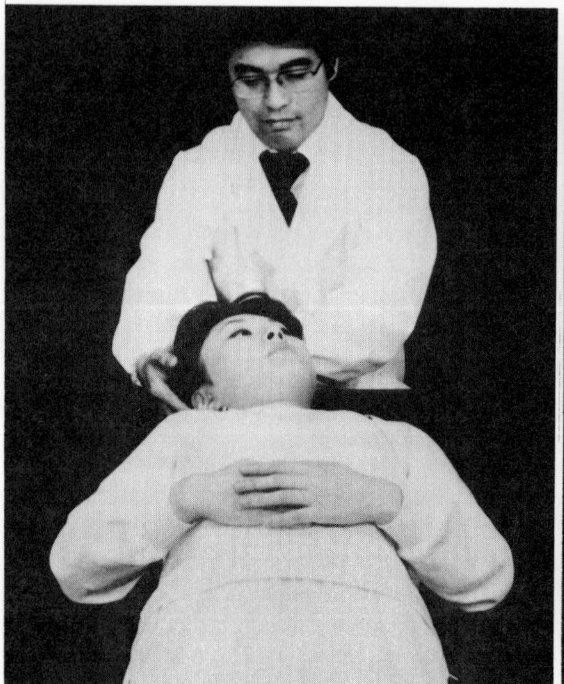

Fig. 142 Supine L-2–2

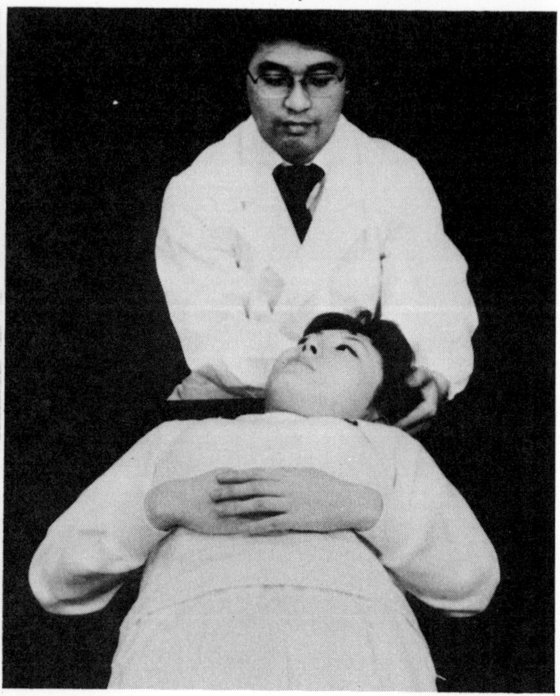

142). The therapist inquires about sensation of comfort and discomfort, comparing that of movement to the right and to the left.

Sōtai: The patient flexes her head laterally from right to left. The therapist gives resistance to this movement by holding the patient's head (Figs. 143 to 145). They maintain tension at a suitable position and release, and then repeat the procedure two or three times.

SupineM-1

Palpation examination: The patient lies in a supine position and relaxes, stretching her entire body. The therapist places his hands under her posterior cervical region and palpates the splenius capitis muscles (Fig. 146). He checks for the presence of pressure sensitive points accompanying abnormal tension in the

Fig. 143 Supine L-2–3

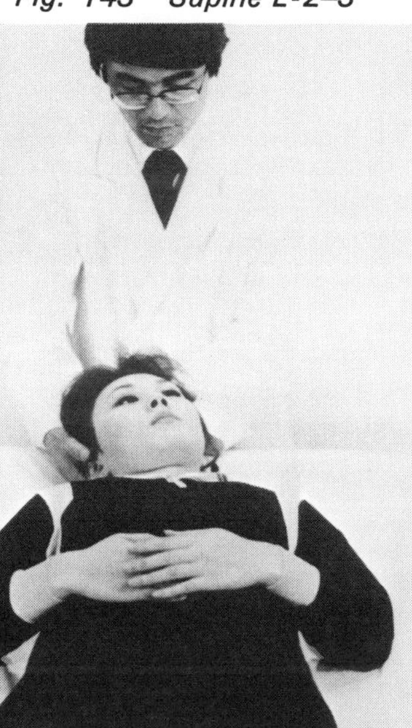

Fig. 144 Supine L-2–4

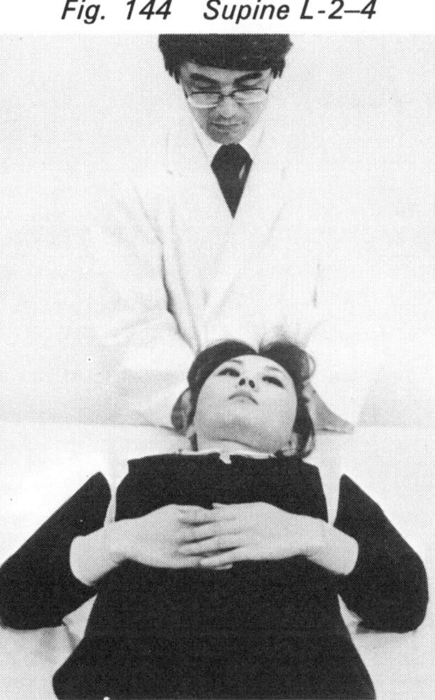

Fig. 145 Supine L-2–5

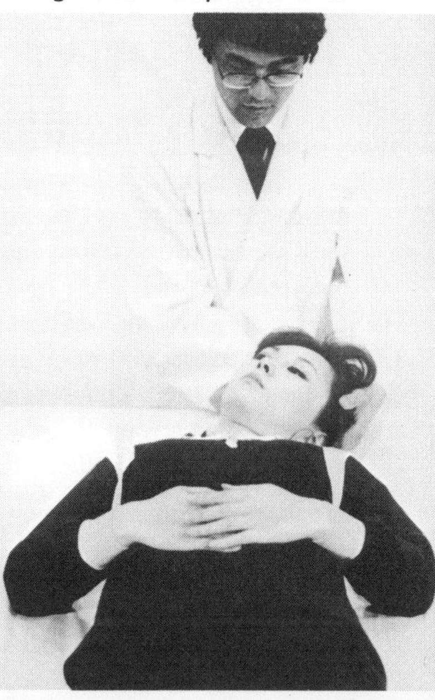

Fig. 146 Supine M-1–1

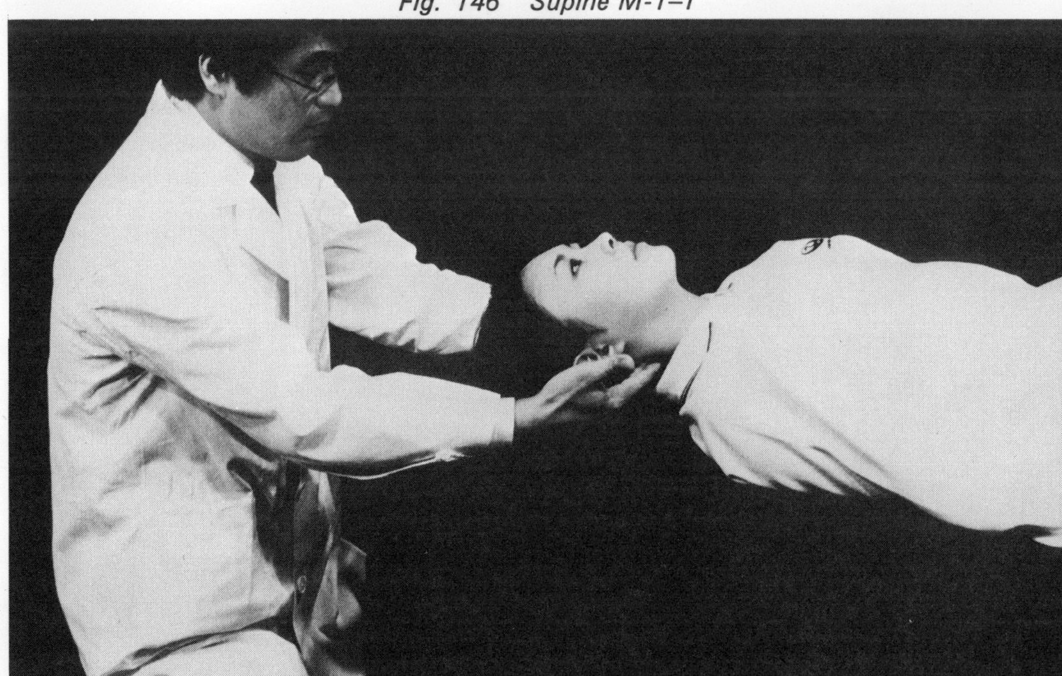

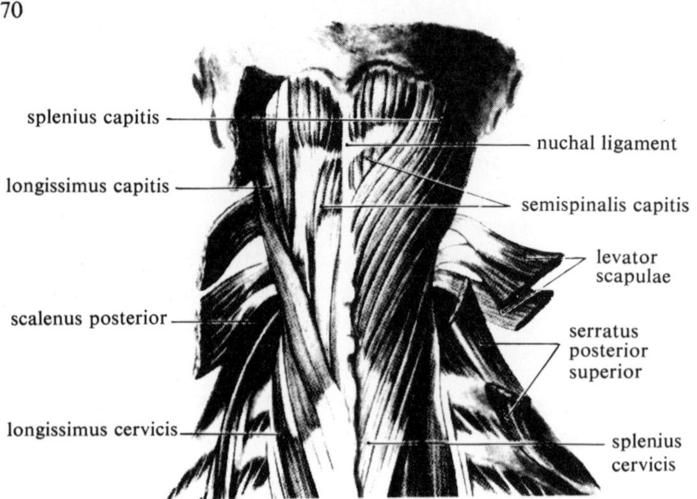

Fig. 147 Anatomical Diagram of Neck

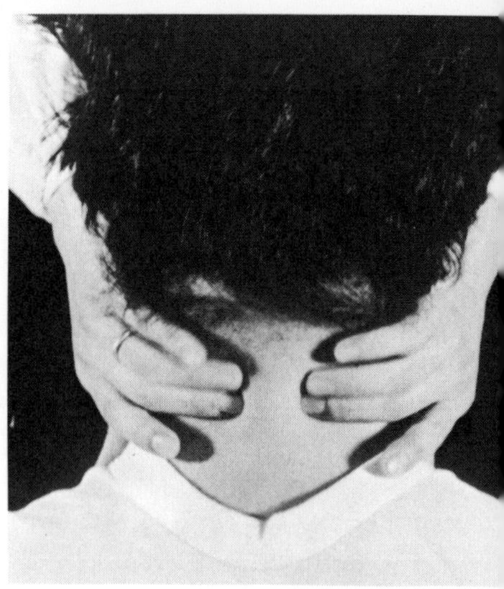

Fig. 148 Area of Palpation

muscle. Figure 147 is the anatomical diagram showing the musculature and Figure 148 shows the area palpated.

Sōtai I: The patient first slowly raises her chin by neck extension (Figs. 149 and 150). Then, using the occipital region as a point of support, she elevates her chest, raising her shoulders and back off the treatment table. The therapist places his hands under the patient's posterior cervical region and applies traction, pulling toward himself (Fig. 151). The motion is stopped and tension is held for three to five seconds at a suitable place. Then the patient lets her shoulders and back fall to the treatment table limply. This procedure is repeated two or three times.

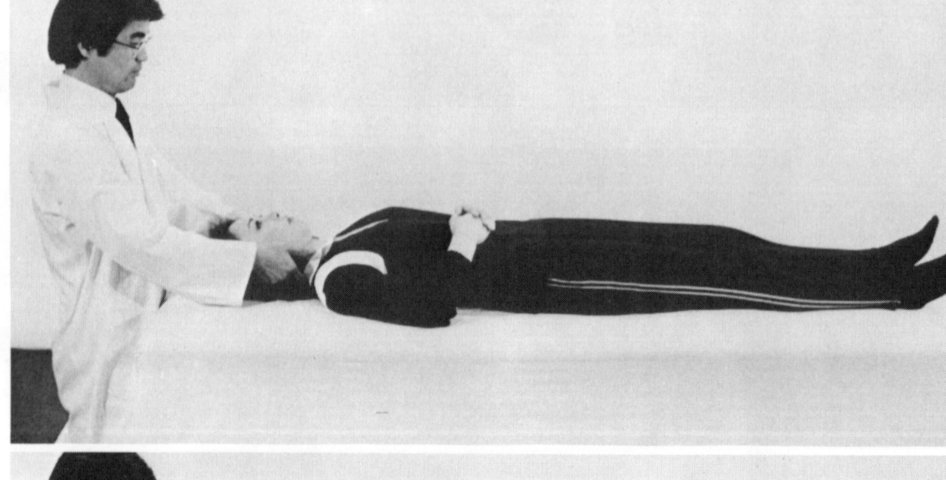

Fig. 149 Supine M-1–2

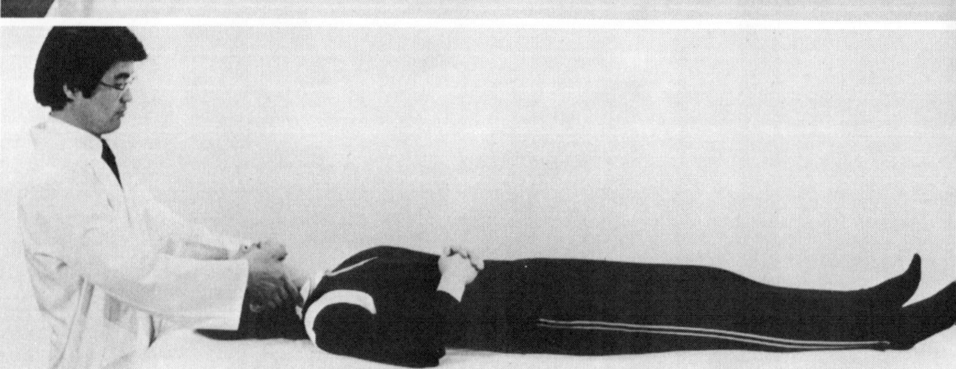

Fig. 150 Supine M-1–3

Fig. 151 Supine M-1–4

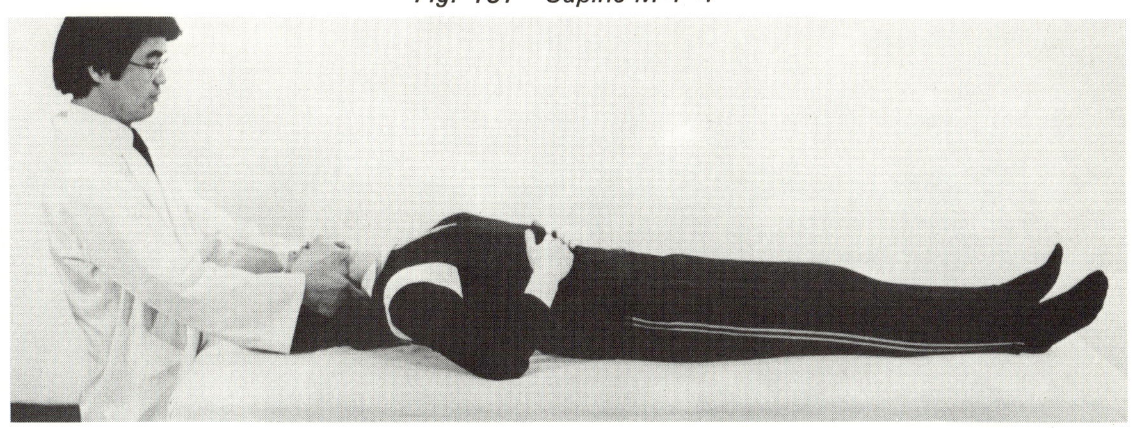

Sōtai II: Sōtai movement M-1–2 through –4 may also be performed actively, that is, by the patient using intrinsic force alone, without aid of a therapist.

In the manner described above, the patient slowly elevates her chin (Figs. 152 and 153). Then, using the occipital region as a point of support, she elevates her chest, raising her shoulders and back above the treatment table (Fig. 154). At a suitable position she stops the motion and holds tension for three to five seconds. She then relaxes and lets her shoulders and back drop down to the table.

Fig. 152 Supine M-1–5

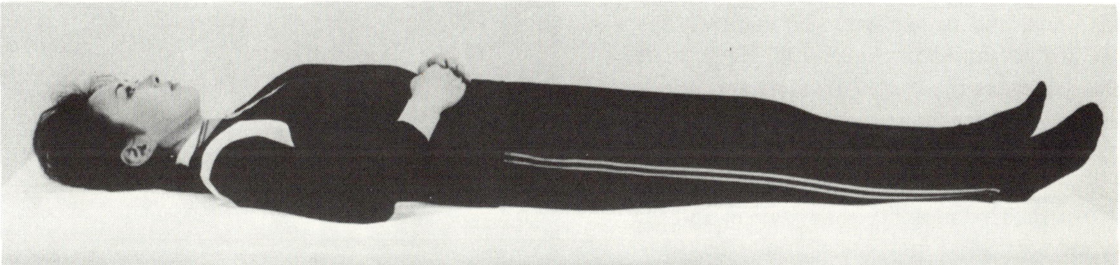

Fig. 153 Supine M-1–6

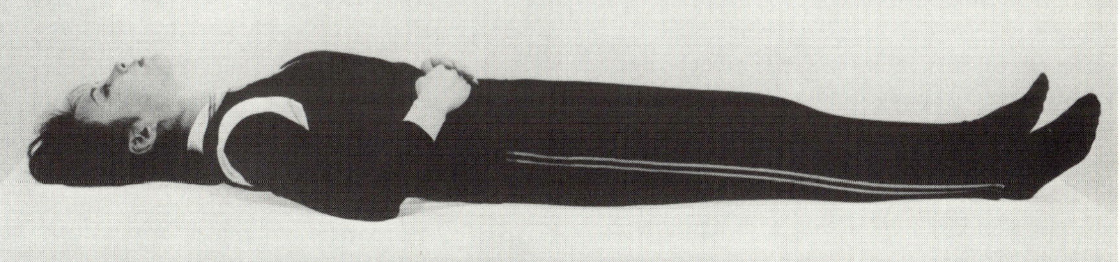

Fig. 154 Supine M-1–7

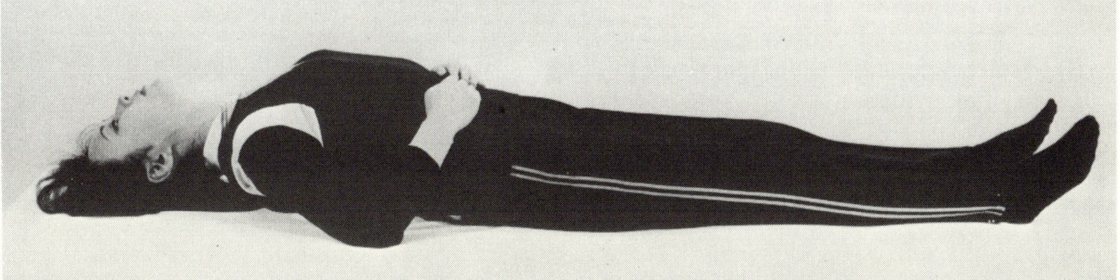

Fig. 155 Supine N-1–1

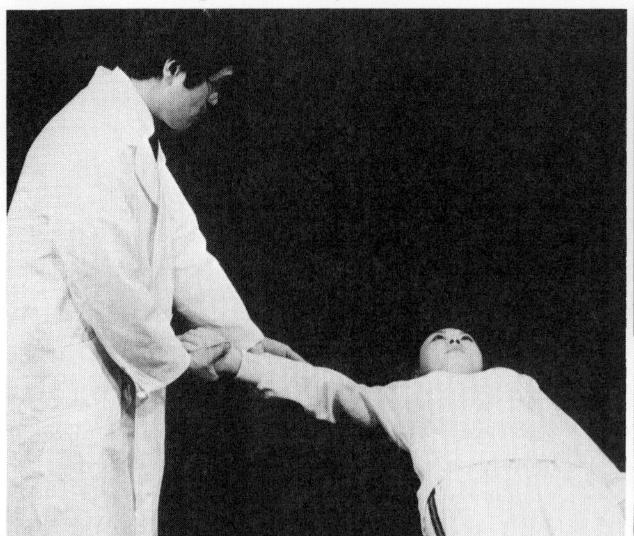

Fig. 156 Supine N-1–2

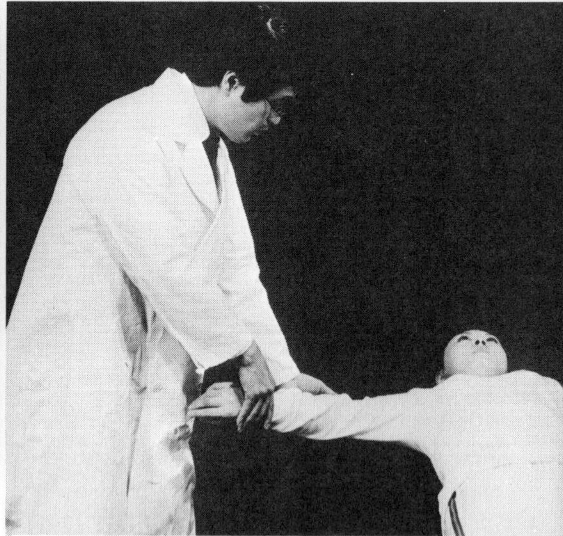

Supine N-1

Dōshin: The patient lies supine and extends both arms out to her side. The therapist holds her arm as shown in Figure 155. He pronates and supinates the arm alternately and questions the patient about accompanying sensations of comfort and discomfort (Fig. 156).

Note: This mobility examination and the subsequent Sōtai movement should be performed with the angle of abduction in the shoulder joint varied, or with the arm in several different positions.

The extent of mobility in the shoulder joint is quite large when revolved on the horizontal, transverse, and sagittal planes. This fact should be kept in mind when Sōtai techniques for the shoulder are performed. Figures 157 and 158 illustrate shoulder joint action with light track photography.

(I) The range of shoulder movement when revolved on the longitudinal (A), sagittal (B), and transverse axes (C)

(II) Entire range of shoulder movement in sagittal revolution

Fig. 157 Shoulder Joint Movement in Standing Position I

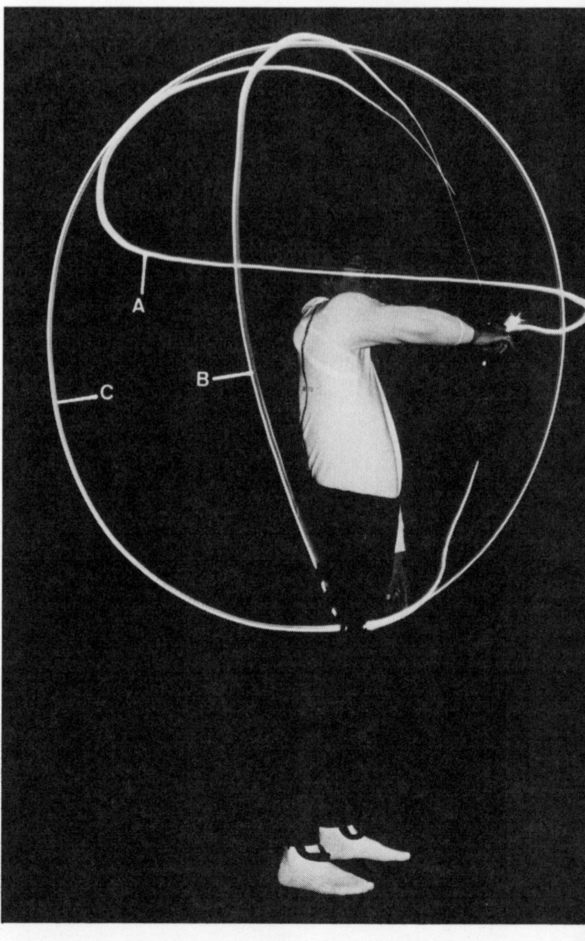

Fig. 158 Shoulder Joint Movement in Standing Position II

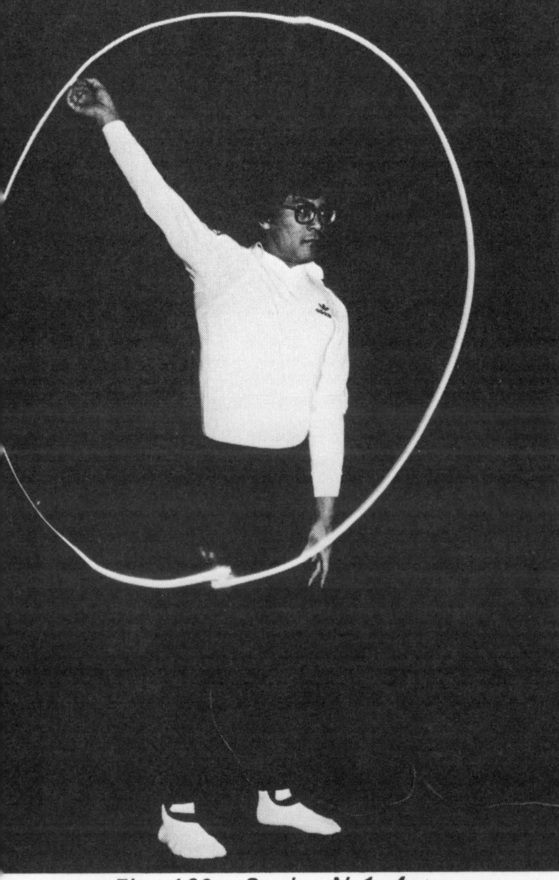

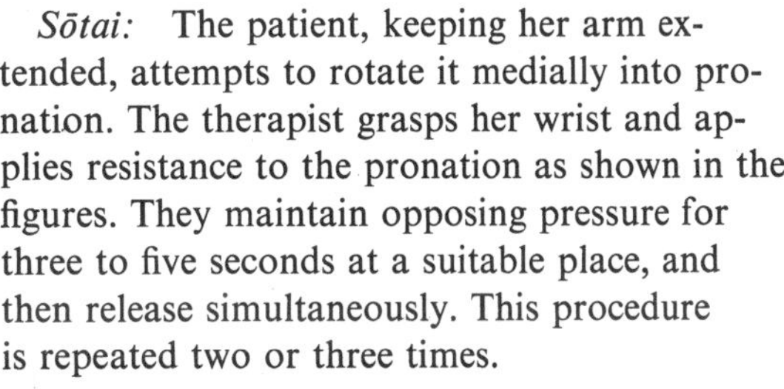

Sōtai: The patient, keeping her arm extended, attempts to rotate it medially into pronation. The therapist grasps her wrist and applies resistance to the pronation as shown in the figures. They maintain opposing pressure for three to five seconds at a suitable place, and then release simultaneously. This procedure is repeated two or three times.

Fig. 159 Supine N-1–3

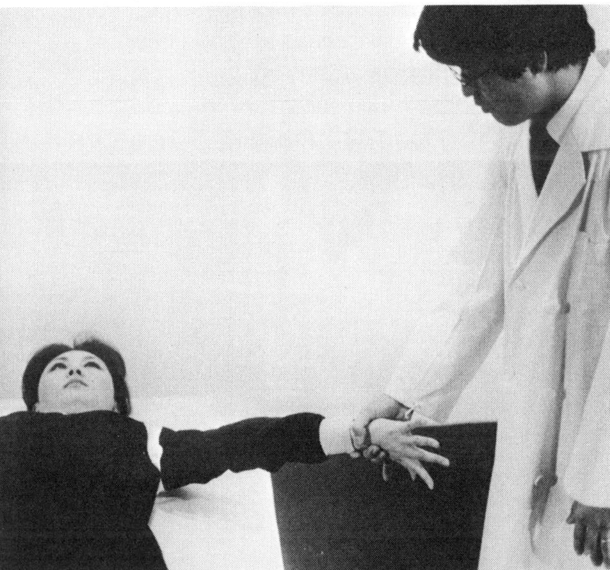

Fig. 160 Supine N-1–4

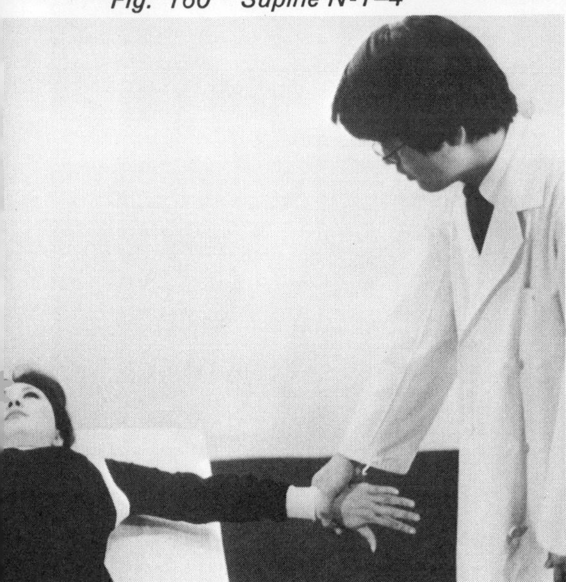

Fig. 161 Supine N-1–5

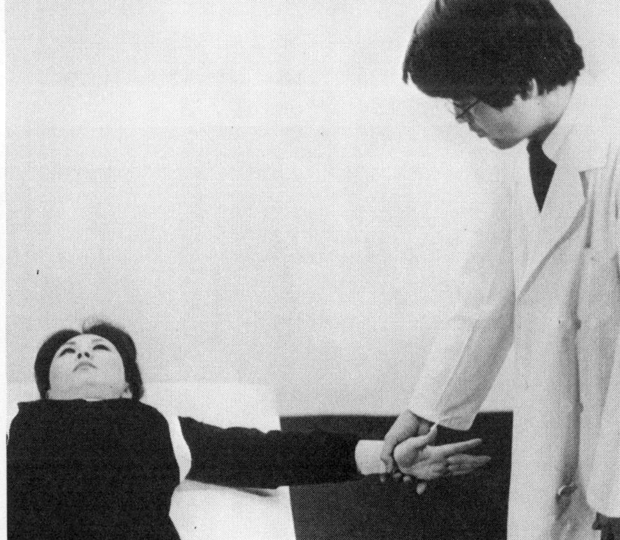

Prone Position

Prone A-1

Palpation examination: The patient assumes a prone posture. Standing at the patient's side, the therapist applies downward pressure on her right and left iliac areas alternately (Figs. 162 and 163). He inquires about sensations of comfort or discomfort produced, and the difference between the right and left sides.

Dōshin I: Standing at the side of the prone patient, the therapist places a hand under the right or left iliac areas and lifts upward alternately (Figs. 164 and 165). He inquires about the sensations of comfort or discomfort produced, and the difference between the left and right sides.

Dōshin II: The therapist stands at the feet of the prone patient. He grasps her ankles, and alternately flexes the right and left legs, pressing the heal to the buttock (Figs. 166 and 167). He checks for sensations of comfort or discomfort, as well as the differences between the right and left sides.

Fig. 162 Prone A-1–1

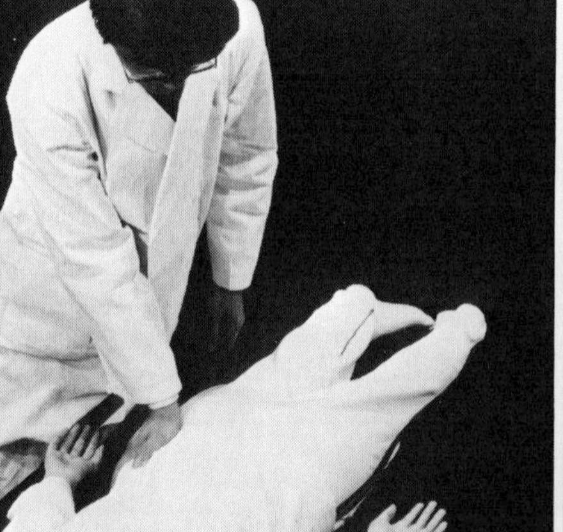

Fig. 163 Prone A-1–2

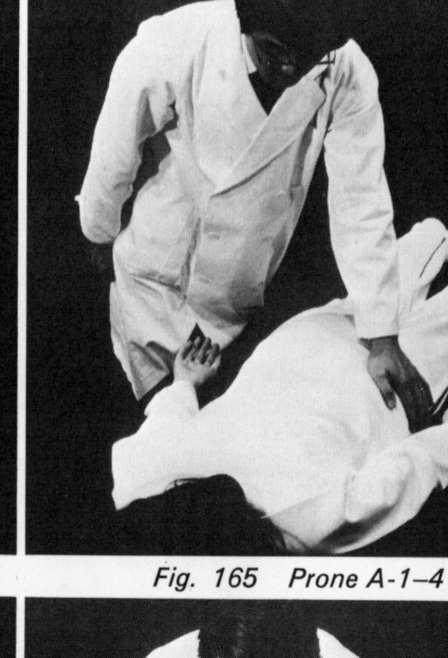

Fig. 164 Prone A-1–3

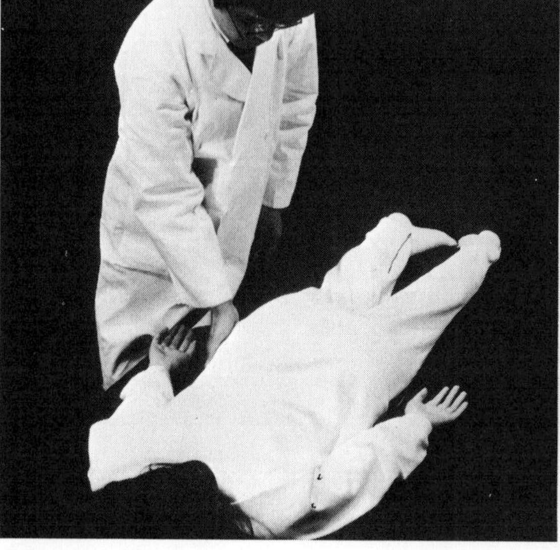

Fig. 165 Prone A-1–4

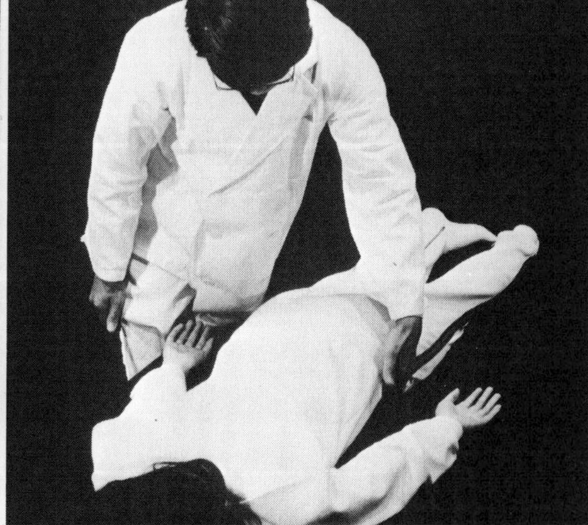

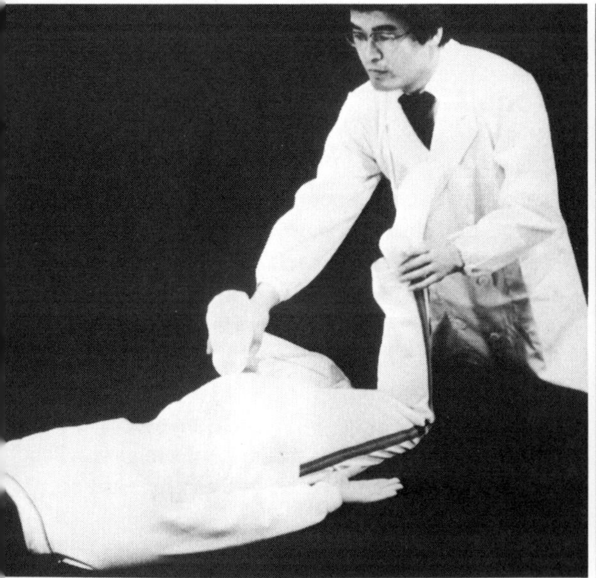

Fig. 166 Prone A-2–1

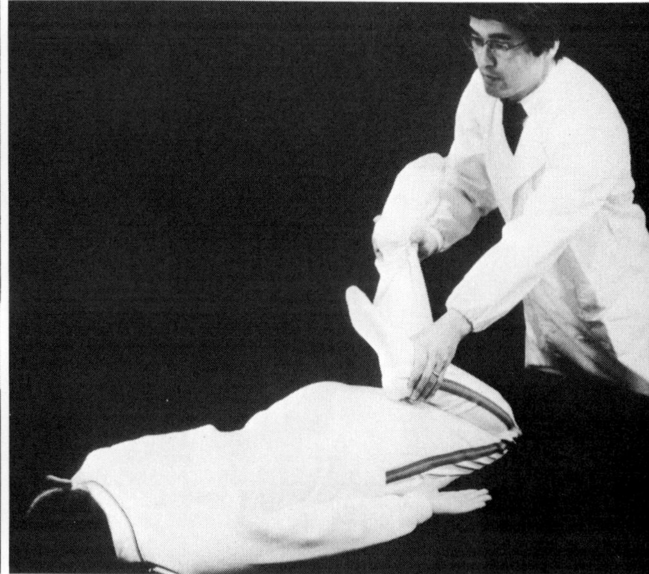

Fig. 167 Prone A-2–2

Fig. 168 Prone A-2-a-3

Prone A-2-a

Sōtai: In a prone position, the patient flexes both knees and draws her heels toward her gluteal region (Fig. 168). Next, from this posture the patient extends both her legs. Holding her ankles, the therapist gives resistance to the leg extension movement (Fig. 169). When they hold opposing pressure at a suitable position, the patient's thighs will rise off the treatment table (Fig. 170). After holding this position for three to five seconds, they both release tension simultaneously. This procedure is repeated two or three times.

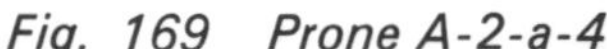

Fig. 169 Prone A-2-a-4

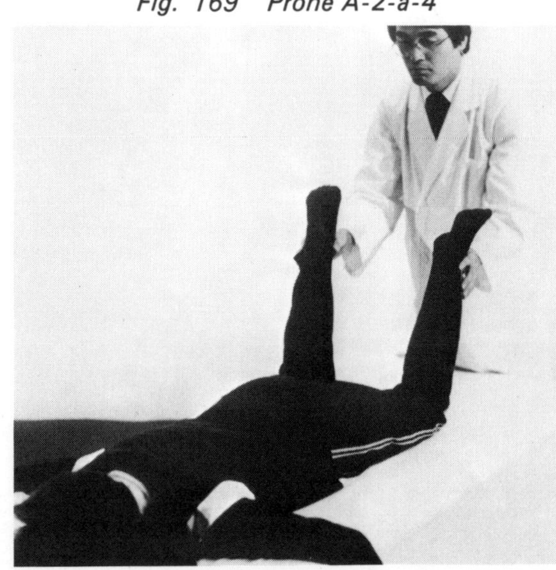

Fig. 170 Prone A-2-a-5

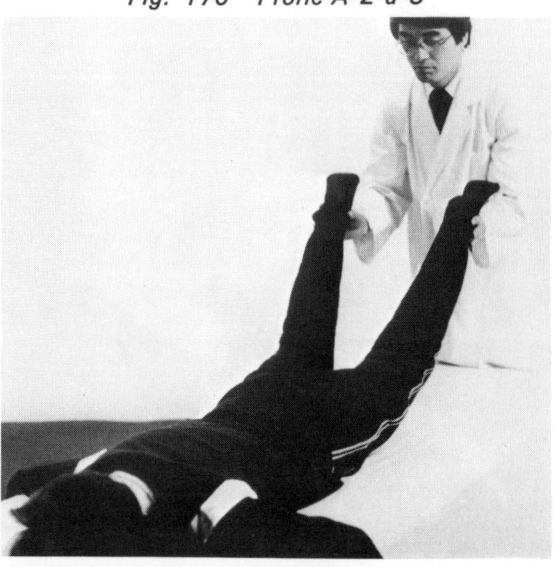

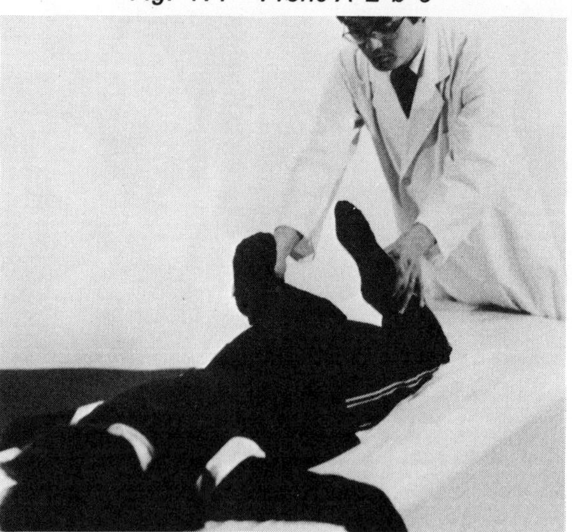

Fig. 171 Prone A-2-b-6

Prone A-2-b

Sōtai: As described above, the patient lies prone, flexes both knees and draws her heels toward her gluteal region. From this posture, the patient extends her left leg only. The therapist applies resistance to this leg extension movement by holding the ankles (Figs. 171 and 172). As they hold tension at a suitable position the patient's extending leg will tend to rise off treatment table (Fig. 173). The position is maintained for three to five seconds and released. This procedure is repeated two or three times.

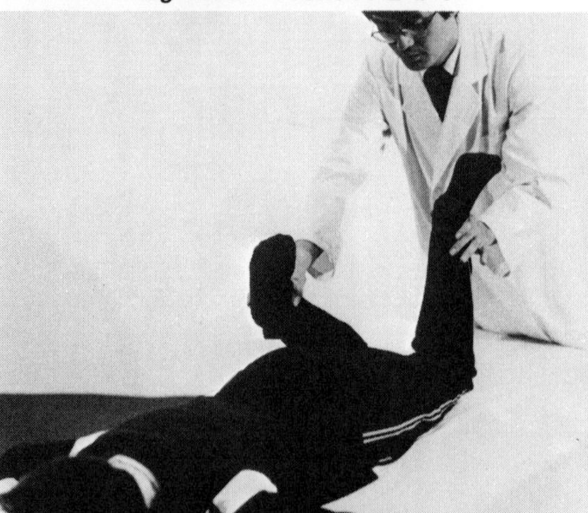

Fig. 172 Prone A-2-b-7

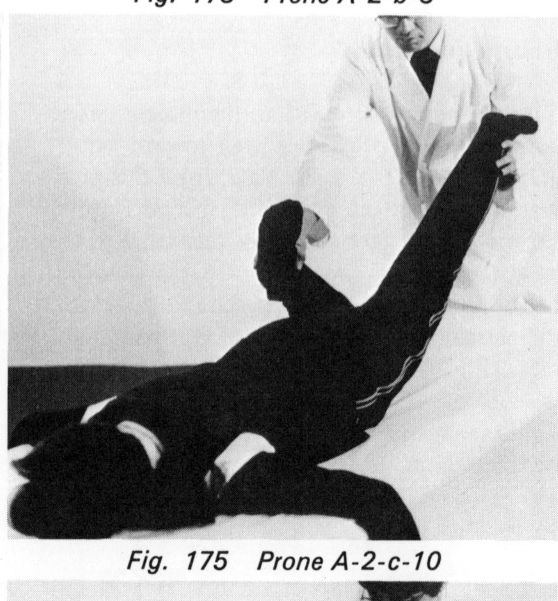

Fig. 173 Prone A-2-b-8

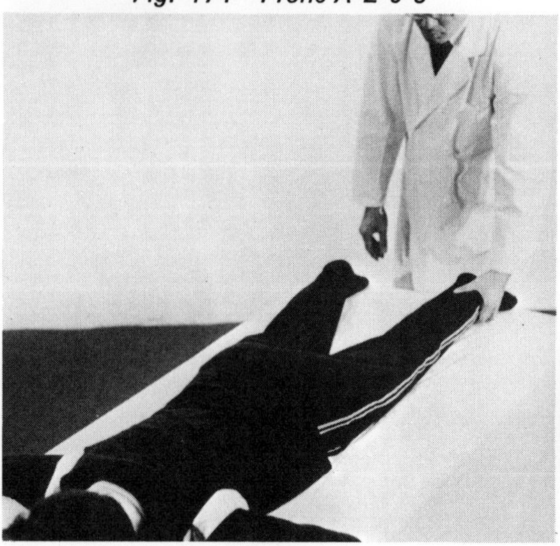

Fig. 174 Prone A-2-c-9

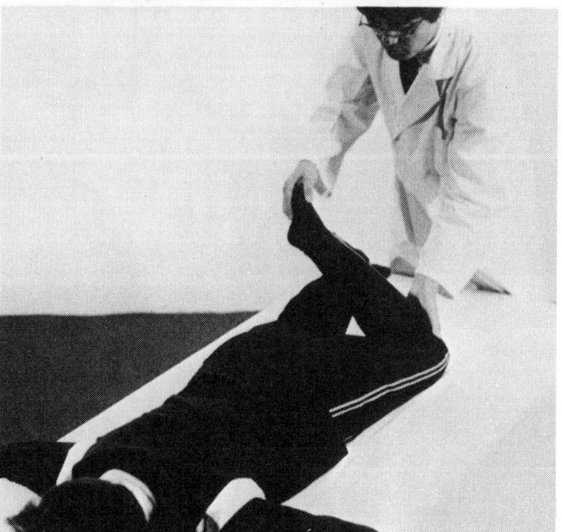

Fig. 175 Prone A-2-c-10

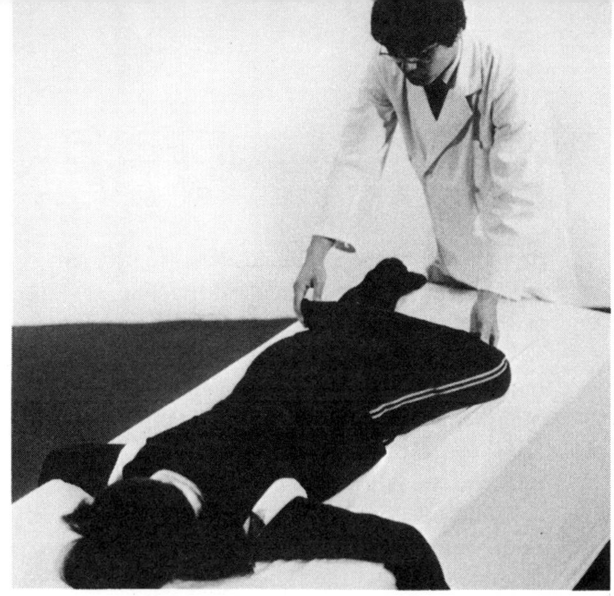

Fig. 176 Prone A-2-c-11

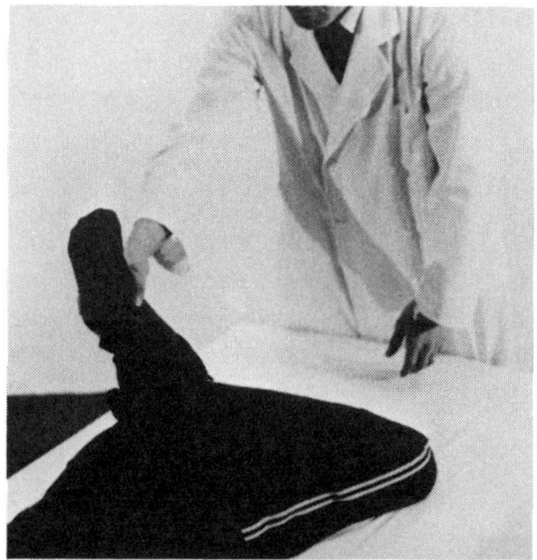

Fig. 177 Prone A-2-c-12

Prone A-2-c

Sōtai: The therapist flexes the patient's left leg at the knee, and places her left foot on her right popliteal region (Figs. 174 and 175). He then flexes her right leg once, then the patient reverses this movement by extending her right leg toward the therapist. The therapist provides resistance to this movement by holding her right ankle (Figs. 177 and 178). As they hold tension in a suitable position, the patient's extending leg will tend to rise off the treatment table. Opposing pressure is maintained for three to five seconds and released, and this is then repeated.

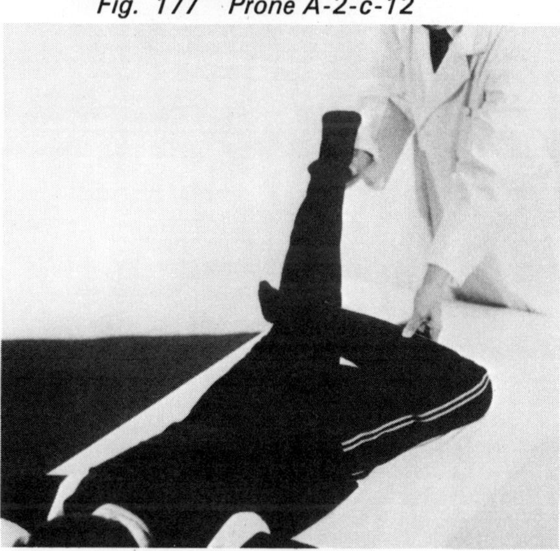

Fig. 178 Prone A-2-c-13

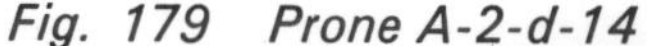

Fig. 179 Prone A-2-d-14

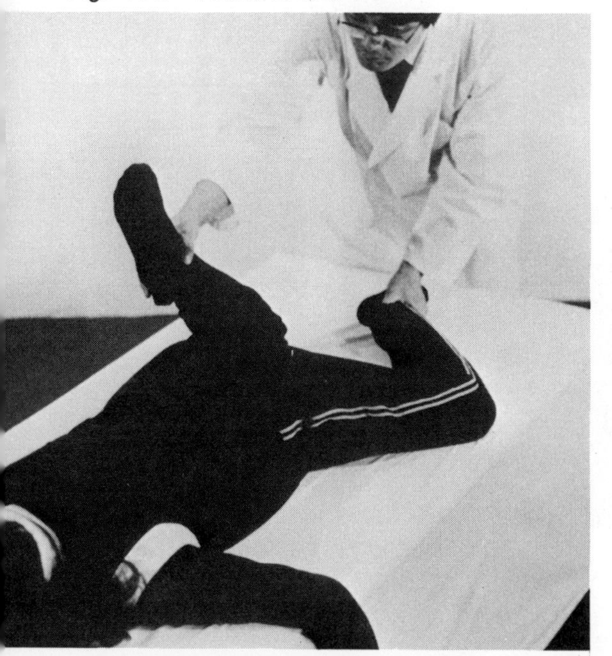

Prone A-2-d

Sōtai: As the therapist flexes the knee of the patient's right leg, he also flexes the left knee out laterally, moving the foot toward the hip while keeping the leg in contact with the table surface (Fig. 179). Next, the patient at the same time as extending her right leg, draws her left knee up toward her side, sliding the right leg on the table. The therapist grasps the patient's right and left ankles and provides resistance against both these movements (Fig. 180). They hold tension at a suitable position for three to five seconds and release, and then repeat the procedure.

Fig. 180 Prone A-2-d-15

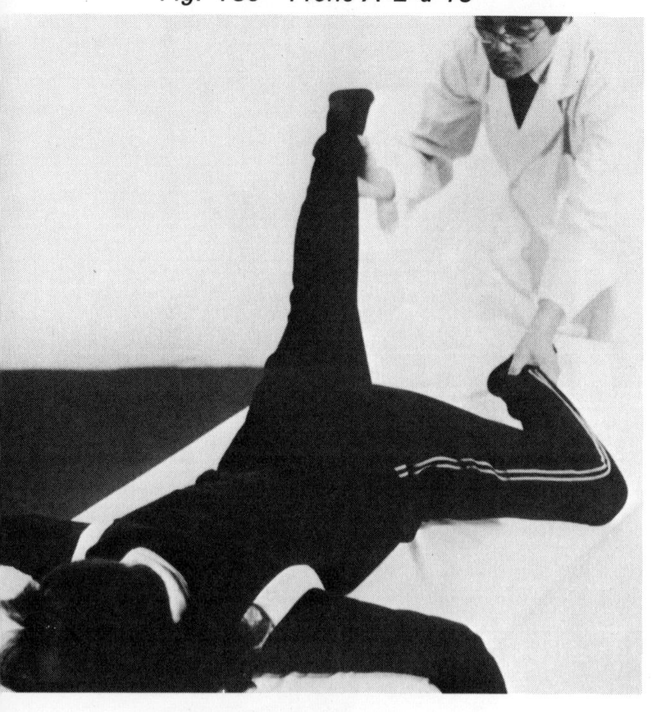

Prone A-2-e

Sōtai: From the prone position, the patient draws her left knee up toward her side, pivoting at the hip joint, and keeping the leg in contact with the table surface. The therapist grasps her left ankle, giving resistance against this movement (Figs. 181 to 183). They maintain tension for three to five seconds at a suitable position and release, and then repeat the procedure.

Upon observing this movement, it can be seen that when the left leg is drawn up to the side of the body, the right leg extends. To take advantage of this linkage action, while grasping the patient's left ankle to resist the abduction of the hip, the therapist should simultaneously apply pressure against her right ankle to provide resistance here also. This will render the technique more effective.

Qualitatively, this Sōtai movement is similar to those movements of Prone C-1 and C-2 which are explained later.

Fig. 181 Prone A-2-e-16

Fig. 182 Prone A-2-e-17

Fig. 183 Prone A-2-e-18

Active movement: Procedure "Prone A-2-e" may also be performed without the help of the therapist. As described before, the patient draws her left knee up toward her side by sliding it over the table surface, pivoting on the hip joint (Figs. 184 and 185, movement of the left leg; Figs. 186 and 187, movement of the right leg). The movement is brought to a stop at a suitable position. After holding tension here for a few seconds, the patient releaxes her body all at once. This exercise should be repeated two or three times.

Fig. 184 Prone A-2-e-19

Fig. 185 Prone A-2-e-20

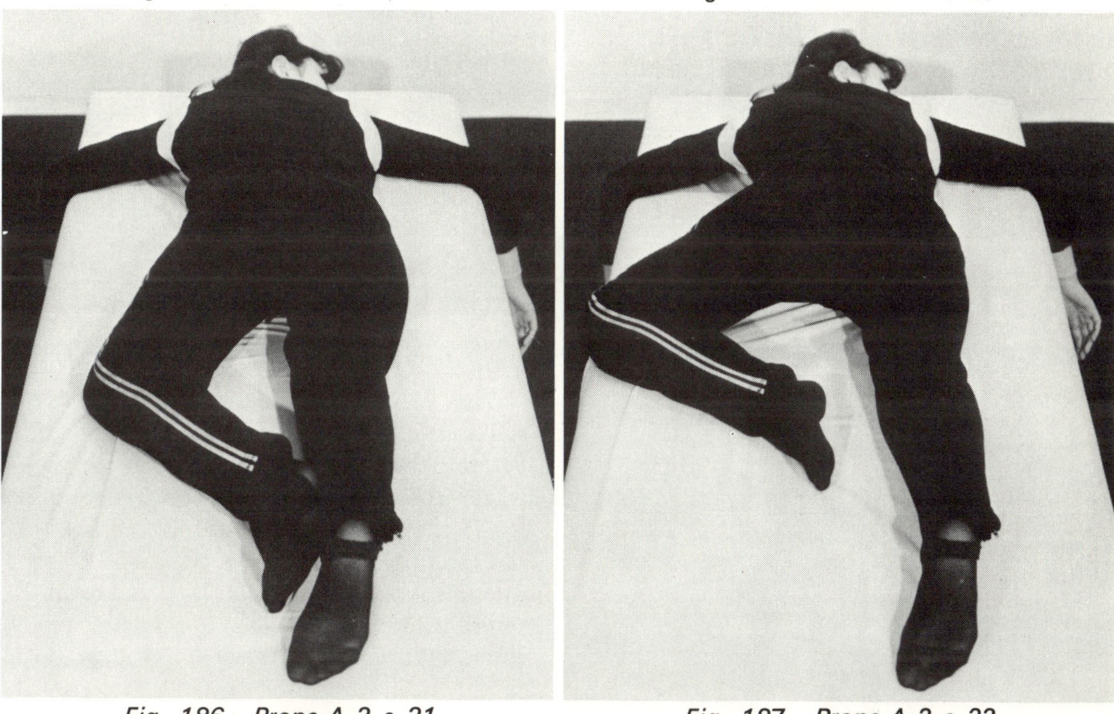

Fig. 186 Prone A-2-e-21

Fig. 187 Prone A-2-e-22

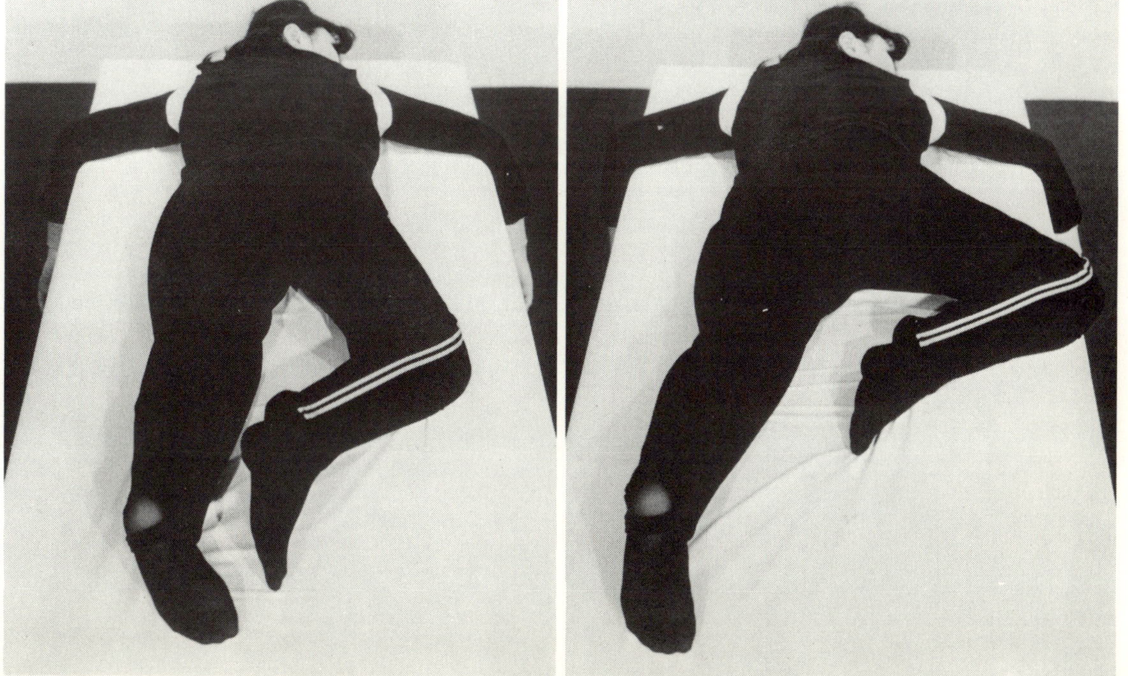

Prone B-1

Dōshin I: The patient lies in the prone position and flexes her knees so that her lower legs extend upward together. The feet are held in dorsiflexion at a right angle to the shins so the plantar aspect of the feet face upward. The therapist holds both feet together at the toes and heels. With the heels as the pivoting point, he rotates the distal ends of her feet to the right and left, inquiring about the resultant sensations of comfort or discomfort (Figs. 188 and 189).

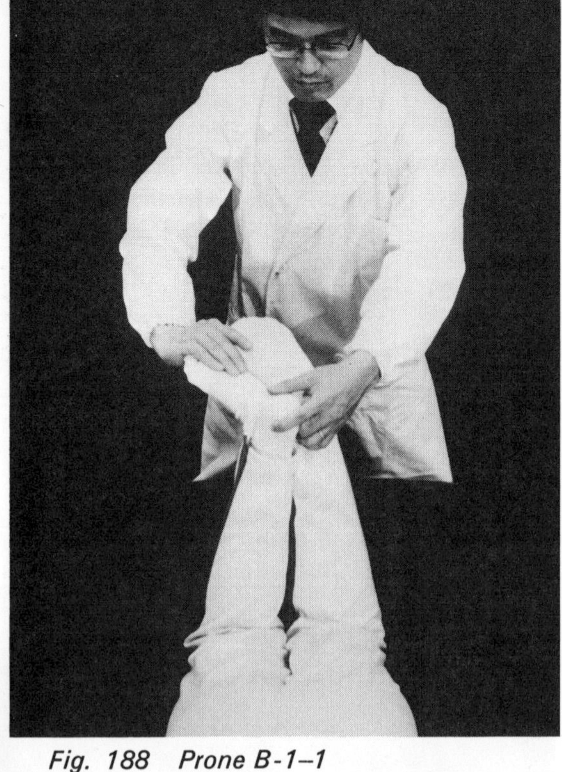

Fig. 188 Prone B-1–1

Fig. 189 Prone B-1–2

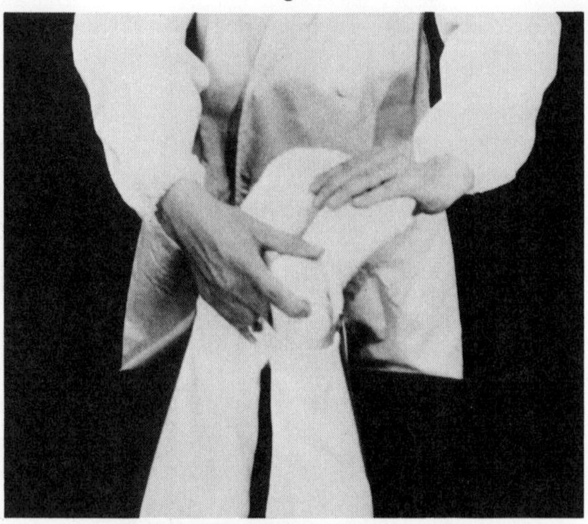

Sōtai I: The patient assumes the same position as in the mobility examination above. Pivoting the movement on her heels, the patient rotates the distal ends of her feet from right to left. The therapist grasps the toes and heels of both feet together and gives resistance to this movement (Figs. 190 and 191). It can be observed while tension is held in a suitable position, that the entire body from the legs to the

Fig. 190 Prone B-1–3

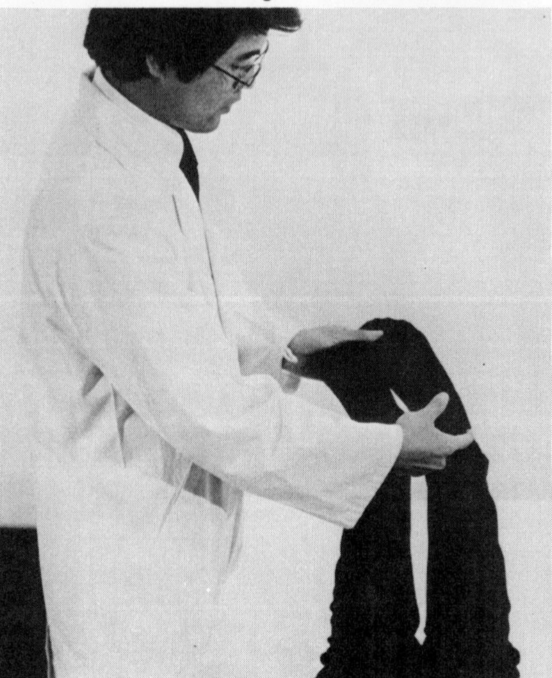

Fig. 191 Prone B-1–4

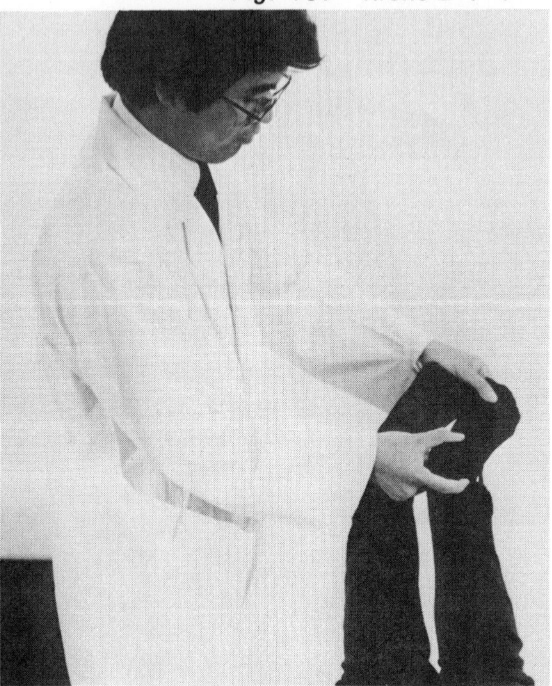

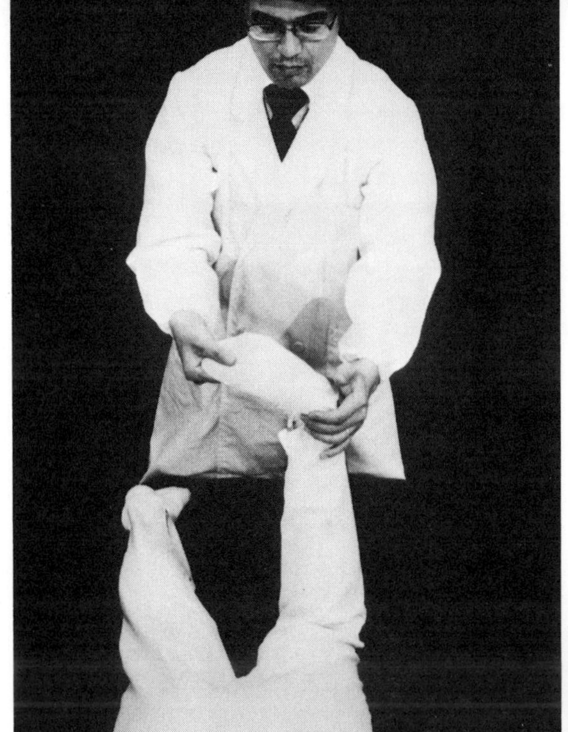

Fig. 192 Prone B-1–5

trunk become twisted with this exertion. Both persons maintain opposing pressure in this manner for a few seconds, and then release this at the same time. This procedure is repeated two or three times.

Dōshin II: In the prone position, the patient flexes either her right or left knee so that the lower leg stands upright. Taking hold of the toes and heel of this raised foot, the therapist rotates the distal end of the foot to the right and to the left, pivoting at the heel (Figs. 192 and 193). He inquires about sensations of comfort and discomfort.

Fig. 193 Prone B-1–6

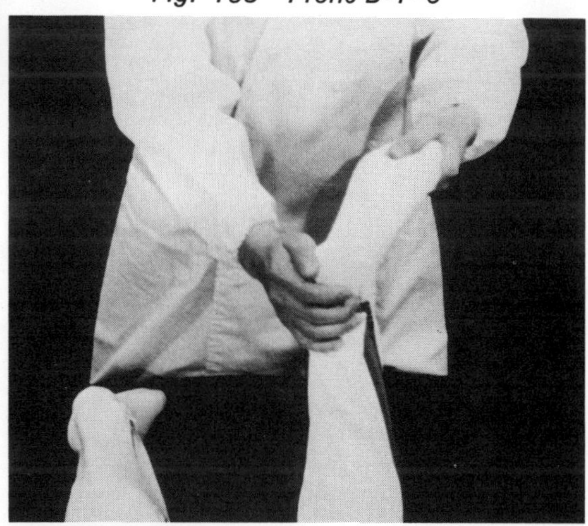

Sōtai II: The patient lies prone and flexes her left knee so that the lower leg stands upright. She then proceeds to rotate this raised foot from right to left, pivoting at the heel. Holding the toes and heel of the patient's raised foot, the therapist gives resistance to her rotation movement (Figs. 194 and 195). They hold tension at a suitable position and release, and then repeat.

Fig. 194 Prone B-1–7

Fig. 195 Prone B-1–8

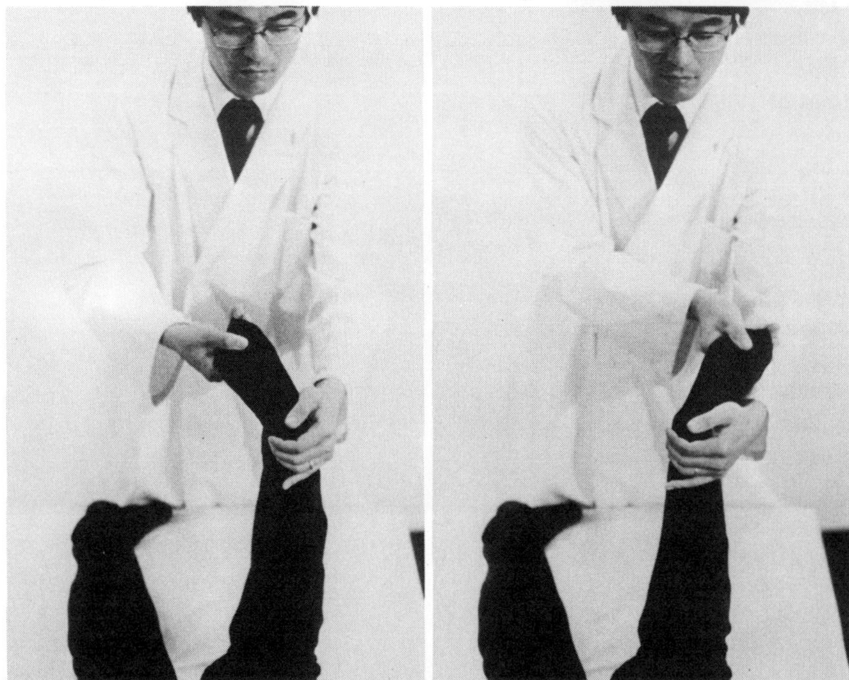

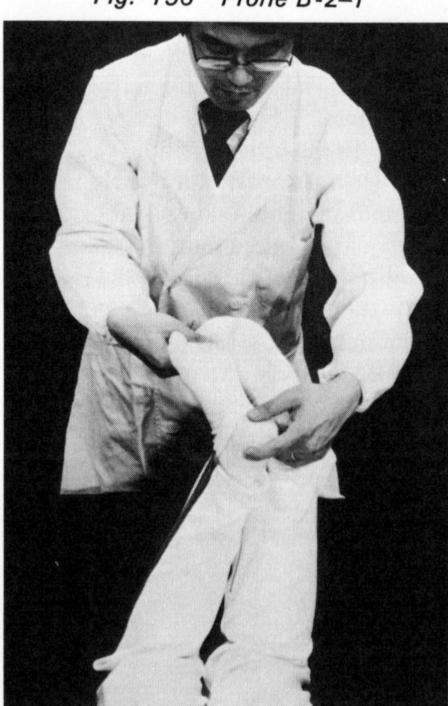
Fig. 196 Prone B-2–1

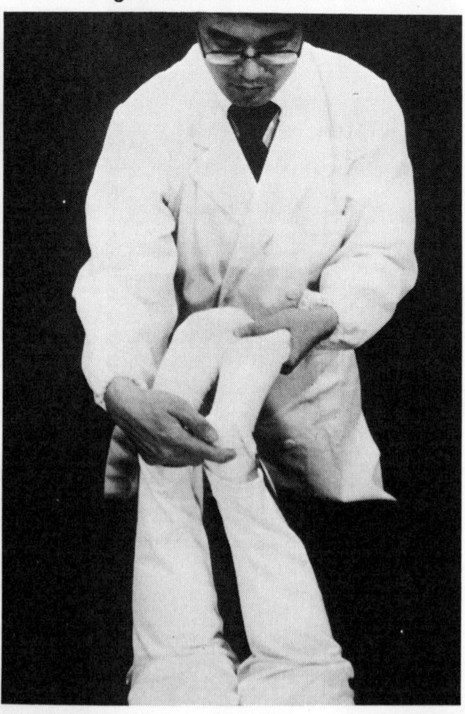
Fig. 197 Prone B-2–2

Prone B-2

Dōshin I: The patient assumes the same position as in Prone B-1. The therapist holds the toes and heels of both feet and rotates the heels to the right and the left, pivoting the motion at the toes (Figs. 196 and 197). He then inquires about any sensations of comfort or discomfort.

Sōtai I: With her feet together and knees flexed, the patient rotates the heels of her feet from right to left pivoting at her toes. The therapist grasps the toes and heels of both feet together and supplies resistance against this movement (Figs. 198 and 199). At a suitable position they hold tension, and release, and then repeat the procedure.

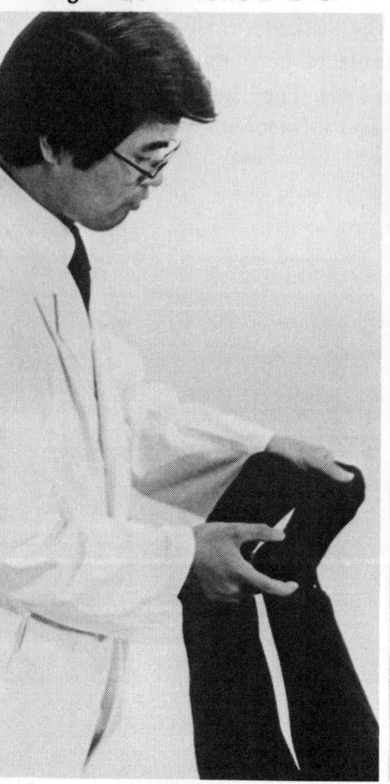
Fig. 198 Prone B-2–3

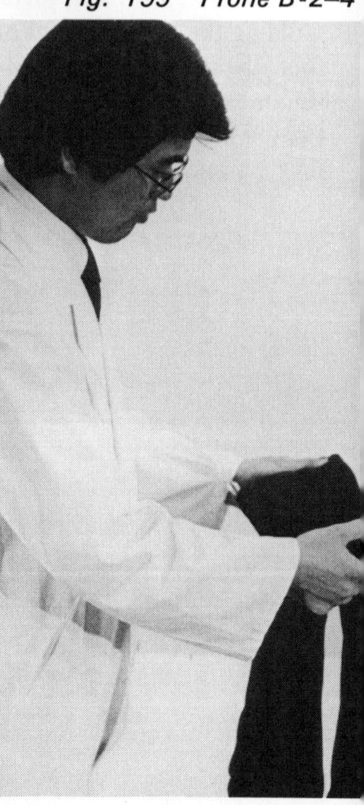
Fig. 199 Prone B-2–4

Fig. 200 Prone B-2–5

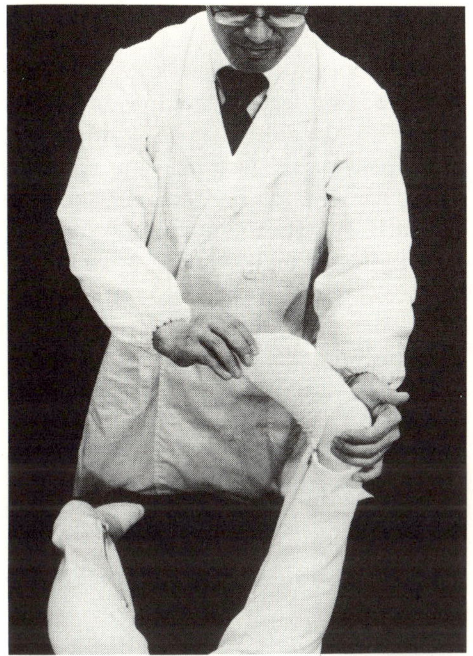

Dōshin II: The patient lies in the prone position and flexes either the right or the left knee so that the lower leg extends upward. Holding the toes and the heel of this raised foot, the therapist rotates the heel of the foot to the right and to the left, pivoting at the toes (Figs. 200 and 201). He inquires about which direction of rotation causes the greater discomfort.

Sōtai II: Lying prone, the patient flexes her left knee so that the lower leg stands upright. She rotates the heel of this foot from left to right, pivoting at the toes. The therapist holds the toes and the heel of this foot, and gives gentle resistance to this rotation (Figs. 202 and 203). They maintain opposing pressure at a suitable position for three to five seconds and then release simultaneously. This procedure is repeated two or three times.

Fig. 201 Prone B-2–6

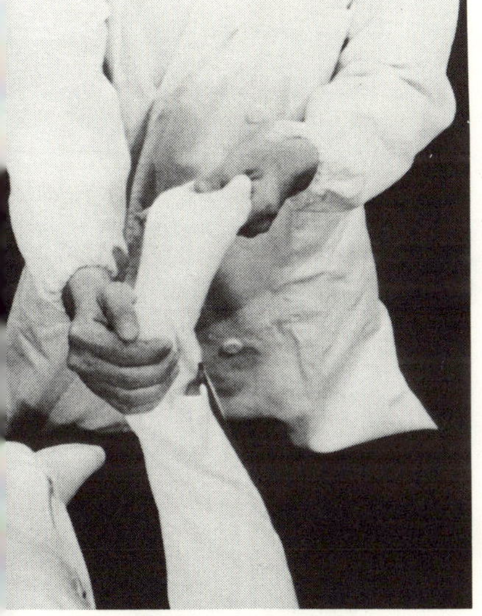

Fig. 202 Prone B-2–7

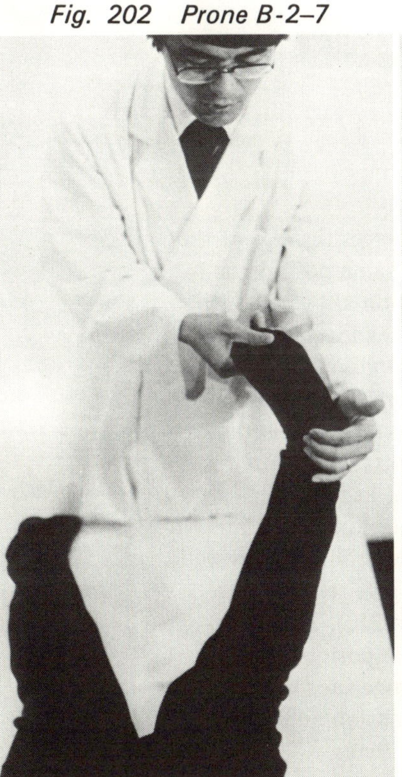

Fig. 203 Prone B-2–8

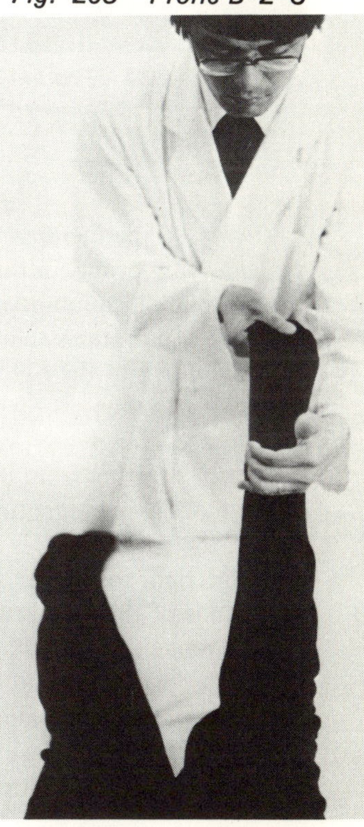

Prone C-1

Morphological observation: The patient lies in the prone position and flexes both knees so that the lower legs extend upward together. Here also, the ankles are flexed to form a right angle between the feet and shins so that the soles face upward. The therapist stands at the patient's feet. He compares the lengths of her legs (indicated by the comparative heights of the heels). He also checks to see whether the center line of the feet line up with the vertebral column (Figs. 204 and 205).

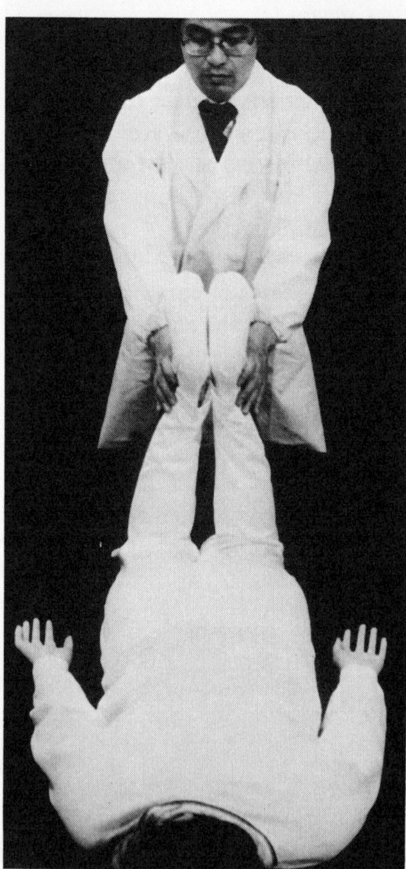

Fig. 204 Prone C-1–1

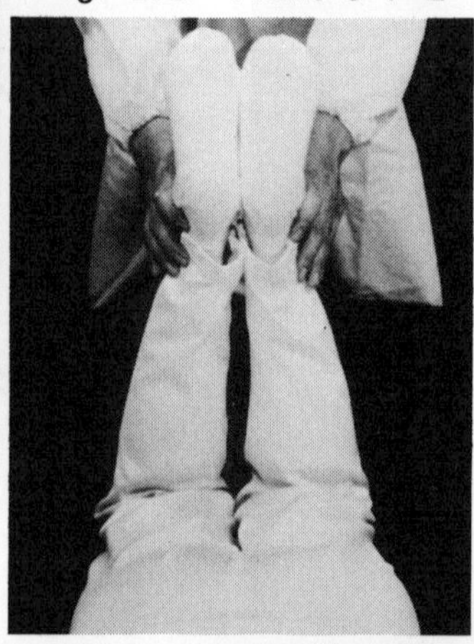

Fig. 205 Prone C-1–2

Dōshin: The therapist places the legs of the patient, lying prone, in the same position as in the morphological observation above. Holding the ankles, he rotates the flexed legs together laterally down to the right and left (Figs. 206 and 207). He then asks which direction of movement causes the greater sensation of discomfort.

Sōtai: Starting from the same posture used in the mobility examination, keeping her feet together, the patient moves her lower legs laterally from the right to the left, describing an arc. The hands of the therapist give resistance to this movement (Figs. 208 to 210). The movement is stopped at a suitable position and opposing pressure is maintained for three to five seconds. They release tension and repeat the movement two or three times.

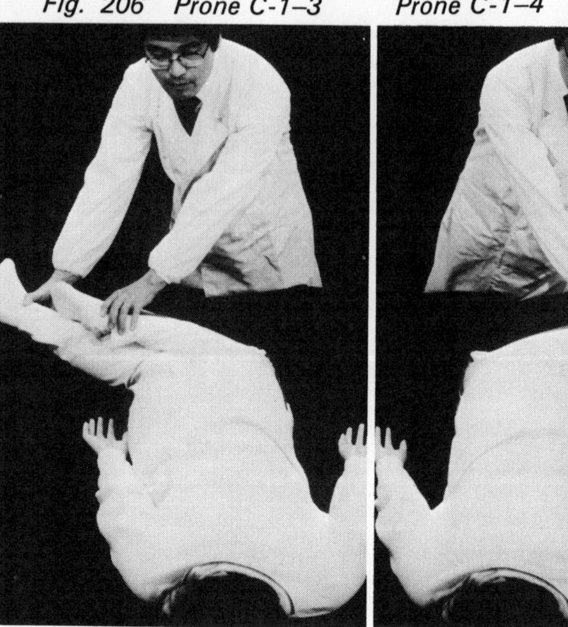

Fig. 206 Prone C-1–3

Fig. 207 Prone C-1–4

Prone C-2

Dōshin: Lying in a prone position with her knees spread slightly apart, the patient again flexes her lower legs into an upright position. Holding her ankles, the therapist rotates her flexed legs laterally downward, pivoting at the knees (Figs. 211 to 213). He asks which direction of movement causes the greater sensation of discomfort.

Fig. 208 Prone C-1–5

Fig. 209 Prone C-1–6 *Fig. 210 Prone C-1–7*

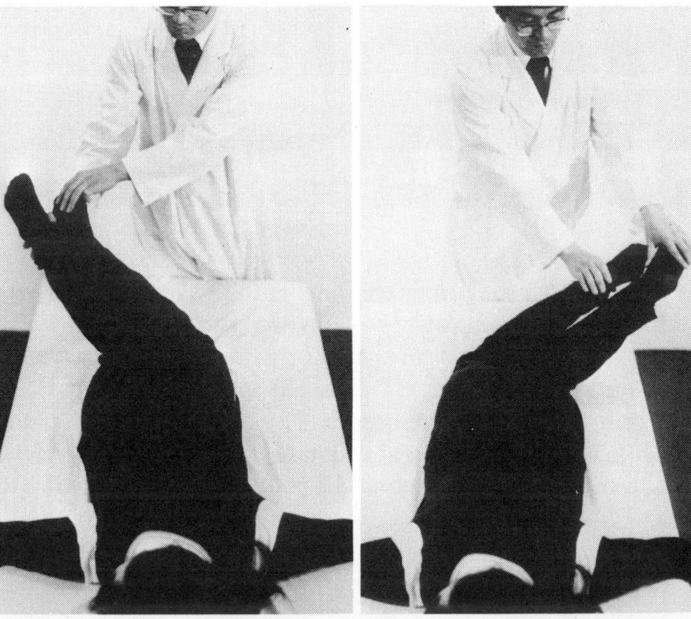

Fig. 211 Prone C-2–1

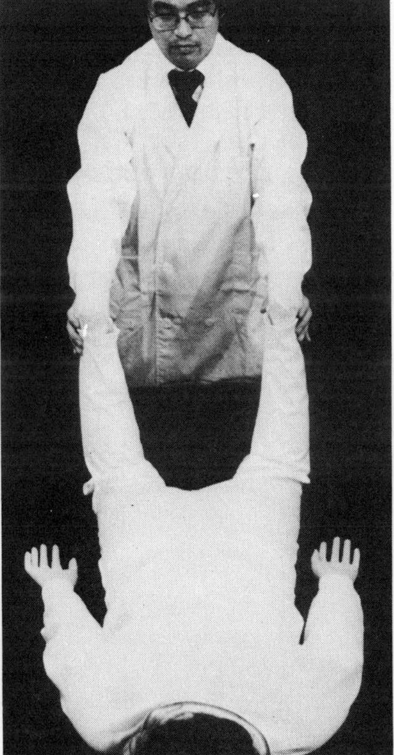

Fig. 212 Prone C-2–2 *Fig. 213 Prone C-2–3*

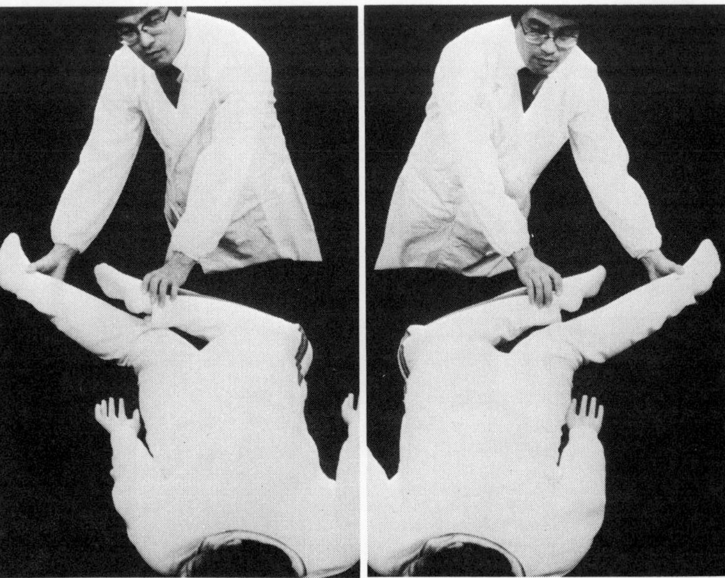

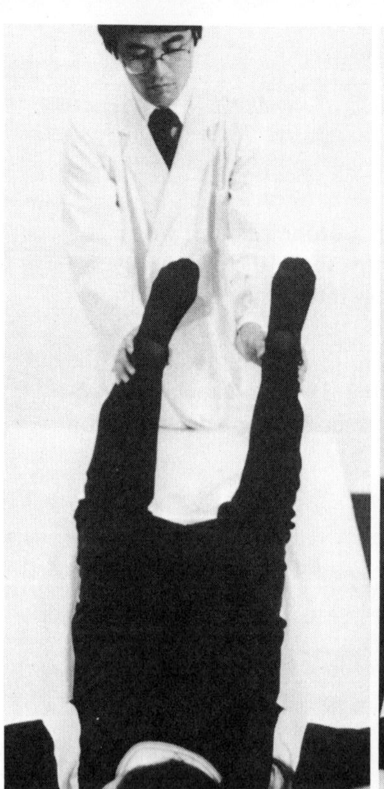

Fig. 214 Prone C-2–4

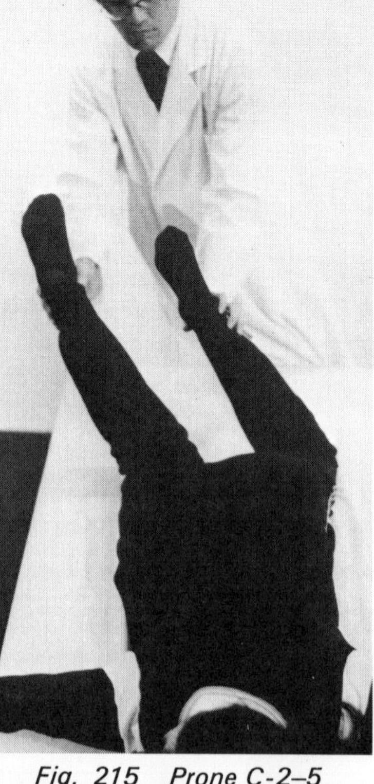

Fig. 215 Prone C-2–5

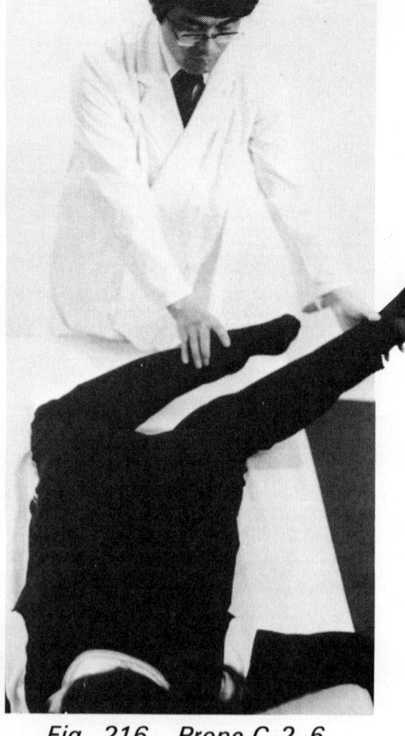

Fig. 216 Prone C-2–6

Sōtai: Starting from the same posture as that used in the mobility examination, keeping her legs spread apart, the patient rotates her lower legs from the right side to the left side. The therapist applies resistance (Figs. 214 to 216). They hold tension at a suitable position and release, and then repeat the procedure.

Prone D-1

Dōshin I: The patient assumes a prone posture and relaxes all tension in her body. Standing opposite the patient's head, the therapist presses down alternately on her right and left shoulders (Figs. 217 and 218). He

Fig. 217 Prone D-1–1

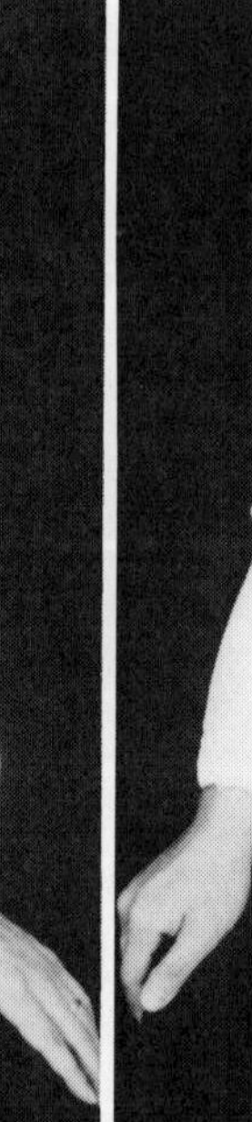

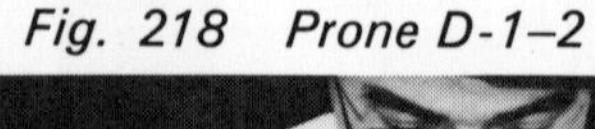

Fig. 218 Prone D-1–2

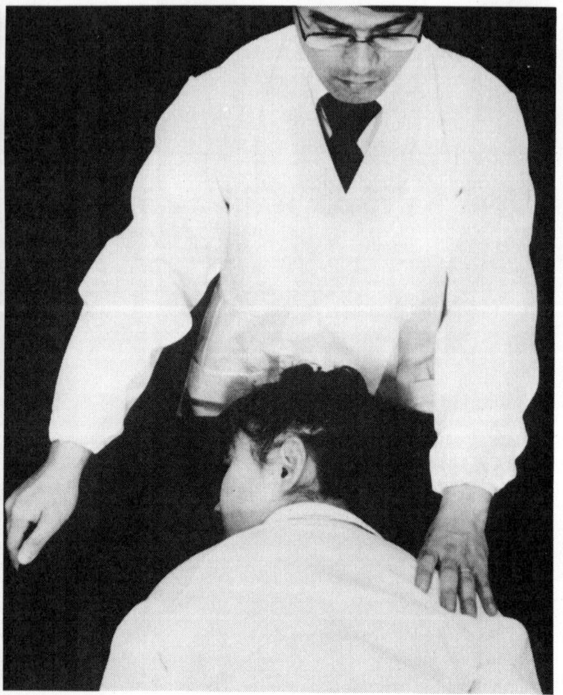

inquires about the resultant sensations of comfort or discomfort as well as about the difference in the sensations between the right and left sides.

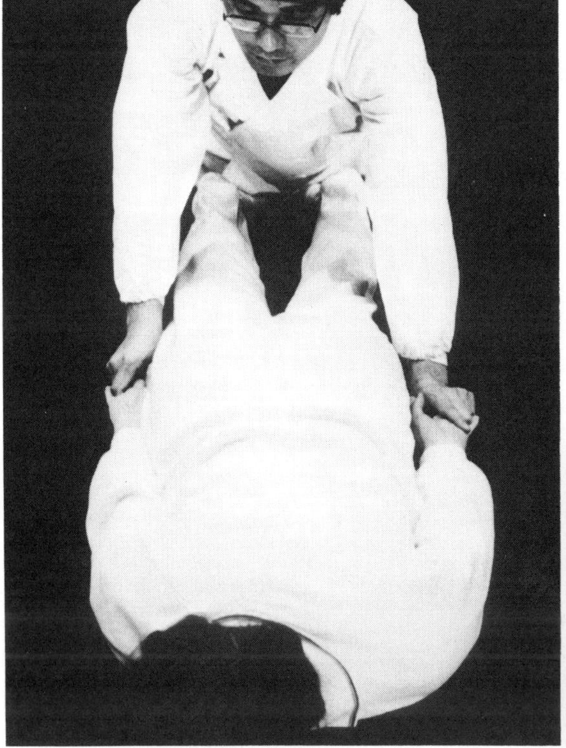

Fig. 219 Prone D-1–3

Dōshin II: The patient assumes the prone position in a state of complete relaxation. Standing opposite her feet, the therapist takes hold of both her wrists. He alternaltely pulls her right and left wrists toward himself while asking about sensations of comfort or discomfort, and of any difference between the right and left arms (Figs. 219 and 220).

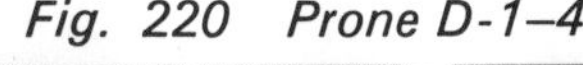

Fig. 220 Prone D-1–4

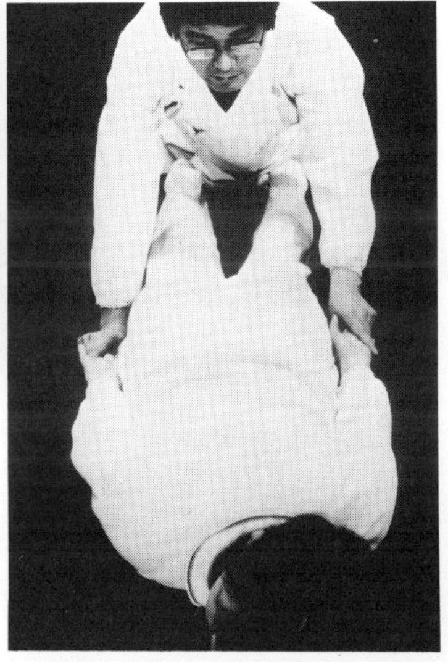

Fig. 221 Prone D-1–5 *Fig. 222 Prone D-1–6*

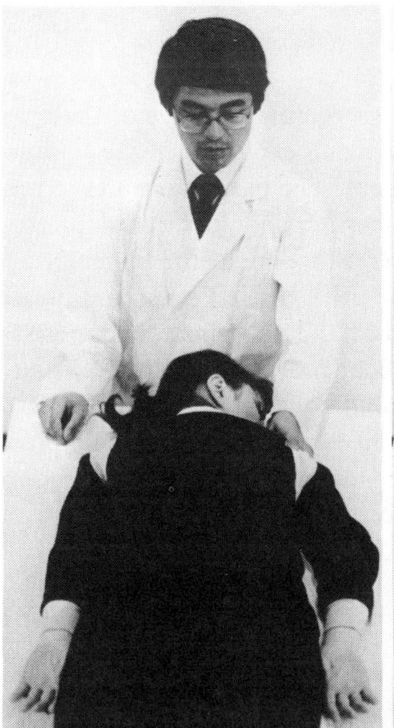

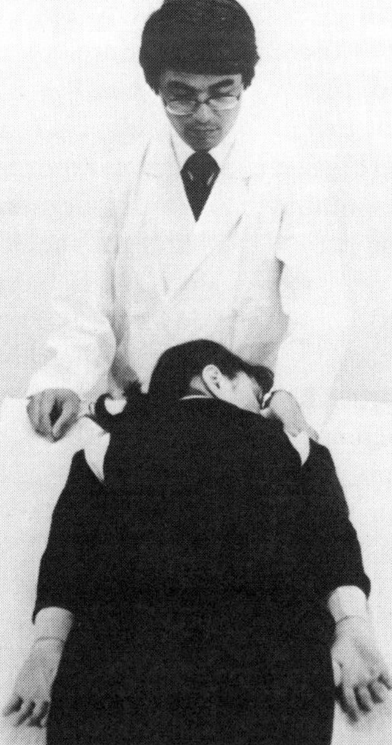

Sōtai I: The patient elevates her right shoulder. Standing at her head, the therapist applies pressure to her right shoulder, gently opposing the movement (Figs. 221 and 222). The movement is stopped at a suitable position and they maintain tension for three to five seconds and release simultaneously. They repeat the procedure two or three times.

Close observation of movement D-1 will reveal that due to structural linkage, the elevation of the right shoulder is accompanied by the depression of the left shoulder. Sōtai movement D-1-7 and -8 take advantage of this linkage.

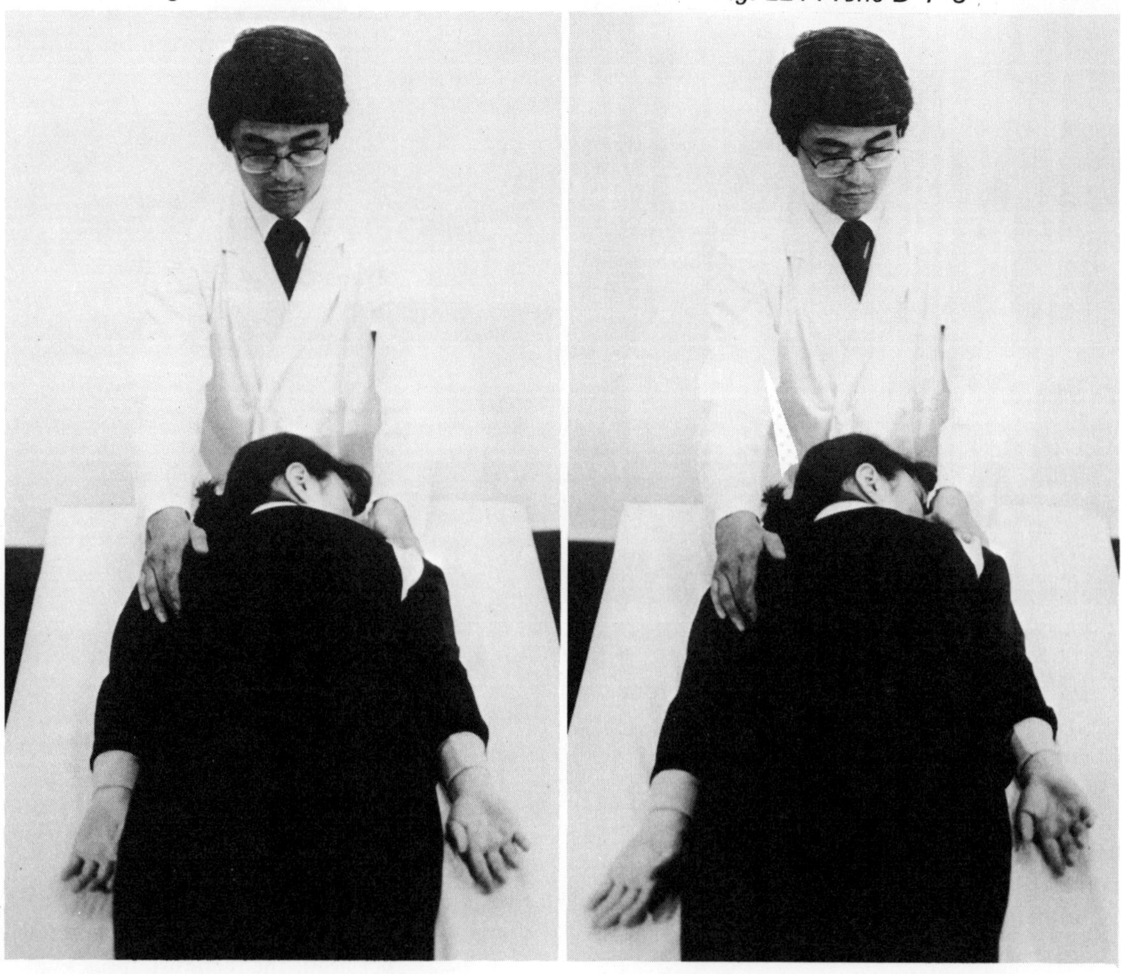

Fig. 223 Prone D-1–7

Fig. 224 Prone D-1–8

Sōtai II: The patient elevates her right shoulder and depresses her left shoulder at the same time. Standing at the patient's head, the therapist holds her right shoulder and left axilla and gives resistance to these movements (Figs. 223 and 224). After holding tension at a suitable position, they release simultaneously. The procedure is repeated two or three times.

Sōtai III: The patient elevates her left shoulder. Standing at the patient's feet, the therapist takes hold of her left wrist in order to give resistance against her shoulder movement (Figs. 225 and 226). At a suitable position, they maintain equal and opposing pressure for three to five seconds and release, and then repeat the procedure.

Sōtai IV: The structural linkage of the shoulders is once again exploited in the following Sōtai movement. The patient simultaneously elevates her left shoulder and depresses her right shoulder. Standing at the patient's feet, the therapist grips her left wrist and presses down on the right hand and gives gentle resistance to the shoulder movement (Figs. 227 and 228). They maintain equal and opposing pressure for three to five seconds at a suitable position, and release simultaneously. The procedure is repeated two or three times.

Fig. 225 Prone D-1–9

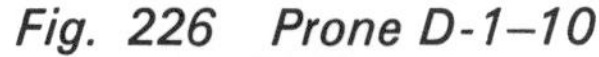

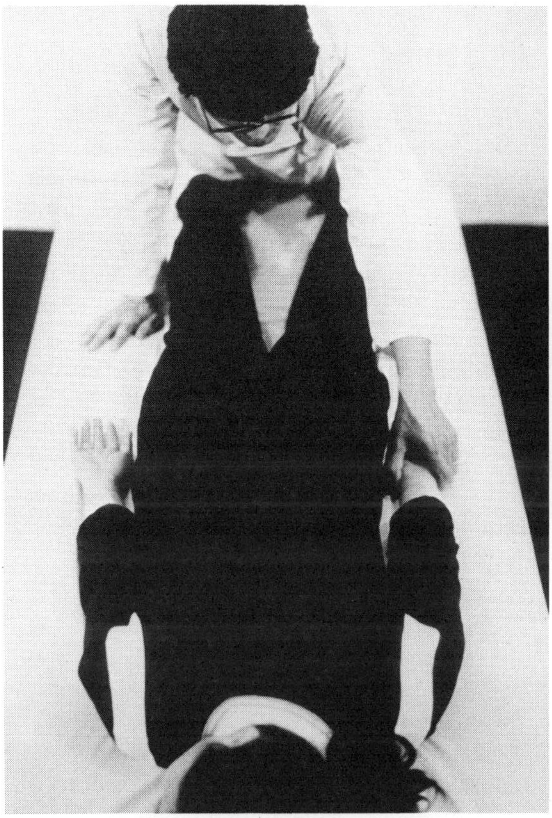

Fig. 226 Prone D-1–10

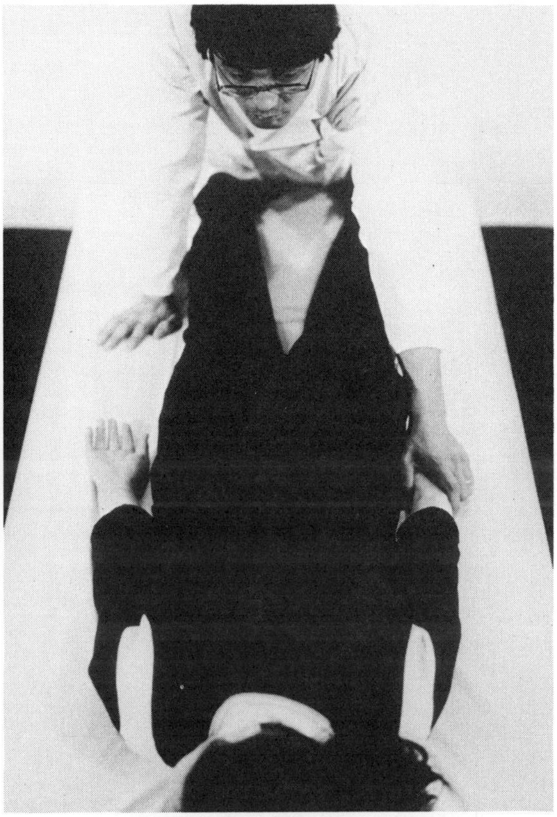

Fig. 227 Prone D-1–11

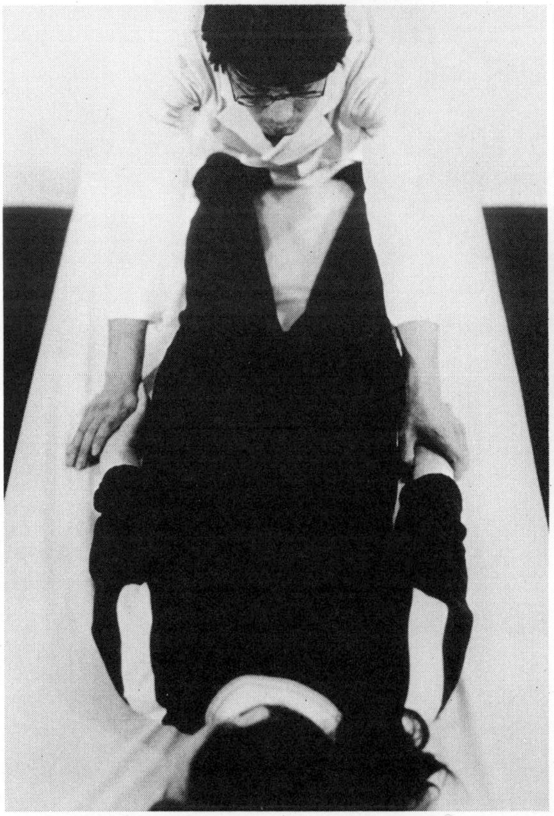

Fig. 228 Prone D-1–12

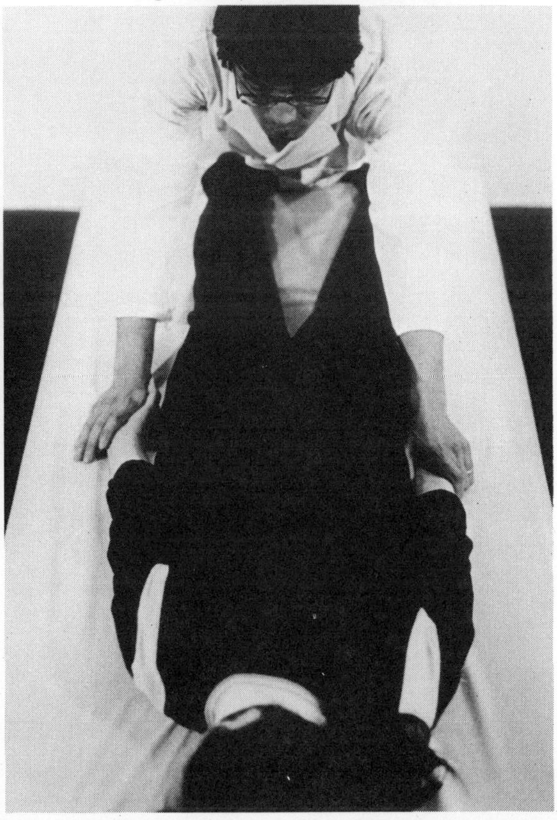

Fig. 229 Seated A-1–1

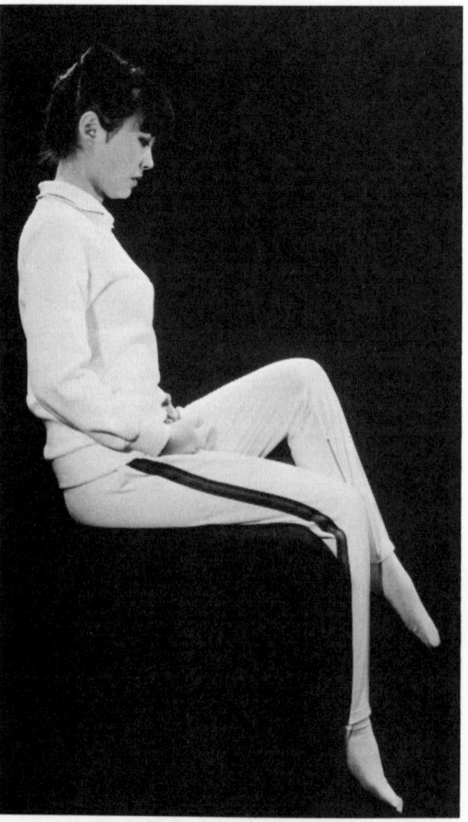

Fig. 230 Seated A-1–2

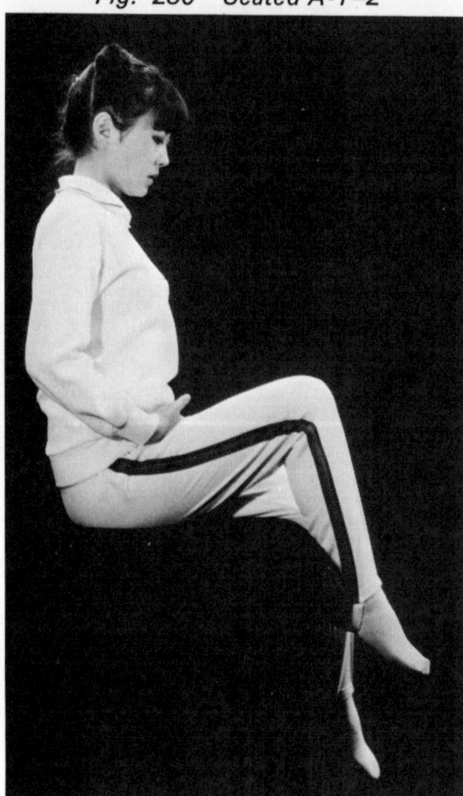

Seated Position

Seated A-1

Dōshin: The patient sits well back on the treatment table. She straightens her back and relaxes her body. She places her hands on her lap with palms facing upward, and fixes her gaze ahead. From this posture, the patient alternately raises one knee at a time, as though bringing each knee up toward her chest (Figs. 229 and 230). Attention is paid to the sensations of comfort and discomfort resulting from the movements, as well as to the difference between the right and left sides.

Sōtai I: When raising the left knee causes more discomfort during the mobility examination, the right leg is raised in the Sōtai movement. The therapist using his hands gives resistance as the patient lifts her right leg (Figs. 231 and 232). They maintain tension bringing the movement to a stop at a suitable position, and then release. This procedure is repeated two or three times.

Sōtai II: This is the same Sōtai movement as performed above except that this is done on the left leg. The patient lifts her left leg and the therapist gives resistance (Figs. 233 and 234). They hold tension after reaching a suitable po-

Fig. 231 Seated A-1–3

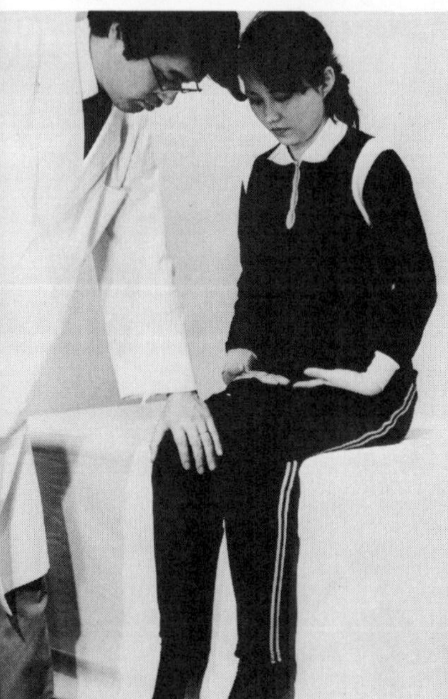

Fig. 232 Seated A-1–4

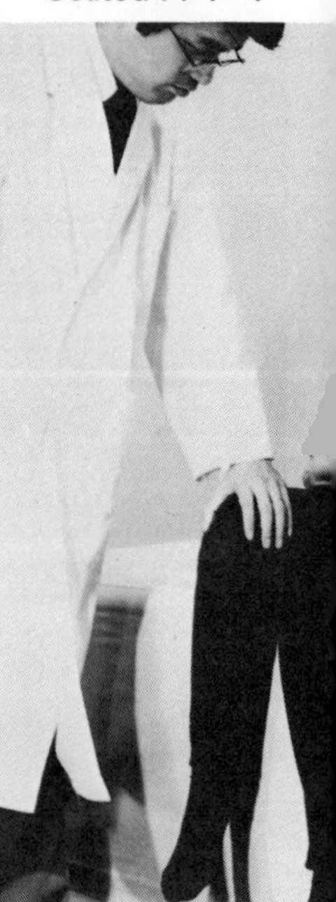

sition and then release this simultaneously. This is repeated two or three times.

Sōtai III: The therapist sits in Seiza fashion at the feet of the seated patient. He raises his right knee slightly so that the patient can rest her left foot on his thigh. From this position, the patient, while lifting her right leg upward, pushes her left foot downward firmly on the therapist's thigh (Fig. 235). The therapist counters both of these movements by giving resistance with his left hand and his right leg (Fig. 236). They maintain opposing pressure after reaching a suitable position, and then release after a few seconds. The procedure is repeated two or three times.

Fig. 233 Seated A-1–5

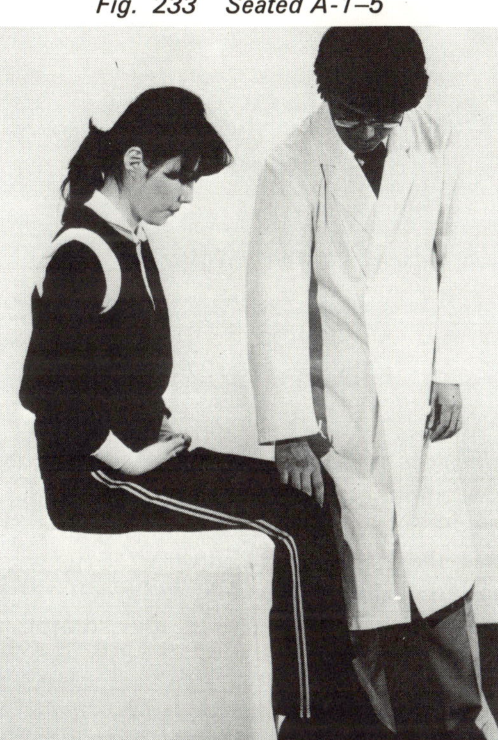

Fig. 234 Seated A-1–6

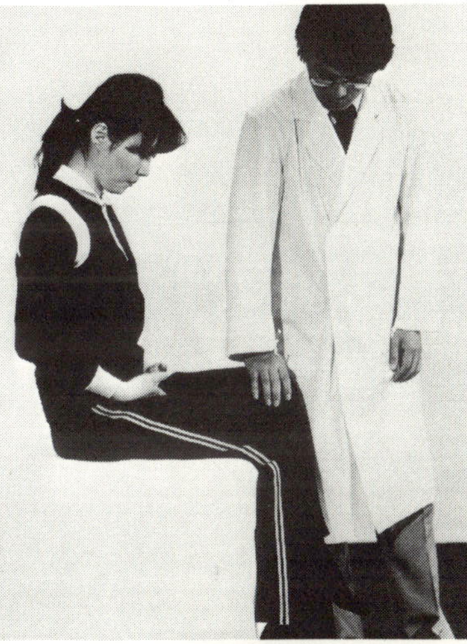

Fig. 235 Seated A-1–7

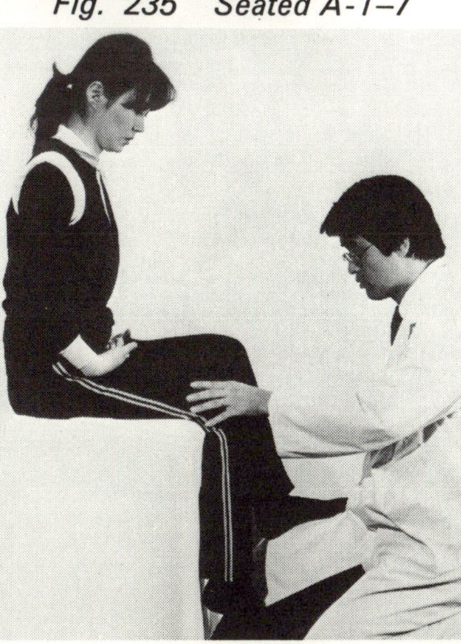

Fig. 236 Seated A-1–8

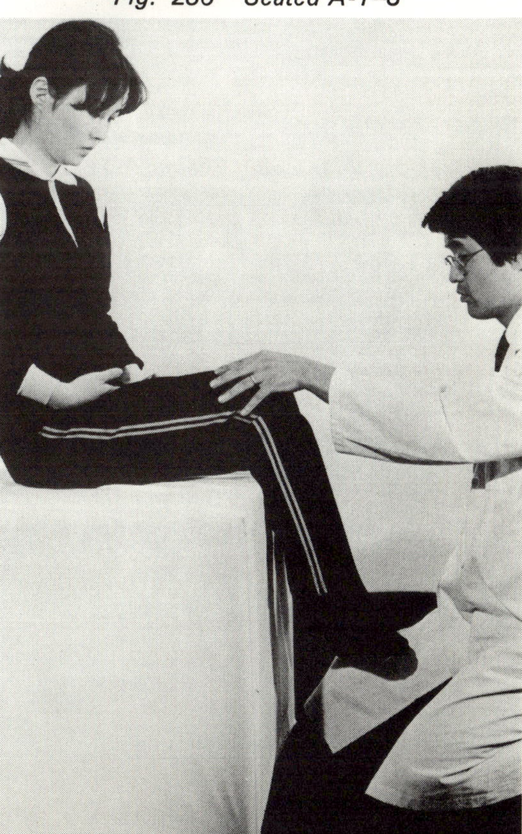

Sōtai IV: Starting from a position with the right knee raised, the patient lowers her right leg while raising her left leg. The therapist gently opposes both these movements by applying pressure on the left knee and holding the right popliteal area (Fig. 237). They hold tension at a suitable position and release, and then repeat the procedure (Fig. 238).

Fig. 237 Seated A-1–9

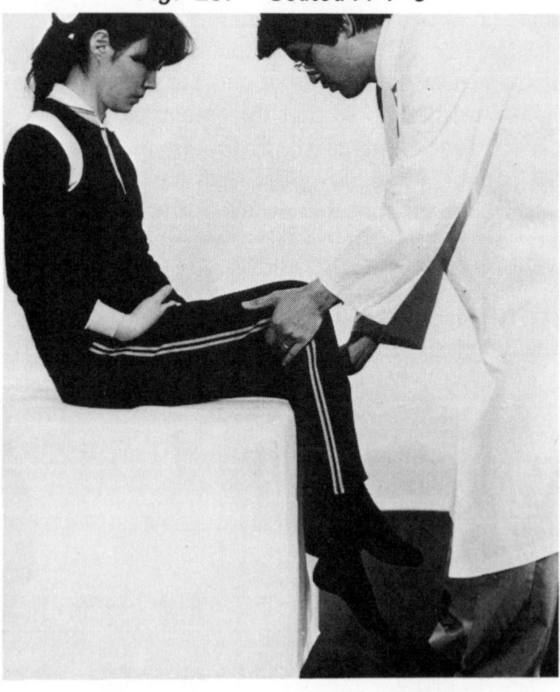

Fig. 238 Seated A-1–10

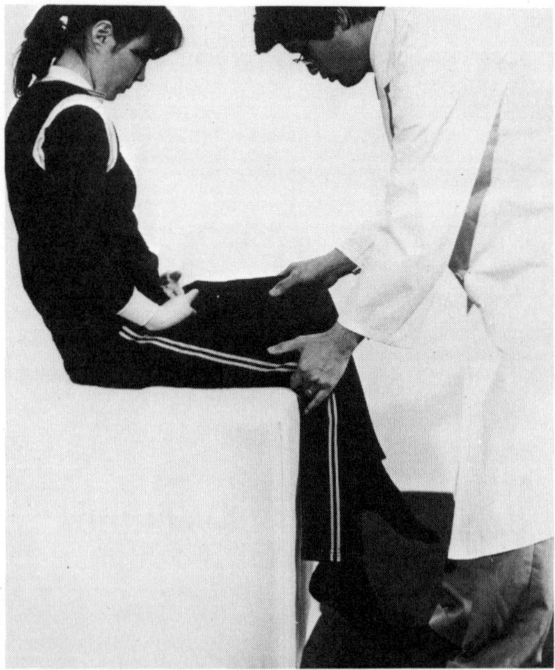

Sōtai V: This is the same procedure as shown above except that it is performed in the opposite manner. Starting with the left knee raised, the left leg is lowered while the right leg is raised, and the therapist gives resistance to both these movements (Figs. 239 and 240).

Fig. 239 Seated A-1–11

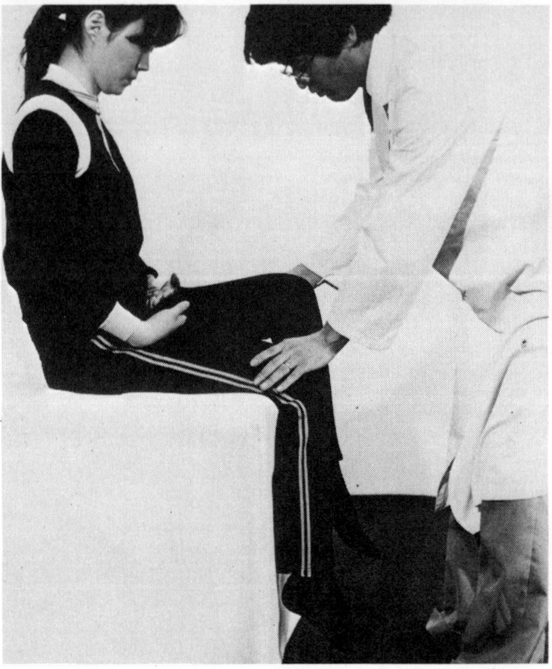

Fig. 240 Seated A-1–12

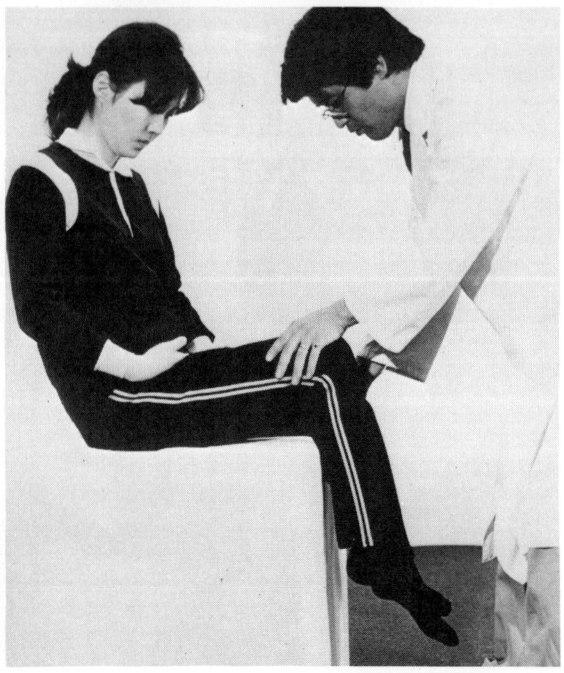

Seated B-1

Dōshin: The patient is seated so her feet are clear of the floor. The therapist turns the patient's feet to the inverted and then the everted position, twisting the feet on the sagittal line connecting the center of the heel with the third toe (Figs. 241 and 242). The other foot is examined in the same manner. He inquires about the resulting sensations of comfort or discomfort.

Fig. 241 Seated B-1–1

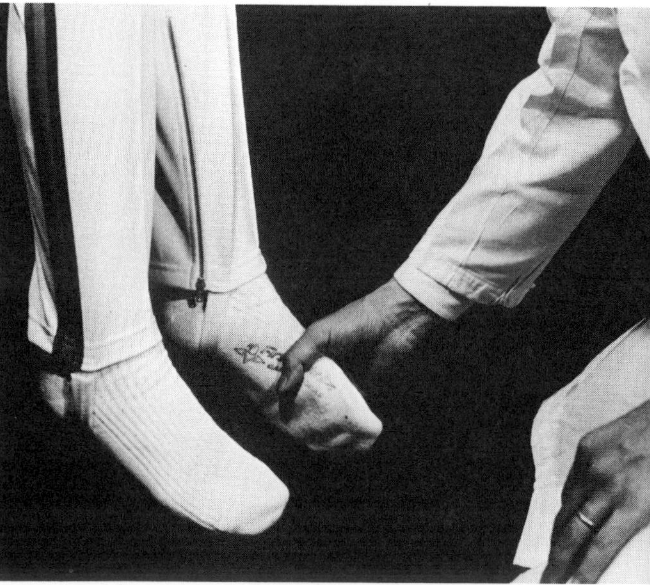

Fig. 242 Seated B-1–2

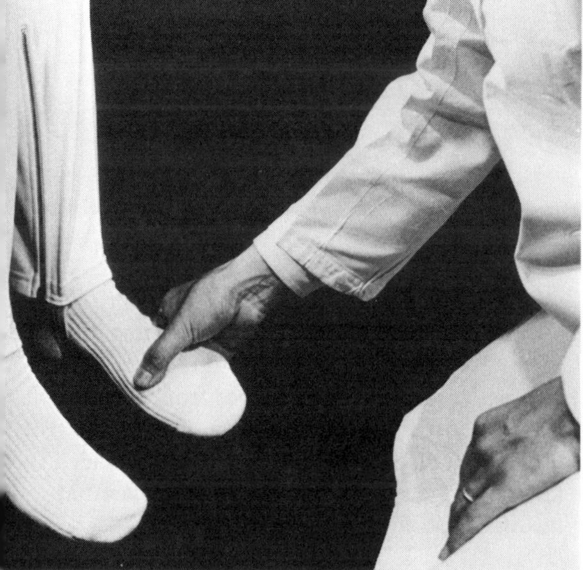

Fig. 243 Seated B-1–3

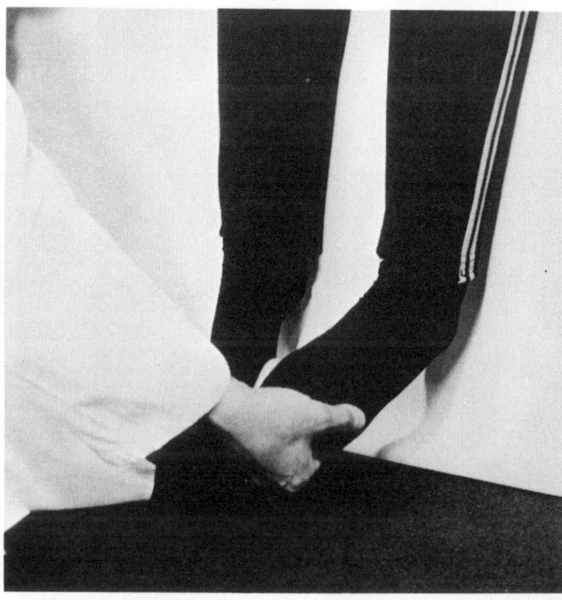

Fig. 244 Seated B-1–4

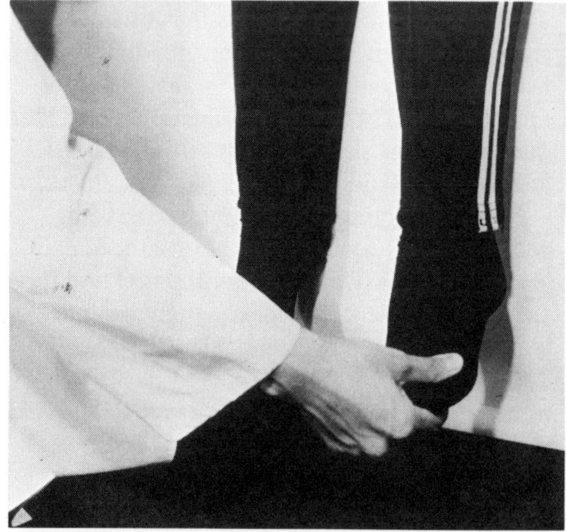

Sōtai I: Turning on the line connecting the heel and the third toe, the patient turns her left foot from the inverted to the everted position. The therapist provides resistance to this movement by grasping her foot (Figs. 243 and 244). They remain motionless and hold tension after reaching a suitable position and release this after a few seconds, and then repeat the procedure.

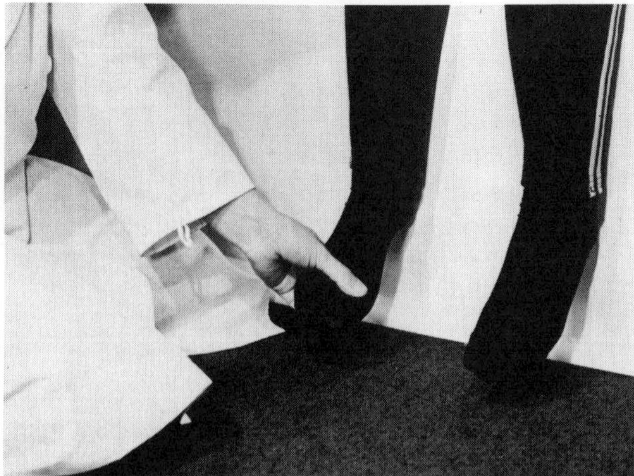
Fig. 245 Seated B-1–5

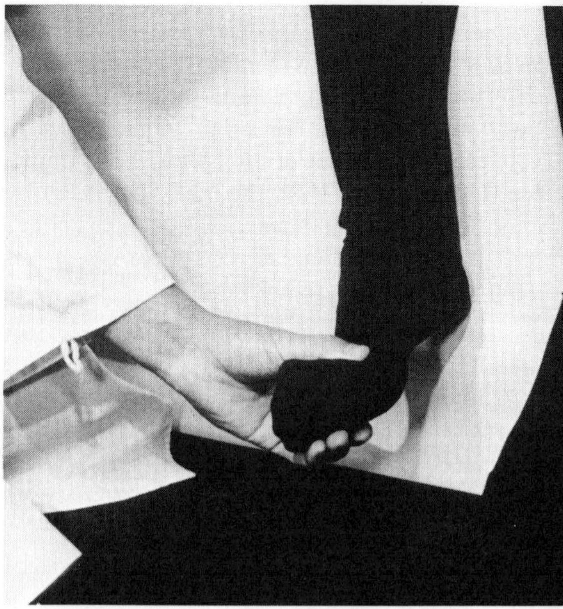
Fig. 246 Seated B-1–6

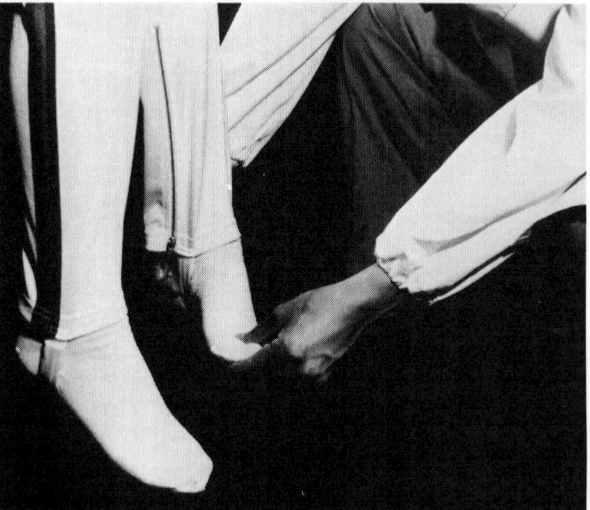
Fig. 247 Seated B-2–1

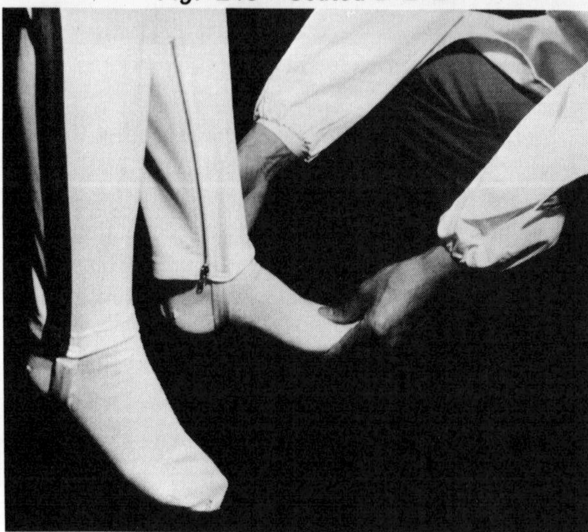
Fig. 248 Seated B-2–2

Sōtai II: This is basically the same procedure as shown above except that it is performed on the right foot with the reverse action. The patient turns her right foot from the everted position to the inverted position. The therapist gives resistance to this movement (Figs. 245 and 246). Tension is held and then released at a suitable position.

Seated B-2

Dōshin: The therapist holds the patient's right or left foot, grasping both the toes and the heel. Pivoting on the heel, he rotates the foot medially (Fig. 247) and then laterally (Fig. 248), questioning the patient about sensations of comfort or discomfort.

Sōtai: Pivoting on her heel, the patient rotates her left foot from the medial to the lateral position. Holding both the heel and the toes of the patient, the therapist gives gentle resistance to the movement (Figs. 249 to 251). After holding tension for three to five seconds at a suitable position, they release together, and then repeat once or twice.

Fig. 249 Seated B-2–3

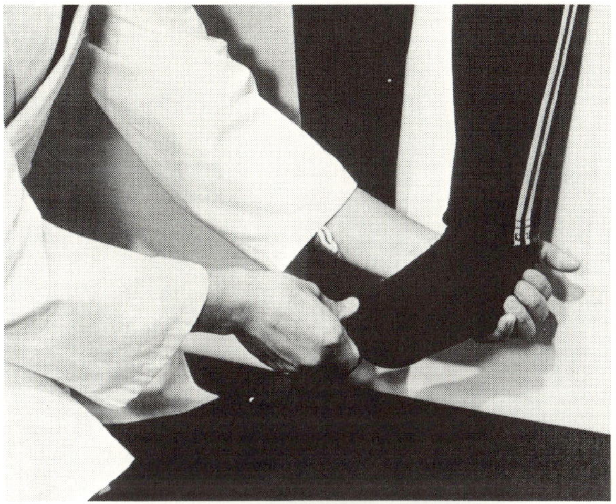

Fig. 250 Seated B-2–4

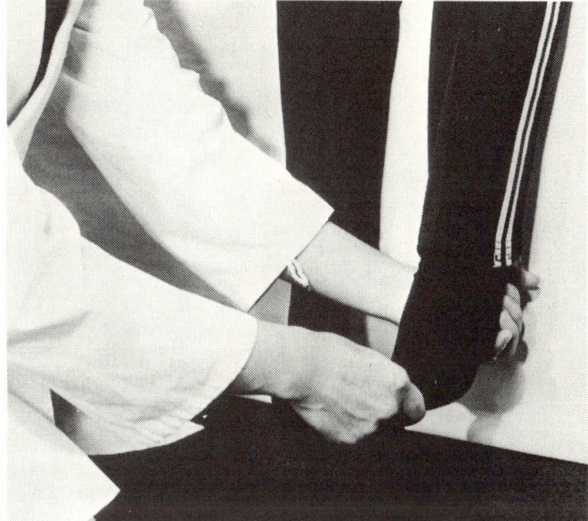

Fig. 251 Seated B-2–5

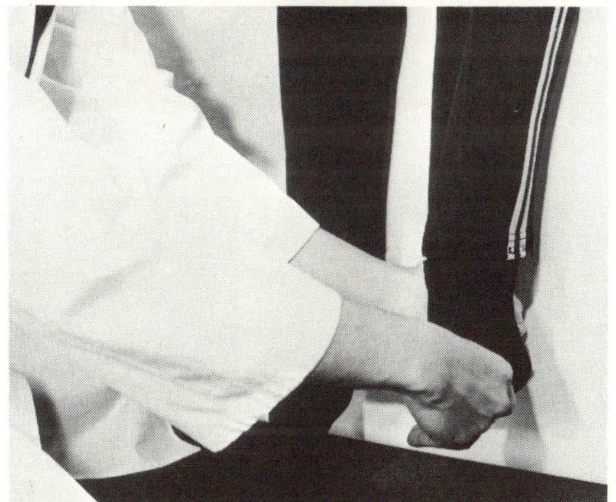

Seated B-3

Dōshin: The patient assumes the basic seated posture. The therapist takes hold of the patient's right or left foot grasping both the toes and the heel. The therapist first raises the toes (dorsiflexion) and then lowers the toes (plantar flexion) pivoting the movement on the heel, and inquires about sensations of comfort or discomfort (Figs. 252 and 253).

Fig. 252 Seated B-3–1

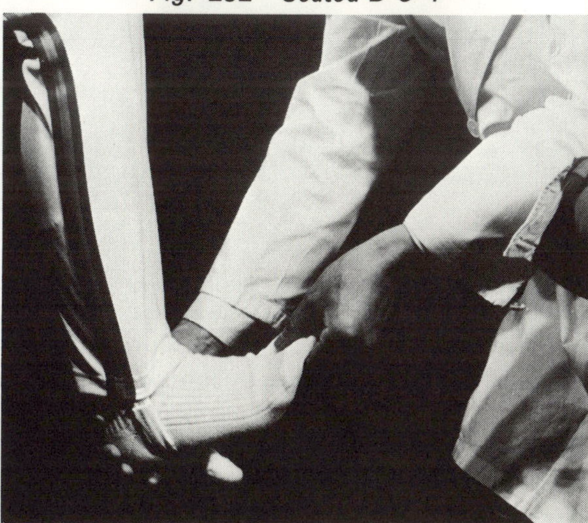

Fig. 253 Seated B-3–2

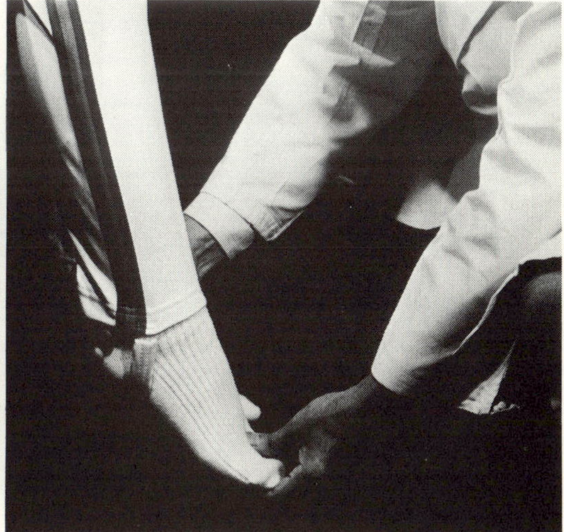

Fig. 254 Seated B-3–3

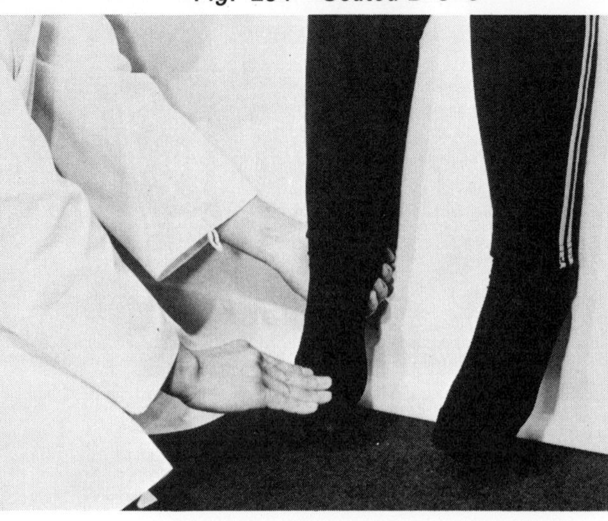

Fig. 255 Seated B-3–4

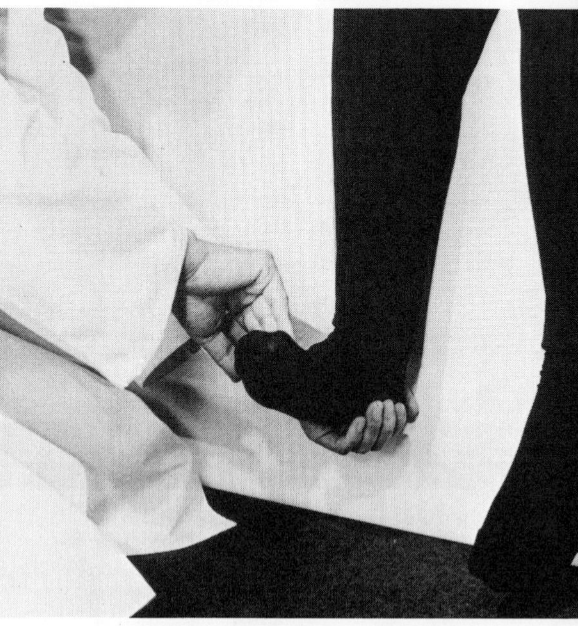

Sōtai I: Pivoting the movement at the heel, the patient raises the toes of her right foot from the plantar flexion position to the dorsiflexion position. Holding both the toes and the heel of their right foot, the therapist provides resistance to this movement (Figs. 254 and 255). After holding tension at a suitable position they both release simultaneously, and then repeat the procedure.

Fig. 256 Seated B-3–5

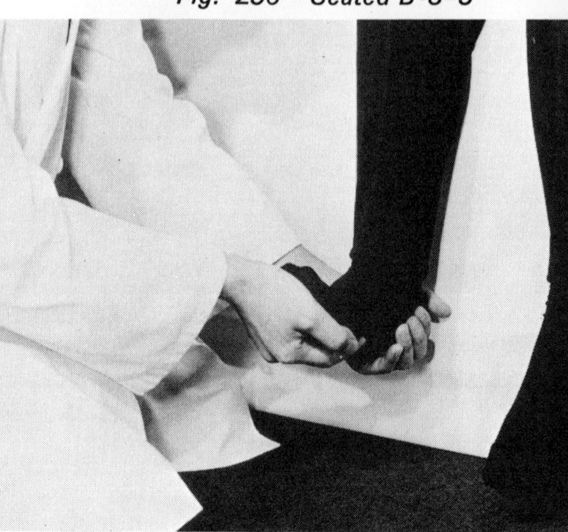

Fig. 257 Seated B-3–6

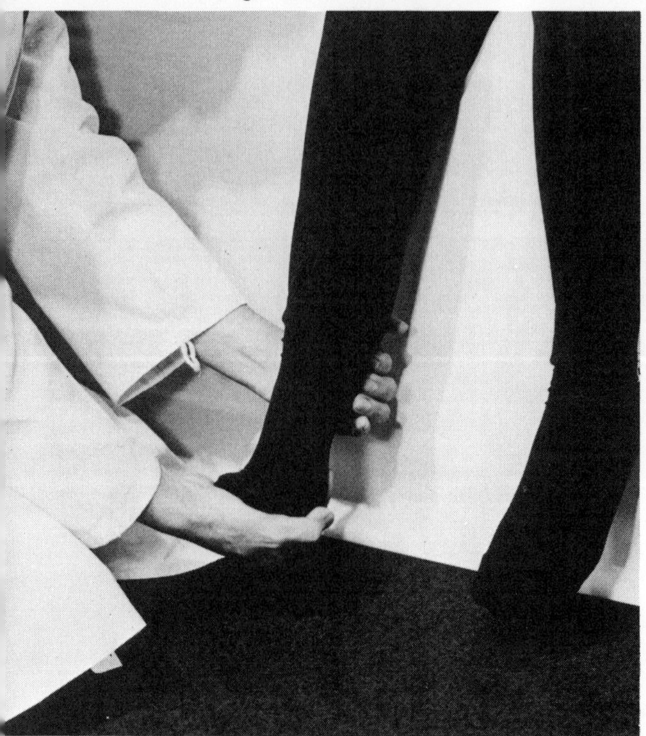

Sōtai II: The patient performs the same movement described above in reverse, lowering the distal ends of her right foot into plantar flexion. The therapist gently resists this movement with his hands until a suitable position is reached (Figs. 256 and 257). After holding tension for three to five seconds they release simultaneously, and then repeat the procedure.

Seated B-4

Dōshin: In this examination, the therapist brings both the patient's feet together and grasps the toes and heels. With the heels stabilized, he rotates the distal ends of her feet together to the right (Fig. 258) and to the left (Fig. 259), inquiring about sensations of comfort or discomfort.

Sōtai: The seated patient places her feet together and rotates the distal ends of her feet from right to left, pivoting on the heels. The therapist grasps both heels and both feet in order to give resistance to this movement (Figs. 260 to 262). They hold tension at a suitable position for a few seconds and release it, and then repeat the procedure.

Fig. 258 Seated B-4–1

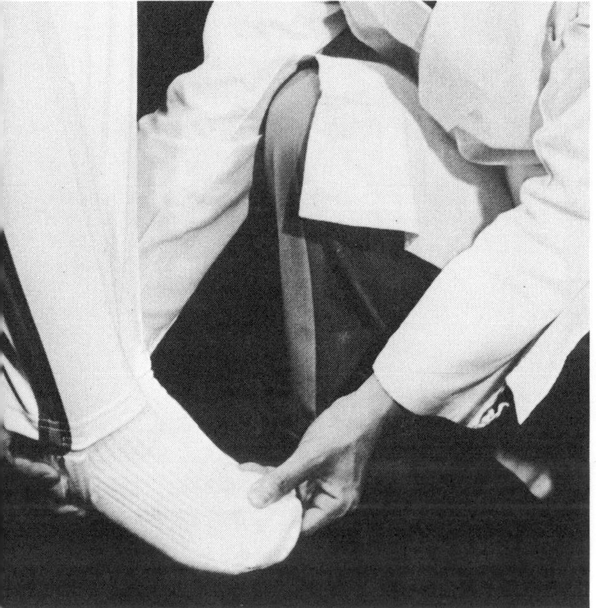

Fig. 259 Seated B-4–2

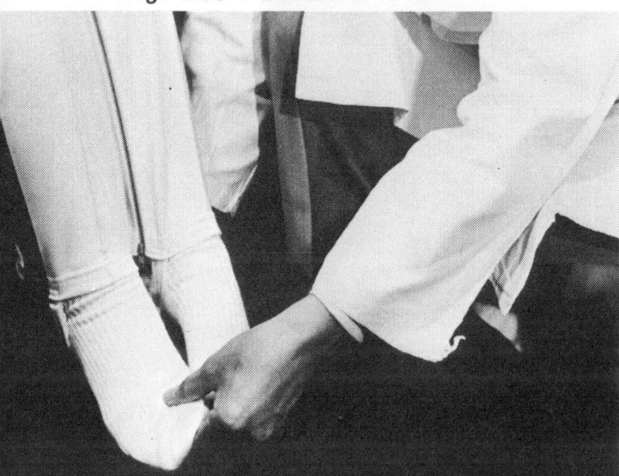

Fig. 260 Seated B-4–3

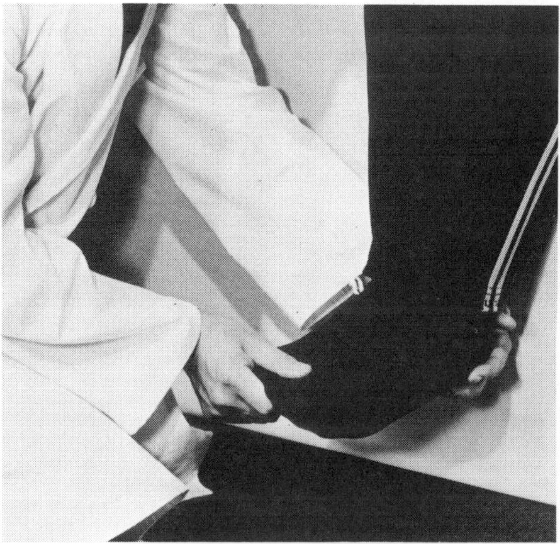

Fig. 261 Seated B-4–4

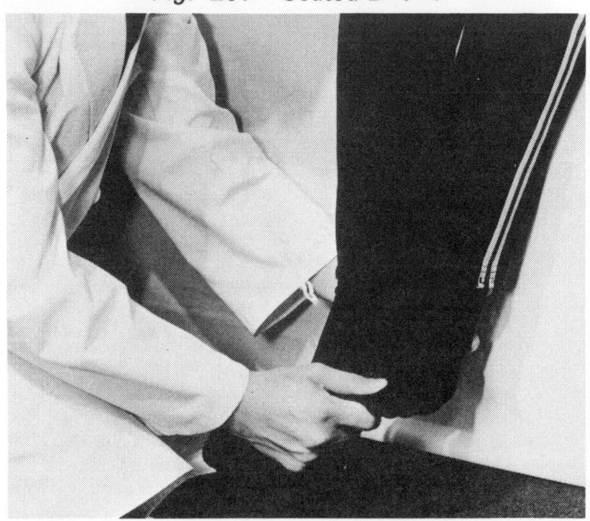

Fig. 262 Seated B-4–5

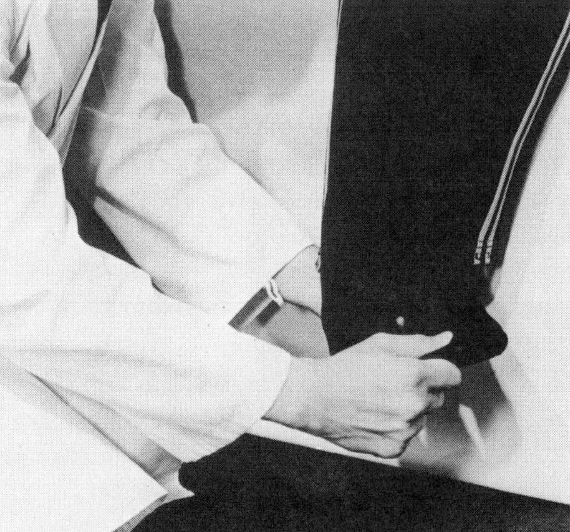

Fig. 263 Seated C-1–1

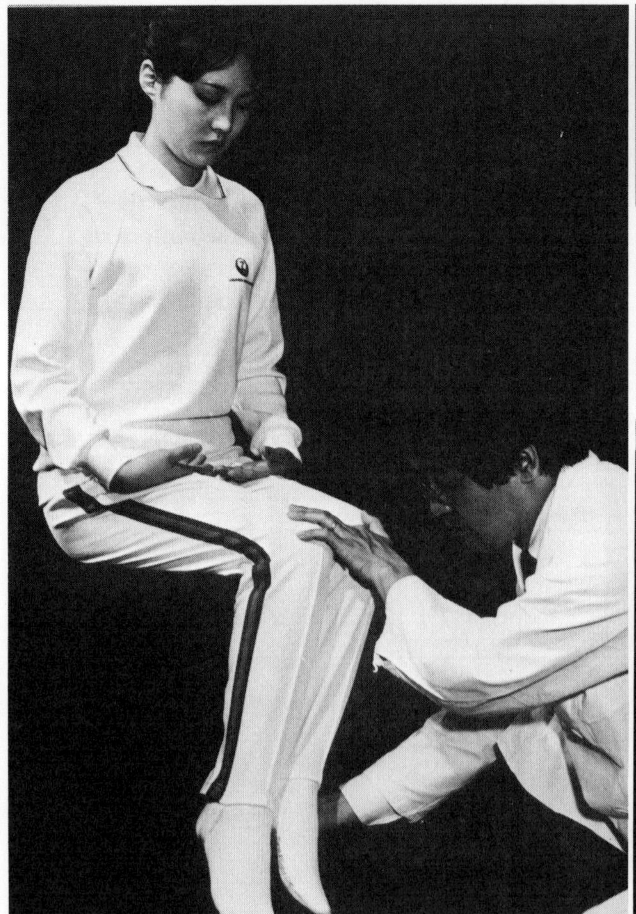

Fig. 264 Seated C-1–2

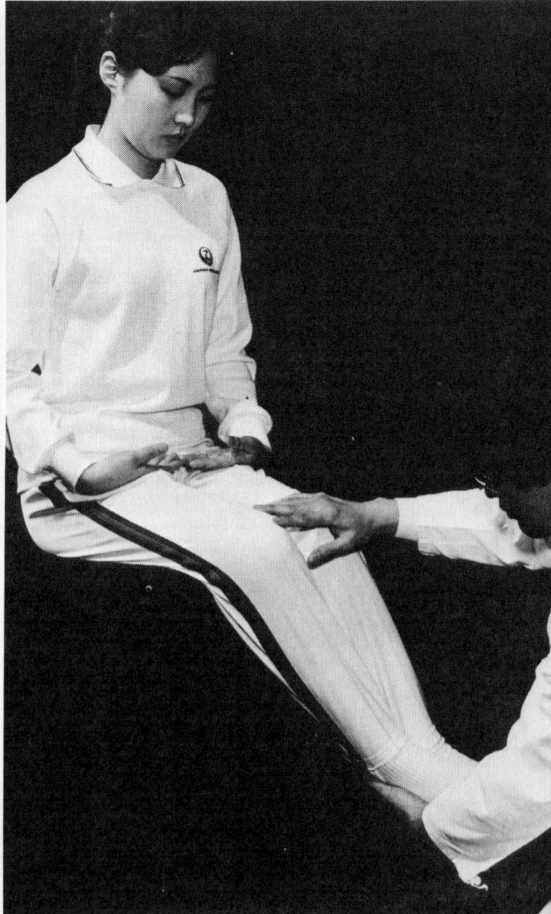

Fig. 265 Seated C-1–3

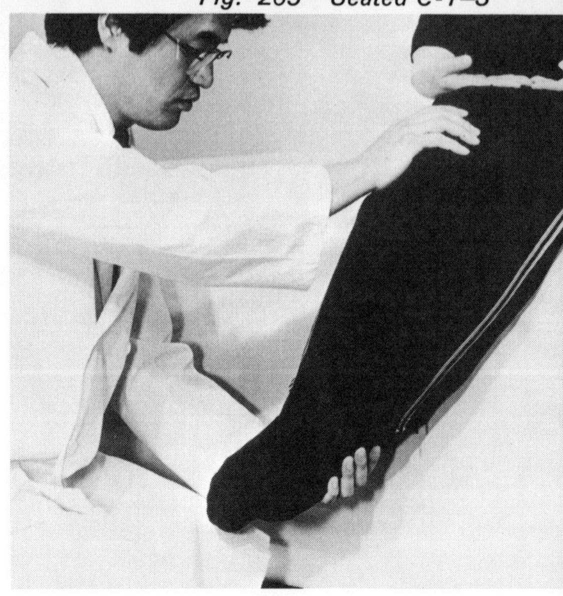

Seated C-1

Dōshin: The therapist takes hold of the seated patient's knees and feet. Keeping the patient's legs together, he swings the lower legs to the right and to the left, pivoting at the knees (Figs. 263 and 264). He inquires about sensations of comfort or discomfort.

Sōtai: The patient swings her lower legs from right to left, pivoting at the knees. By pushing on the knees and pulling the feet toward him, the therapist gives resistance to her movement (Figs. 265 to 267). They hold tension at a suitable place for three to five seconds and then release. This procedure is repeated two or three times.

Seated C-2

Dōshin: The therapist takes hold of the knee and foot of the seated patient's right (or left) leg. He swings the lower legs medially and laterally, pivoting at the knee (Figs. 268 and 269). He asks about sensations of comfort or discomfort produced.

Fig. 266 Seated C-1–4

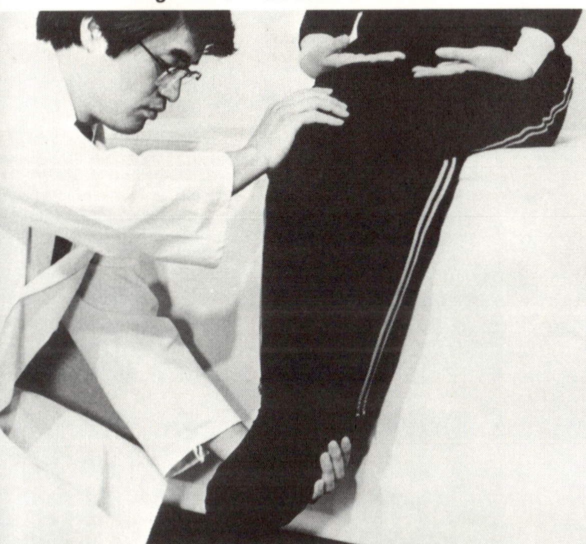

Fig. 267 Seated C-1–5

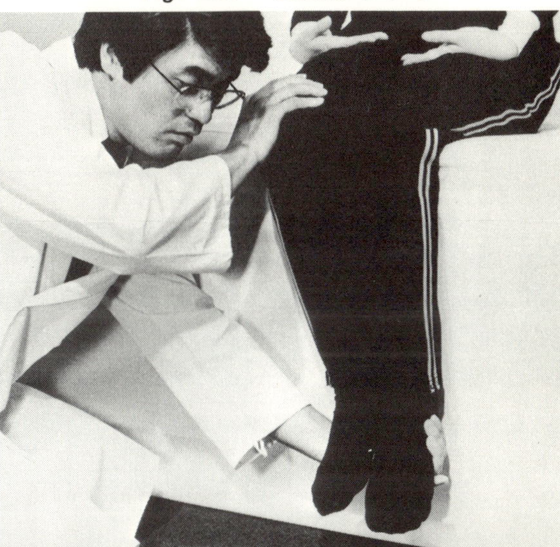

Fig. 268 Seated C-2–1

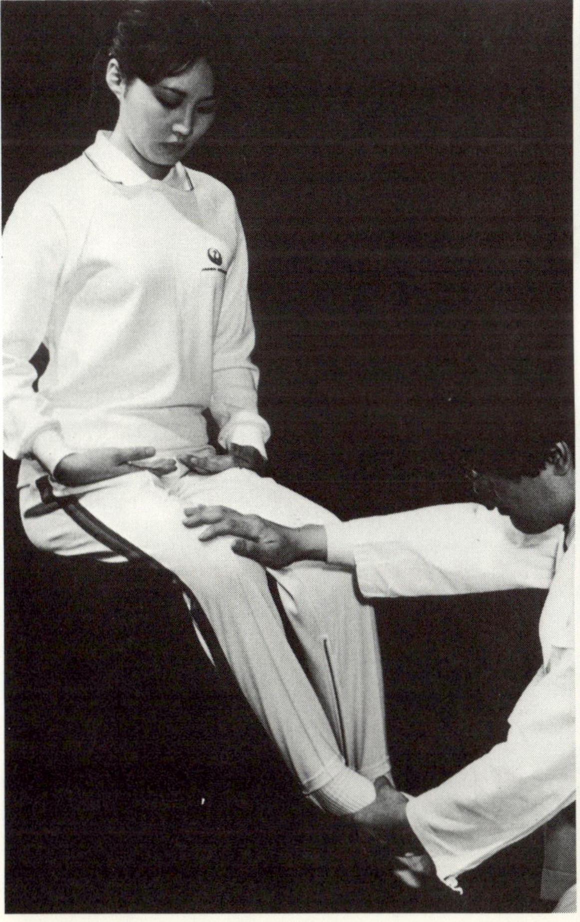

Fig. 269 Seated C-2–2

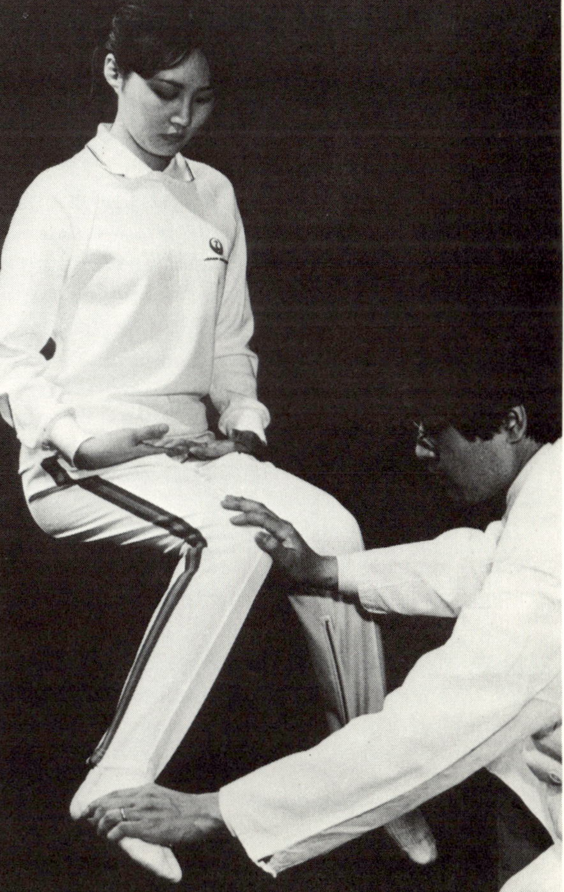

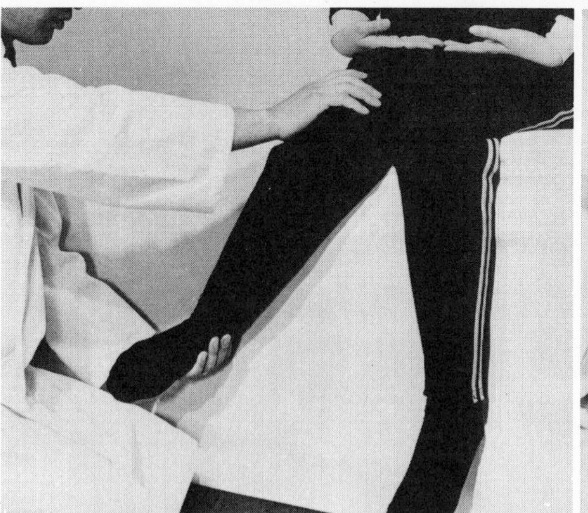

Fig. 270 Seated C-2–3

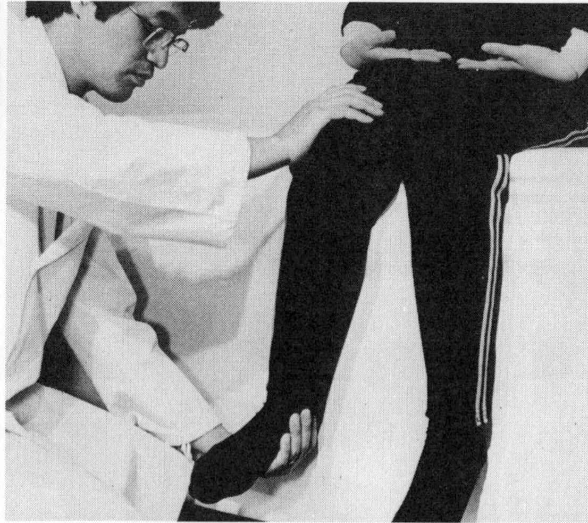

Fig. 271 Seated C-2–4

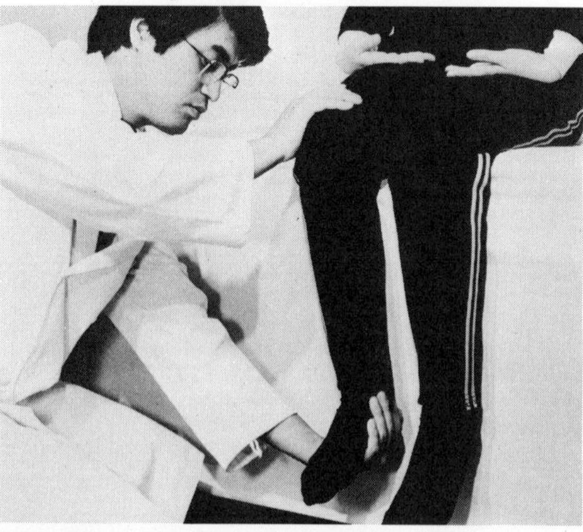

Fig. 272 Seated C-2–5

Sōtai: Using her right knee as a pivoting point, the patient swings her right lower leg from the outside toward the median. Holding her knee and foot, the therapist gently resists the movement (Figs. 270 to 272). They hold tension at a suitable position and release, and then repeat the procedure.

Seated D-1

Dōshin: In the seated position, the patient clasps both her hands behind her head. Standing behind her back, the therapist grasps both of her elbows in order to rotate her upper trunk to the right and to the left (Figs. 273 and 274). He asks which direction of rotation causes more discomfort.

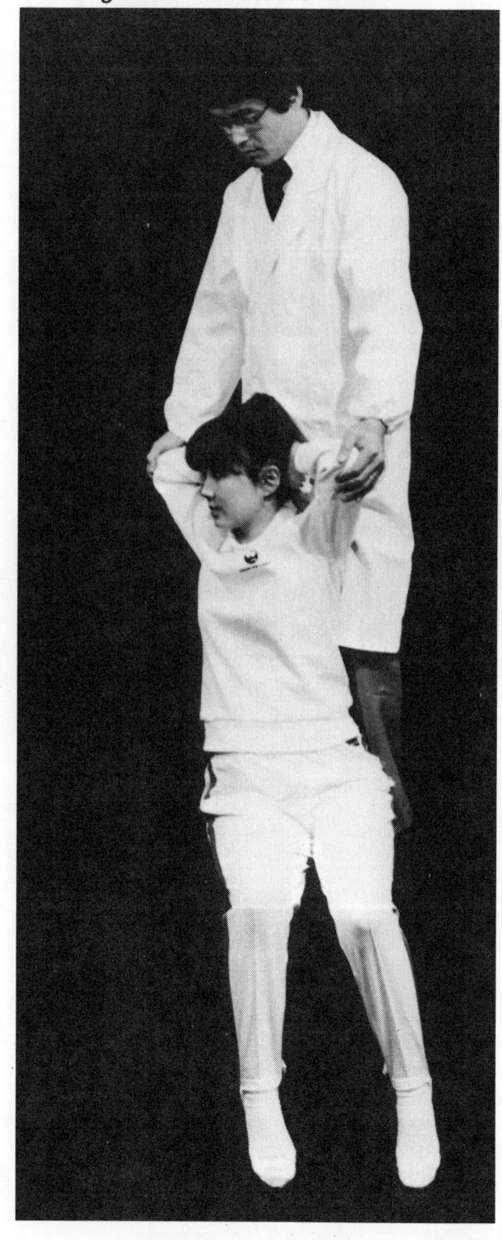

Fig. 273
Seated D-1–1

Sōtai: The patient rotates her upper trunk from right to left facing positions. Holding both of her elbows, the therapist gives resistance to her movement (Figs. 275 to 277). After maintaining tension for three to five seconds at a suitable position, they both release the tension simultaneously. The procedure is repeated two or three times.

To increase effectiveness, the therapist should stabilize the patient's back by supporting it with his knees. This will help prevent the patient's rotation movement from getting off center.

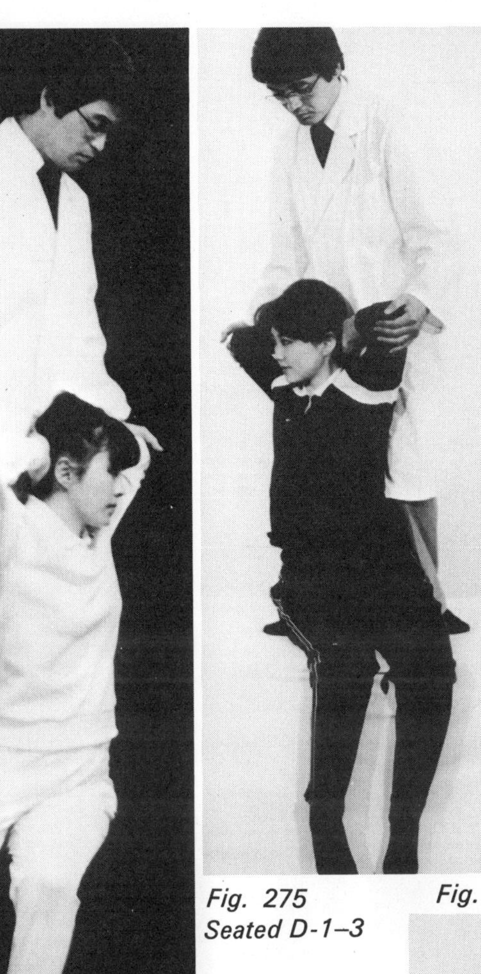

Fig. 274 Seated D-1–2

Fig. 275 Seated D-1–3

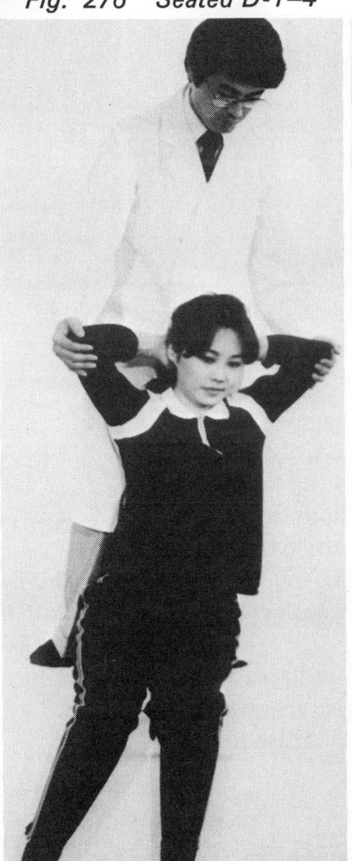

Fig. 276 Seated D-1–4

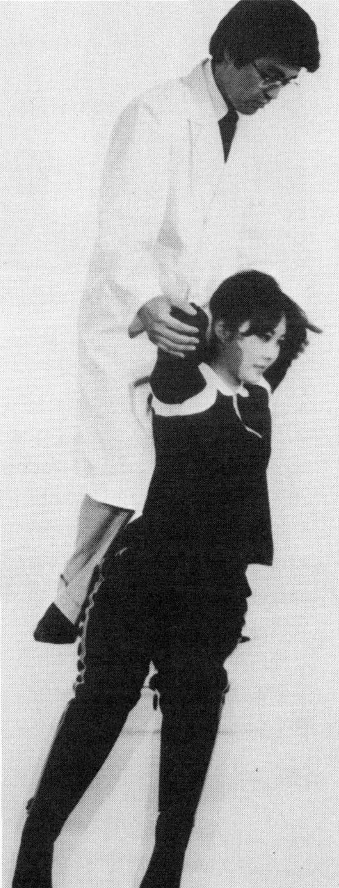

Fig. 277 Seated D-1–5

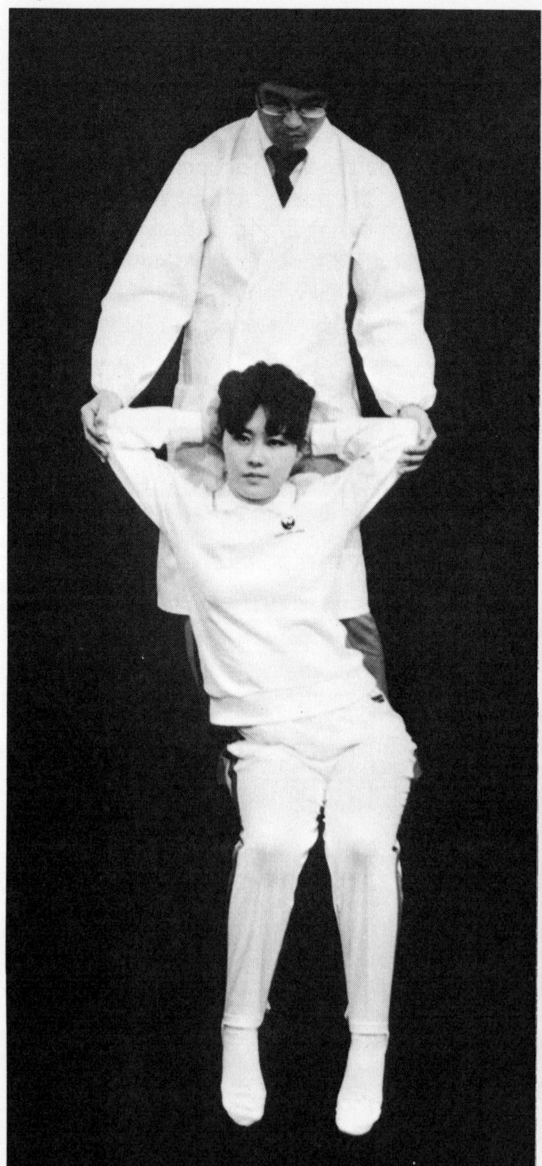

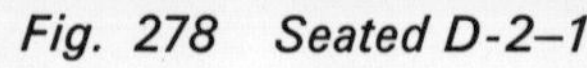

Fig. 278 Seated D-2–1

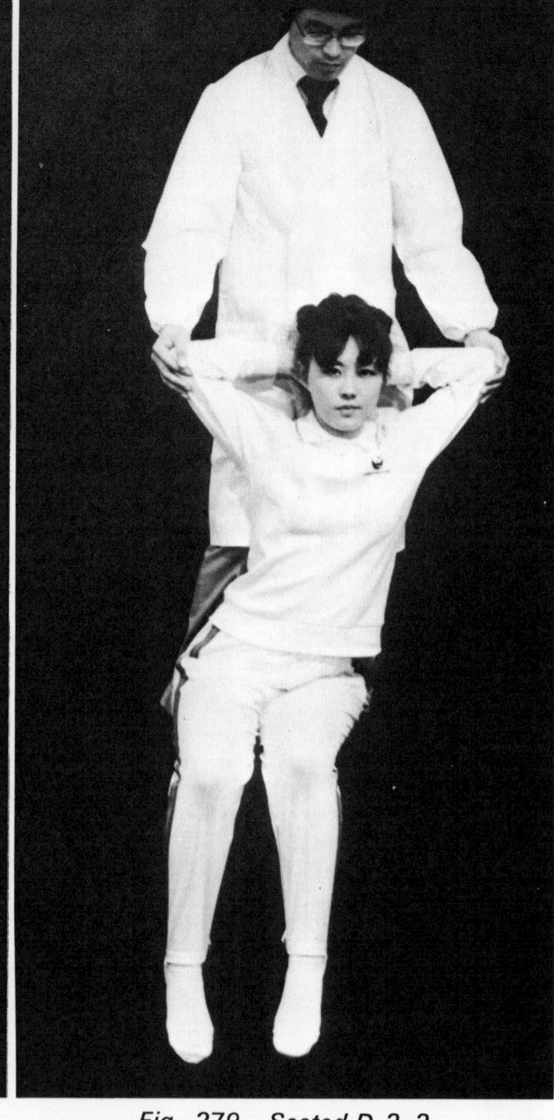

Fig. 279 Seated D-2–2

Dōshin: In the seated position, the patient again clasps her hands behind her head. Standing behind her and grasping both her elbows, the therapist shifts the upper torso to the right and left (transverse movement), inquiring about sensations of comfort and discomfort (Figs. 278 and 279).

Sōtai: The patient shifts her upper torso from right to left. The therapist grasps both of her elbows in order to give resistance to her movement (Figs. 280 to 282). They hold tension for a few seconds in a suitable position and release, and then repeat the procedure.

Seated E-1

Dōshin: The therapist holds the head of the seated patient. He rotates her head to the right and to the left, inquiring about which direction of movement produces more discomfort (Figs. 283 and 284).

Fig. 280 Seated D-2–3

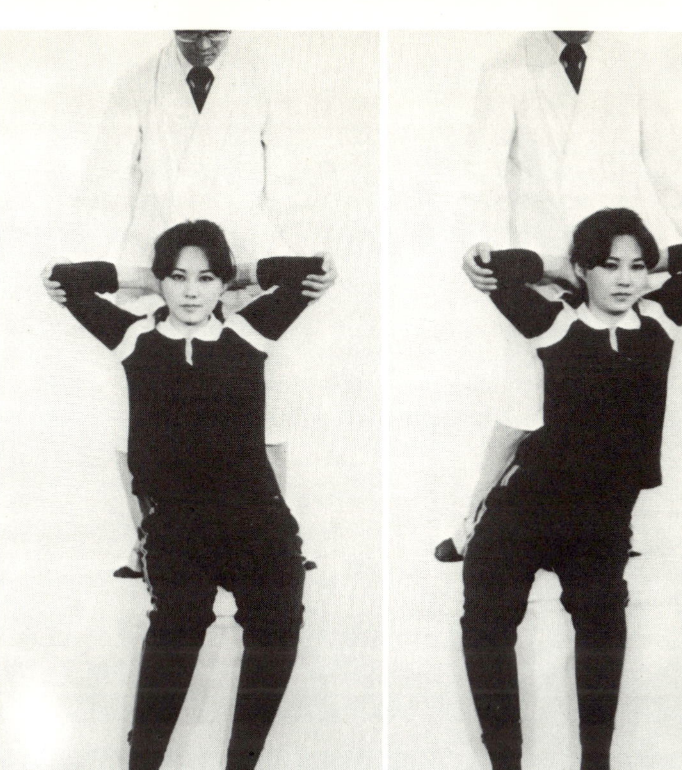

Fig. 281 Seated D-2–4

Fig. 282 Seated D-2–5

Fig. 283 Seated E-1–1

Fig. 284 Seated E-1–2

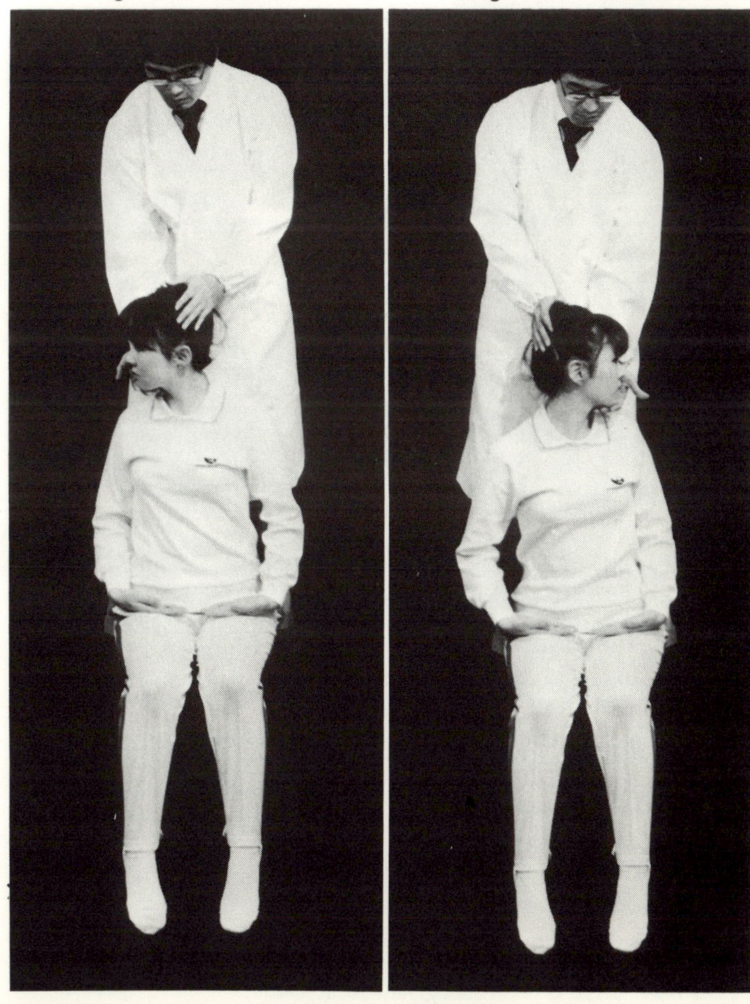

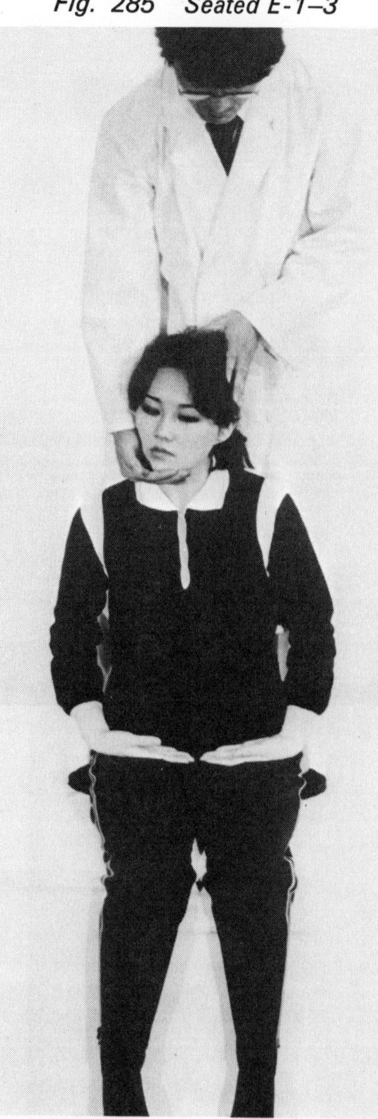

Fig. 285 Seated E-1–3

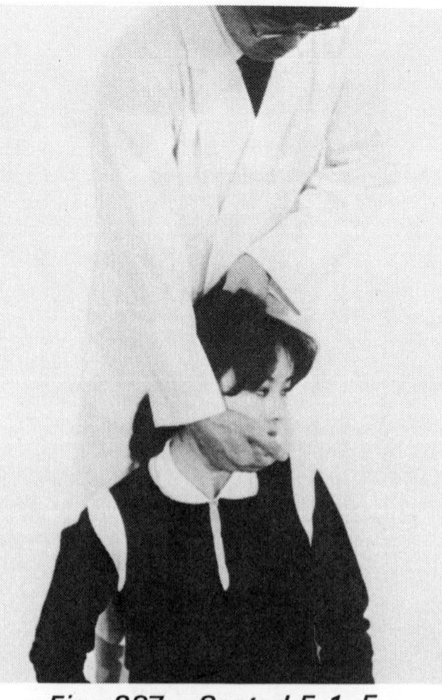

Fig. 286 Seated E-1–4

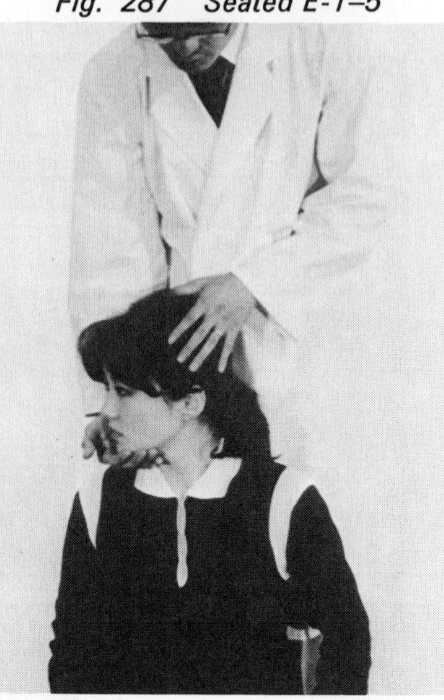

Fig. 287 Seated E-1–5

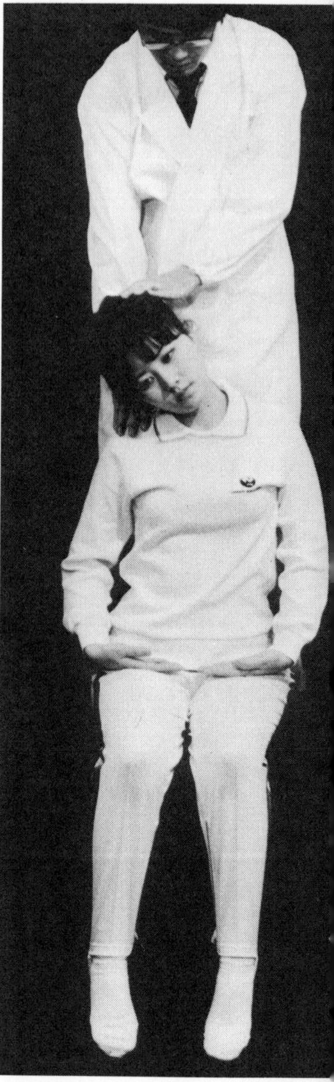

Fig. 288 Seated E-2–1

Sōtai: The patient rotates her head from left facing to right facing positions. The therapist gives resistance by holding the patient's occiput and cheek (Figs. 285 to 287). They hold tension at a suitable position and release, and then repeat the procedure.

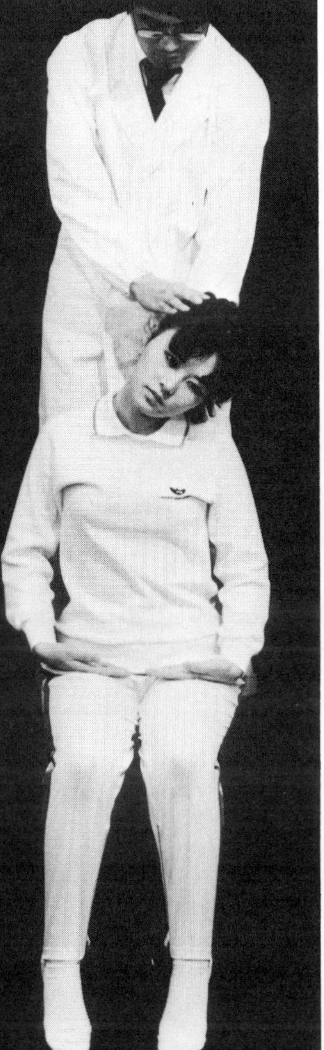

Fig. 289 Seated E-2–2

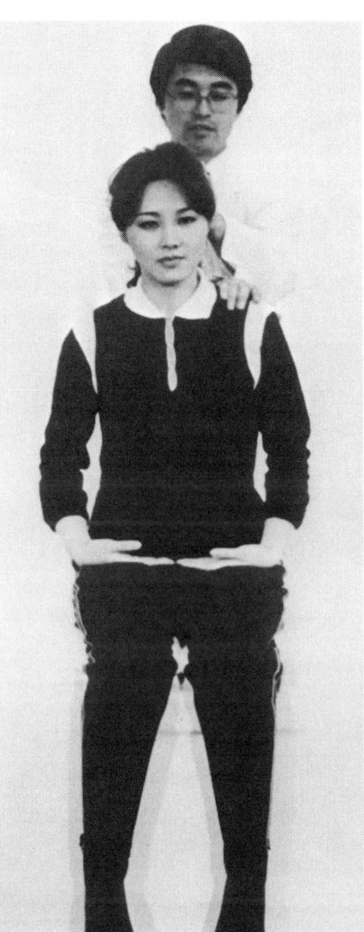

Fig. 290 Seated E-2–3

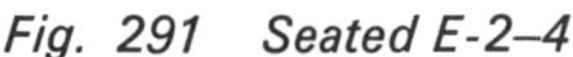

Fig. 291 Seated E-2–4

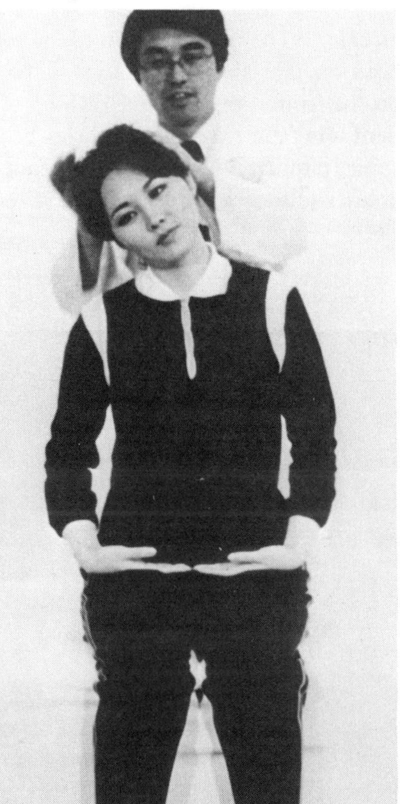

Fig. 292 Seated E-2–5

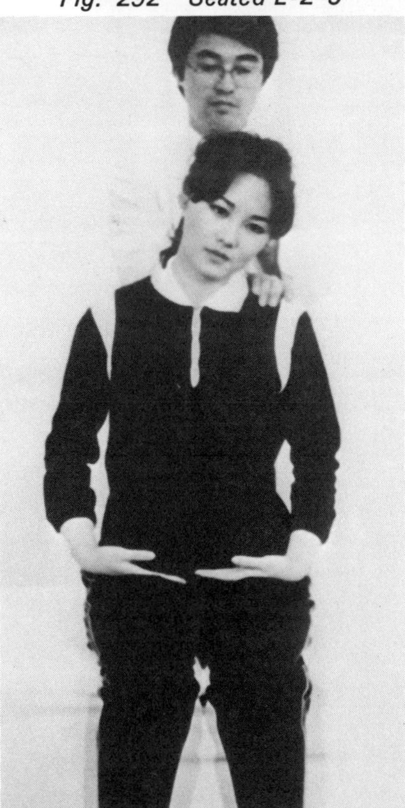

Seated E-2

Dōshin: The therapist holds the head of the patient. He flexes the patient's head laterally to the right and left, asking which direction of movement causes more discomfort (Figs. 288 and 289).

Sōtai: The patient moves her head from right lateral flexion through the upright position into left lateral flexion. The therapist places his hands upon her left shoulder and left temporal region to give resistance to the movement of her head (Figs. 290 to 292). They hold tension at a suitable position for several seconds and release, and then repeat.

Seated E-3

Dōshin: The patient assumes the basic seated position. The therapist places his hands either on the frontal or occipital regions of the patient. He then extends and flexes her cervical spine, inquiring which motion produces the greater sensation of discomfort (Figs. 293 and 294).

Fig. 293 Seated E-3–1

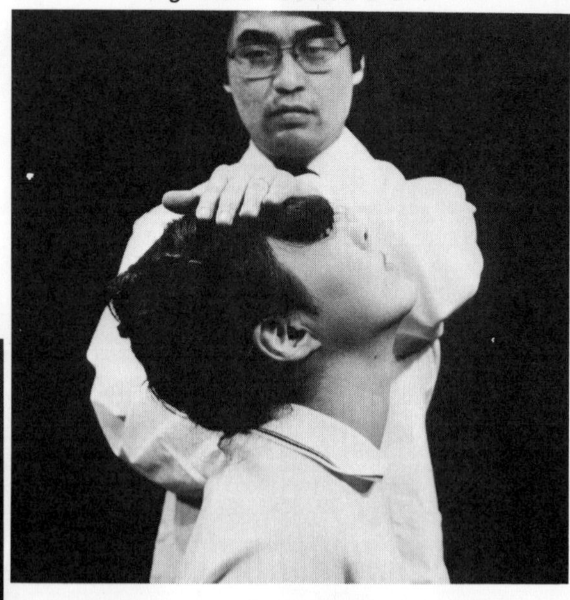

Fig. 294 Seated E-3–2

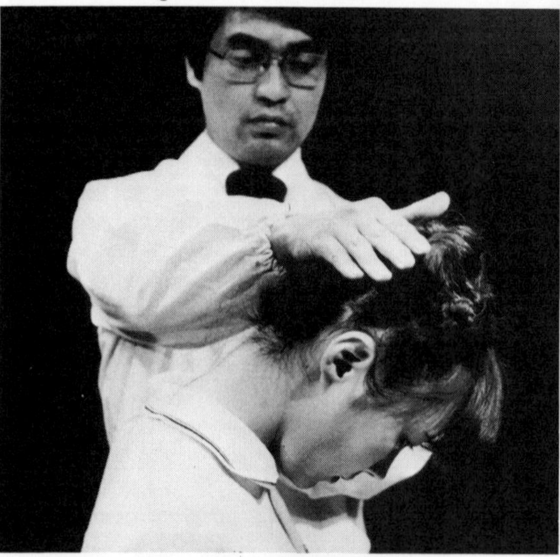

Sōtai I: The patient flexes her neck forward bringing her chin to her chest. The therapist gives resistance by supporting her chin (Figs. 295 and 296). They hold tension at a suitable position for three to five seconds and release, and then repeat the procedure.

Fig. 295 Seated E-3–3

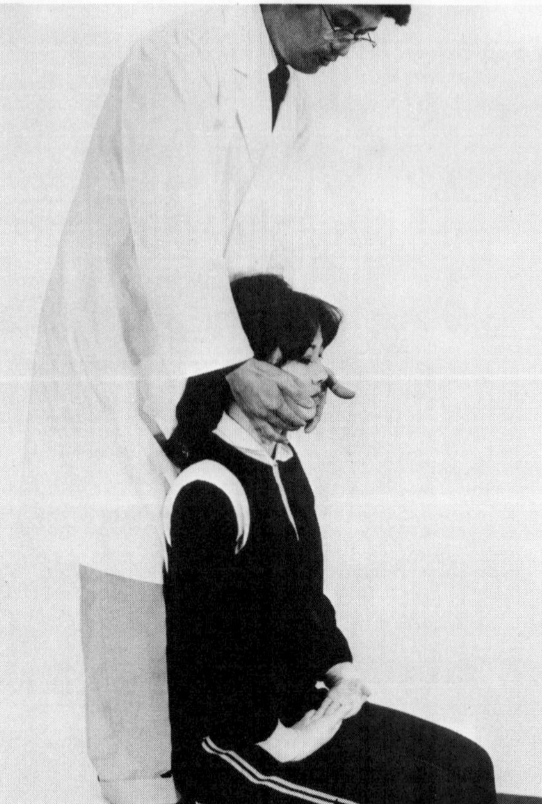

Fig. 296 Seated E-3–4

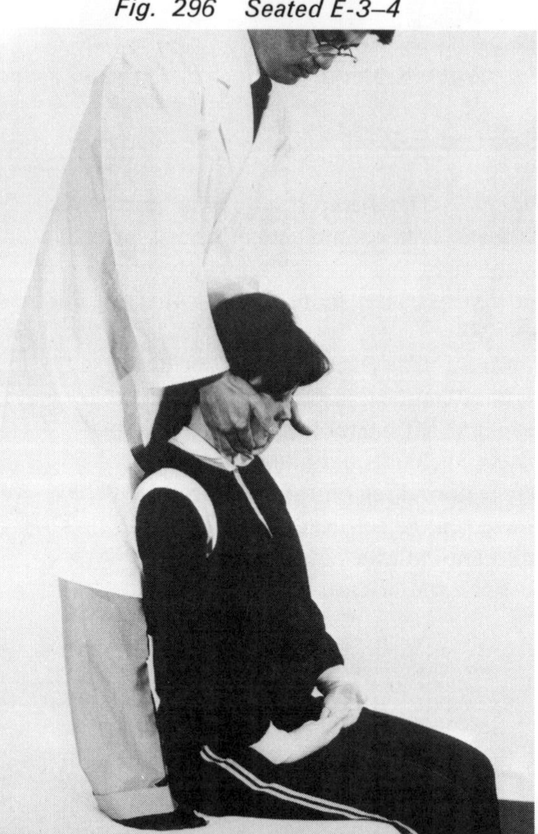

Fig. 297 Seated E-3–5

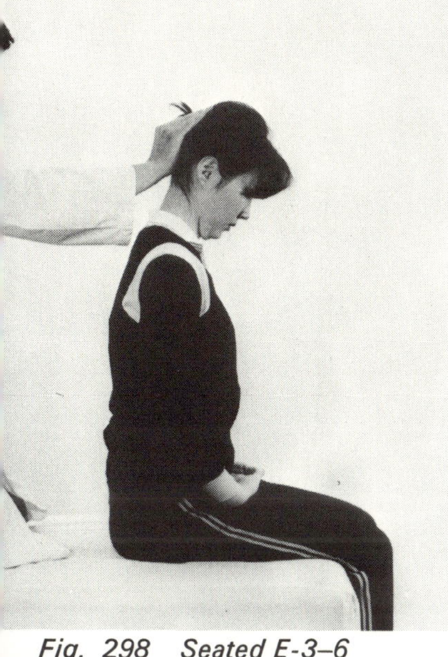

Fig. 298 Seated E-3–6

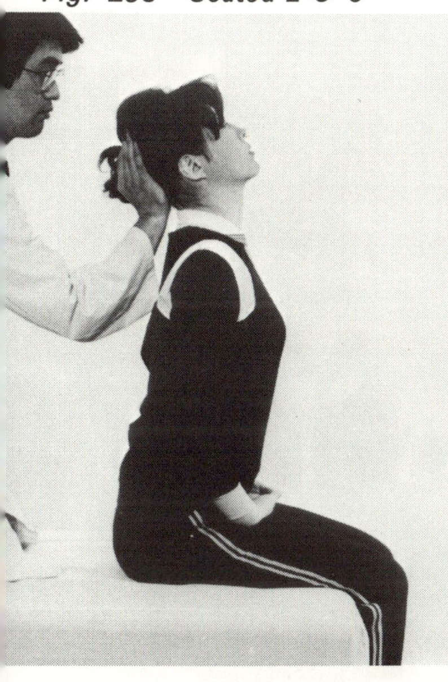

Fig. 299 Seated F-1–1

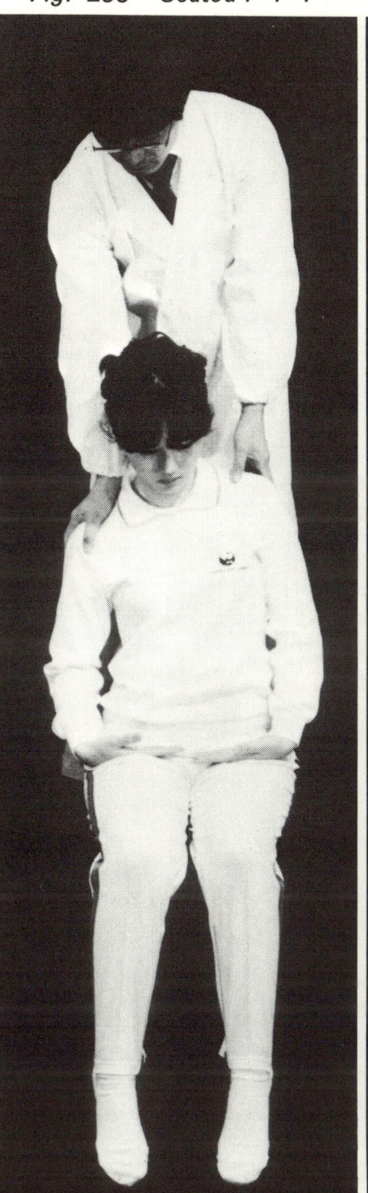

Fig. 300 Seated F-1–2

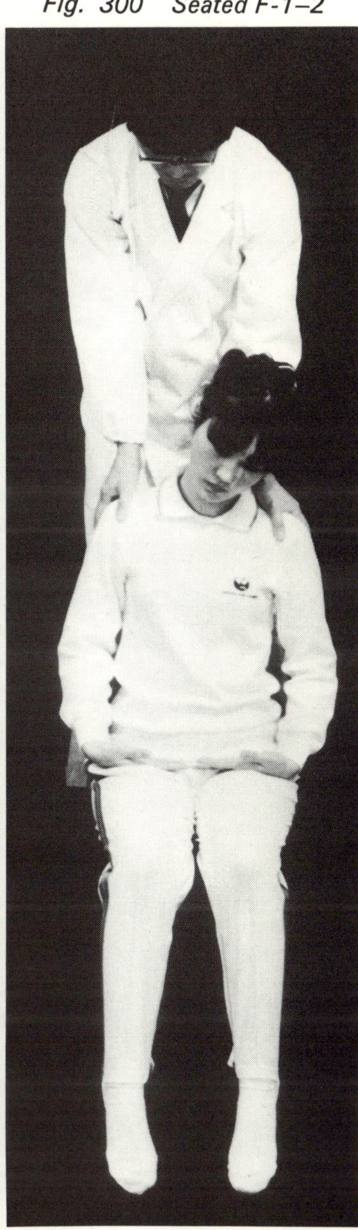

Sōtai II: The patient extends her neck, tilting her neck back. The therapist supports her occipital region and resists her head movement (Figs. 297 and 298). After holding tension for three to five seconds at a suitable position they release, and then repeat the procedure.

Seated F-1

Dōshin: The therapist depresses the patient's right and left shoulders alternately, questioning her about the resultant sensations of comfort or discomfort, as well as the differences between the right and left sides (Figs. 299 and 300).

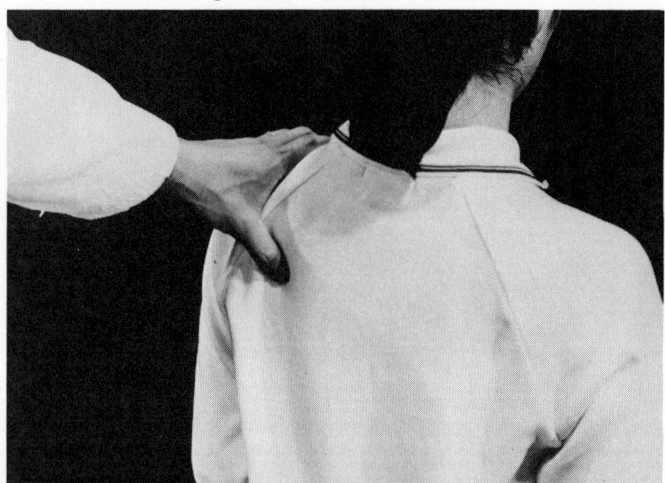

Fig. 301 Seated F-1–3

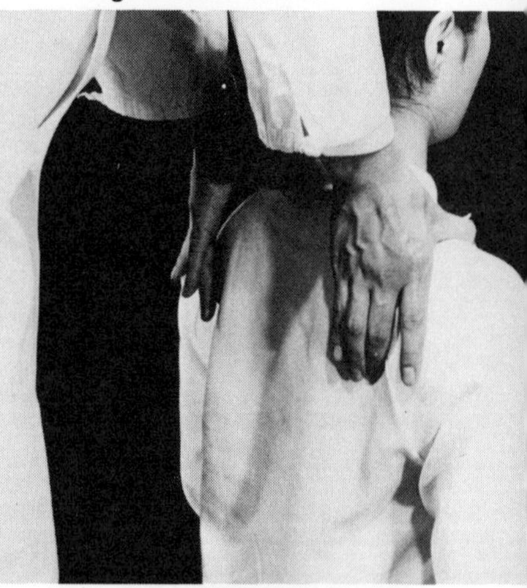

Fig. 302 Seated F-1–4

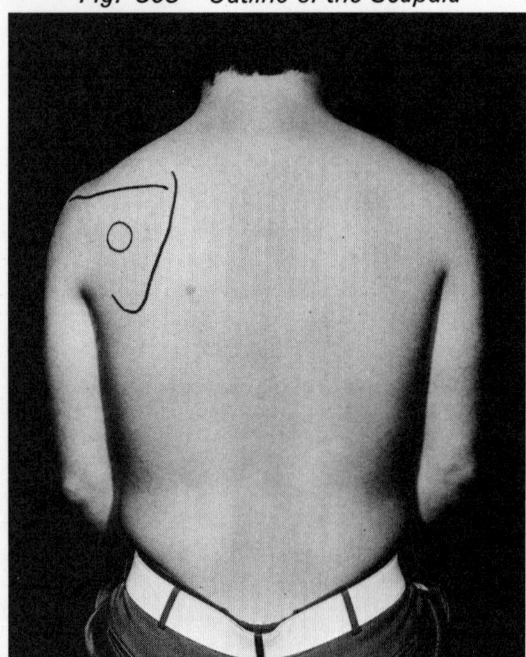

Fig. 303 Outline of the Scapula

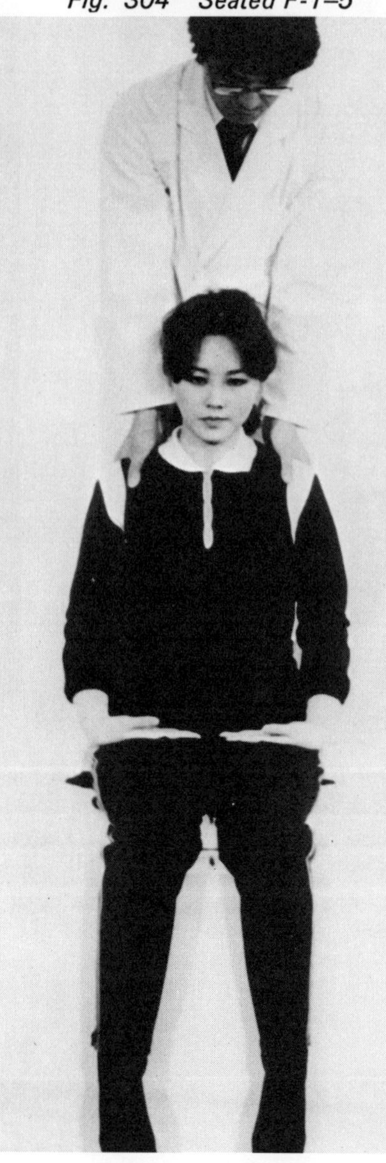

Fig. 304 Seated F-1–5

Palpation examination: The therapist palpates the region inferior to the spine of the scapulae from behind the seated patient, one side at a time (Fig. 301), or both sides together (Fig. 302), checking for the locations of pressure sensitive points. Figure 303 shows the outline of the scapula and the location of the point most likely to be sensitive. (See also Fig. 111 on p. 60.)

Sōtai I: The patient elevates her right shoulder. The therapist places his hands on her shoulders in order to resist this movement (Figs. 304 and 305). They hold tension at a suitable position and release, and then repeat the procedure.

Close observation of the patient's movements reveals that the elevation of the right shoulder is accompanied by a slight depression of the left shoulder. The following Sōtai movement takes advantage of this linkage.

Sōtai II: The patient elevates her right shoulder while simultaneously depressing her left shoulder. The therapist places one hand on her right shoulder and places the other hand inside the left axilla (Fig. 306). He gives gentle resistance against her shoulder movements (Fig. 307). They maintain opposing pressure at a suitable position and release after a pause. This procedure is repeated two or three times

Fig. 305 Seated F-1–6

Fig. 306 Seated F-1–7

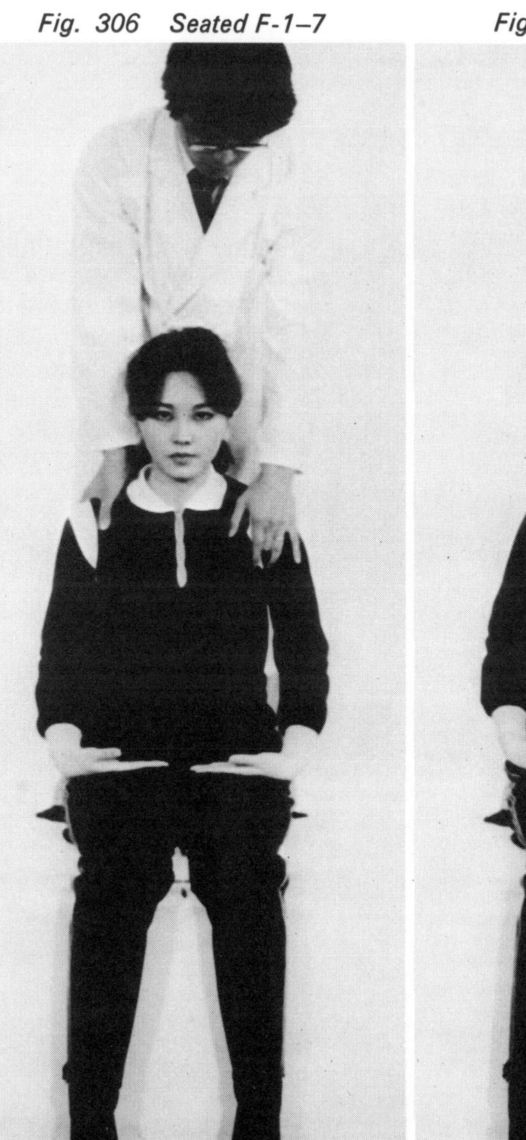

Fig. 307 Seated F-1–8

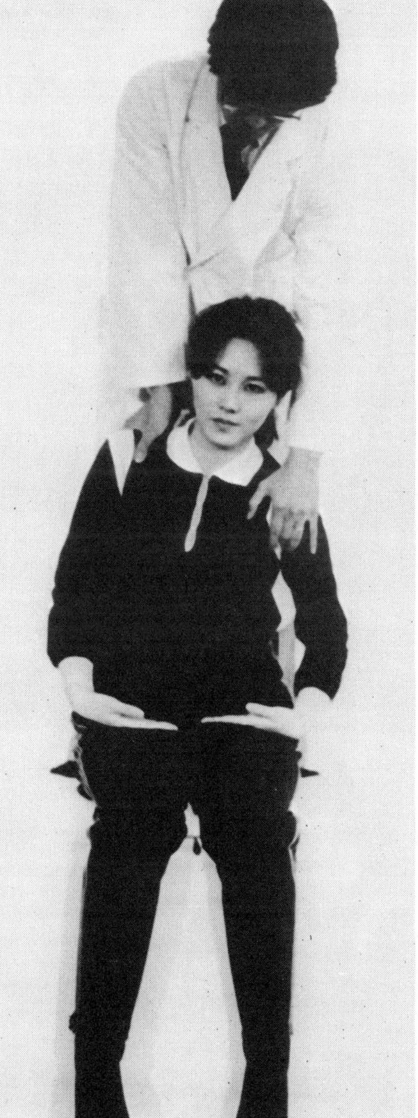

Fig. 308 Seated G-1–1

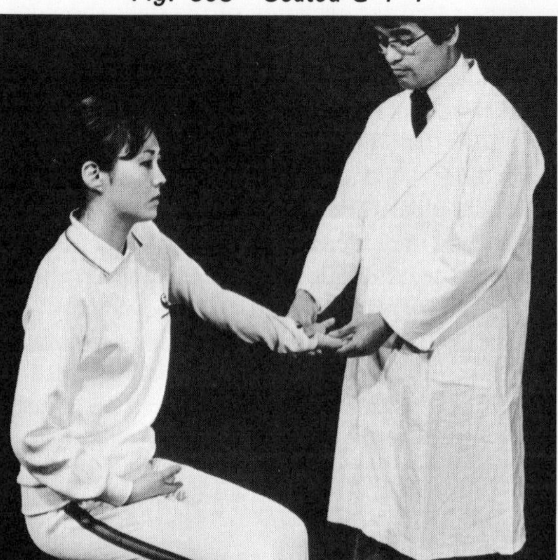

Fig. 309 Seated G-1–2

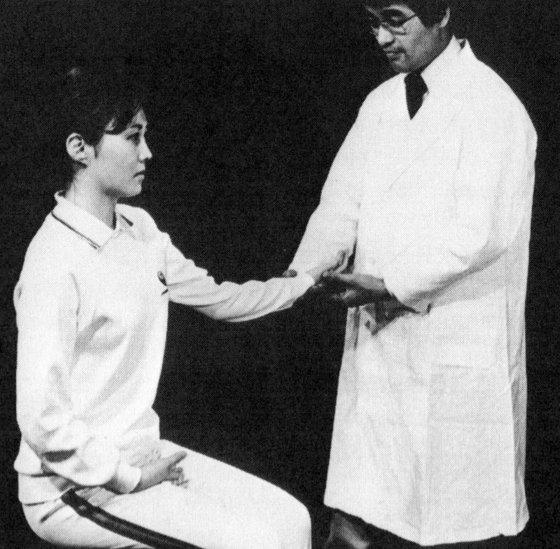

Fig. 310 Seated G-1–3

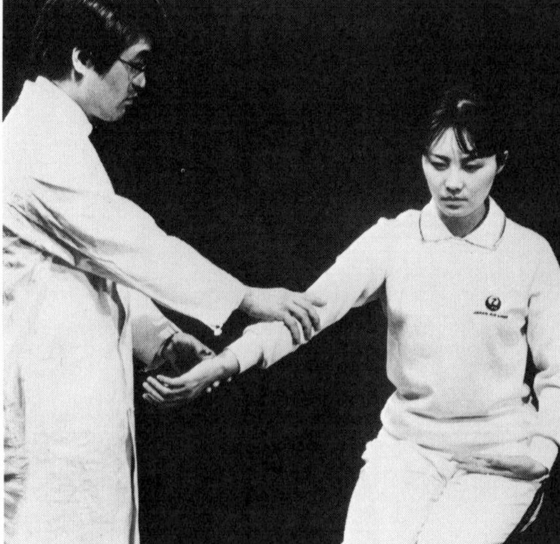

Seated G-1

Dōshin: The patient takes the seated posture and extends her right or left arm forward at a diagonal (anterolaterally). The therapist takes hold of the wrist of the extended arm and rotates it into the pronated and supinated positions, inquiring about the sensations of comfort or discomfort (Figs. 308 to 310).

Seated G-1-a

Sōtai I: The patient with her left arm extended, rotates it from the supinated to the

Fig. 311 Seated G-1-a-4

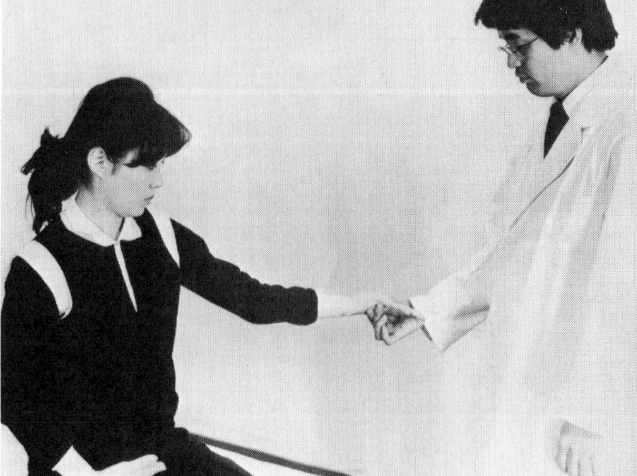

Fig. 312 Seated G-1-a-5

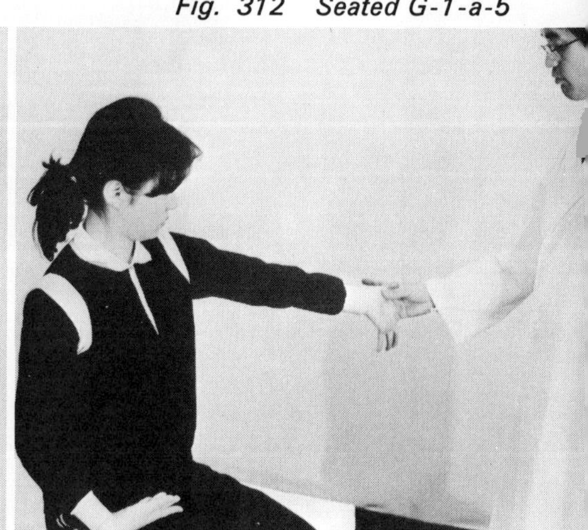

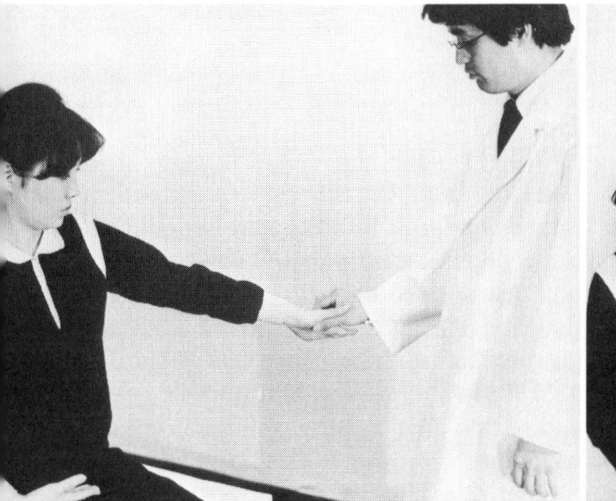

Fig. 313 Seated G-1-a-6

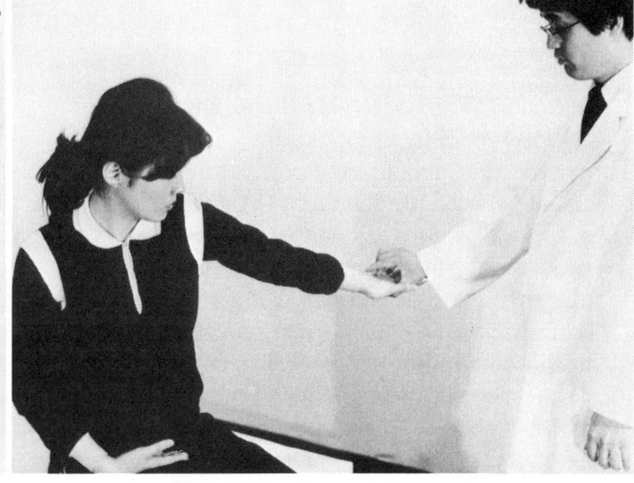

Fig. 314 Seated G-1-a-7

pronated position. The therapist holds her left hand in the manner illustrated in Figures 311 through 314. They hold tension at a suitable position and release after a pause. They repeat the procedure two or three times.

Sōtai II: The Sōtai movement in this procedure is simply the reverse of the preceding movement described. The patient rotates her arm from the pronated to the supinated position (Figs. 315 through 318).

Fig. 315 Seated G-1-a-8

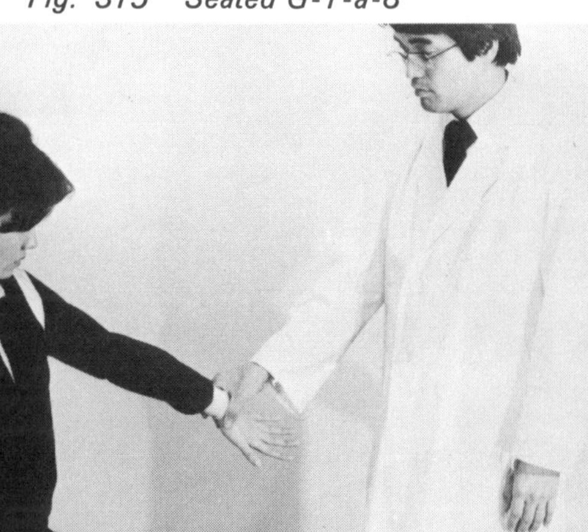

Fig. 316 Seated G-1-a-9

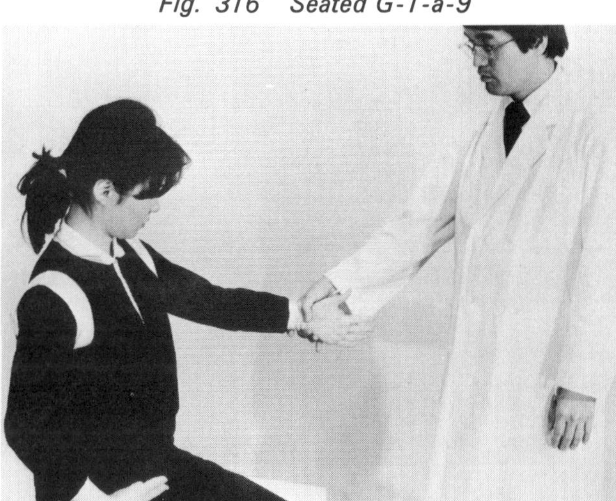

Fig. 317 Seated G-1-a-10

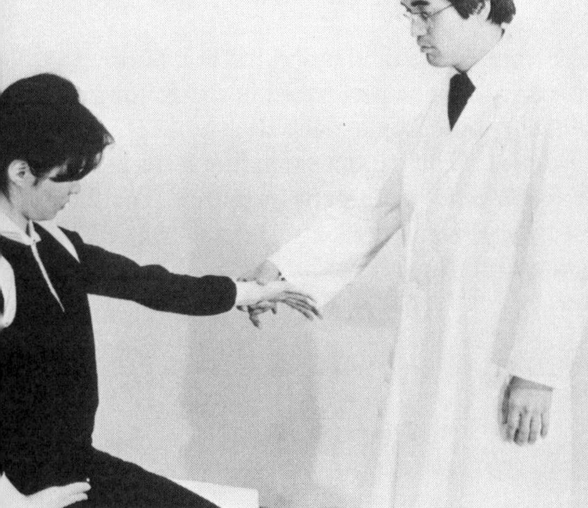

Fig. 318 Seated G-1-a-11

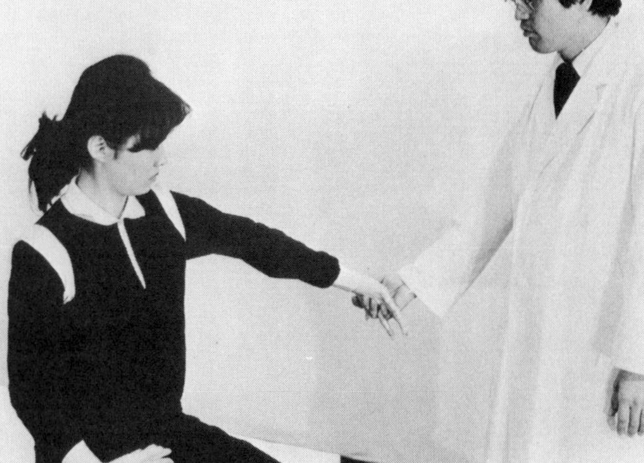

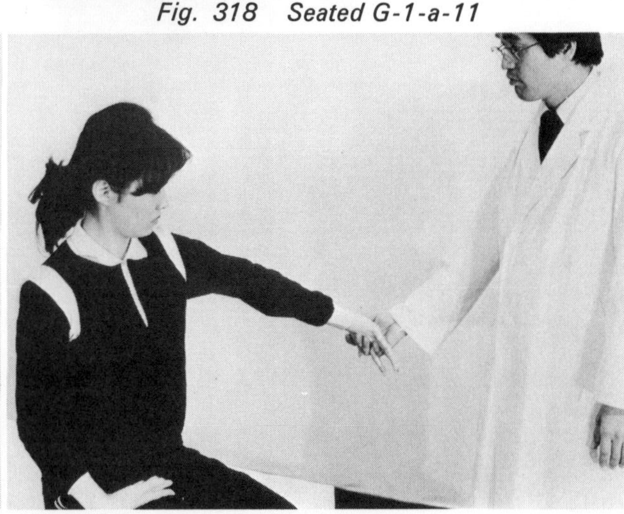

Note: When observing the results of the one arm mobility examinations just described, in most cases a consistent correlation can be found between the right and left arms in regard to sensations of comfort and discomfort produced during their rotation. Usually, if lateral rotation of one arm is more comfortable (compared to its medial rotation), then the medial rotation of the other arm conversely will be the more comfortable direction of rotation. When both medial rotation of the right arm and lateral rotation of the left arm are comfortable in both cases, the following Sōtai movements can be performed.

Seated G-1-b

Sōtai I: In the seated position, the patient extends her arms forward with her palms together. Keeping the palms in contact, she twists both her arms to the left. The therapist grips the patient's hands, holding them together and gives resistance to her movement (Figs. 319 and 320). They hold tension at a suitable position and release after a pause, and then repeat the procedure.

Sōtai II: This Sōtai movement is simply the reverse of the movement described above. The patient with her arms outstretched and her palms together, twists her arms to her right as the therapist provides resistance to this movement (Figs. 321 and 322).

Fig. 319 Seated G-1-b-12

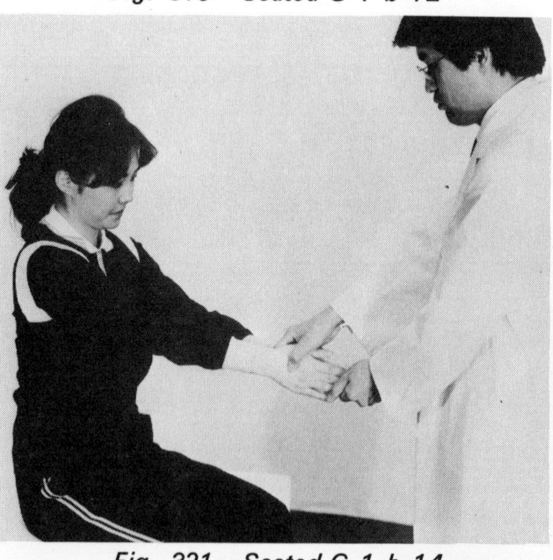

Fig. 320 Seated G-1-b-13

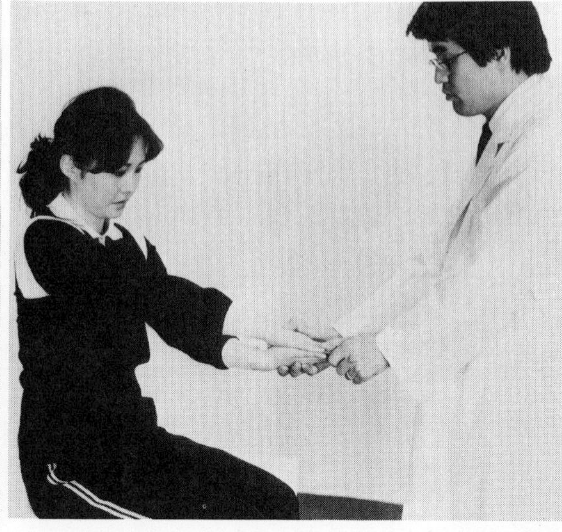

Fig. 321 Seated G-1-b-14

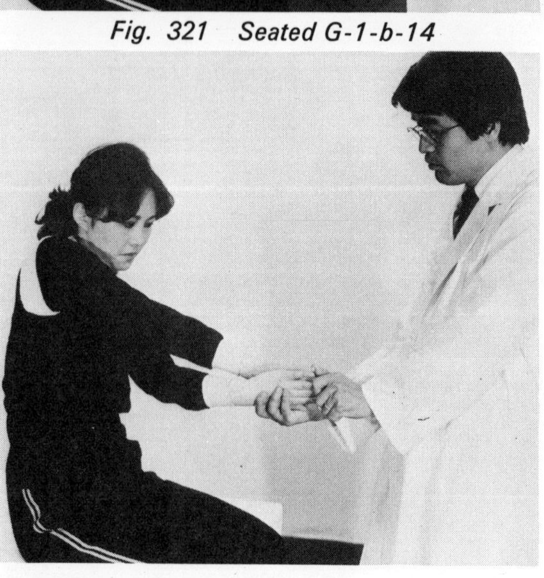

The mobility examination for this Sōtai movement can be performed in the following manner (photographe deleted);

Dōshin: The patient extending both arms to the front, holds both palms together. The therapist twists the patient's arms together to the right and to the left, and inquires about sensations of comfort or discomfort.

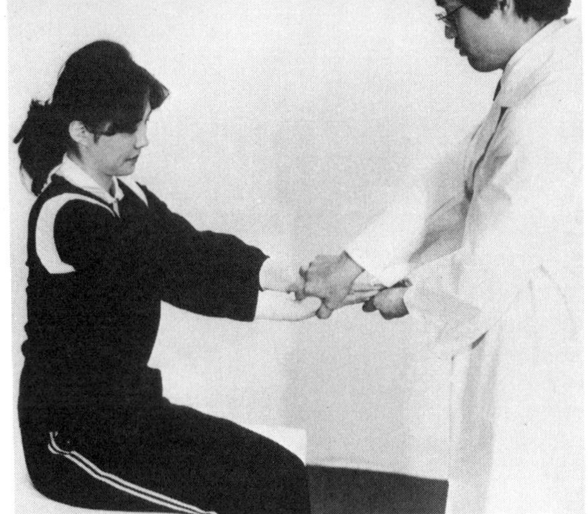

Fig. 322 Seated G-1-b-15

Seated G-2

Dōshin: In the seated position, the patient flexes her right or left arm at the elbow so that her fingertips touch (or approach) her shoulder. Holding the elbow and the shoulder of the patient's flexed arm, the therapist moves the arm to check the shoulder movement in the following manner;

(1) lateral abduction of shoulder by raising elbow (Fig. 323),
(2) lateral adduction of shoulder by lowering elbow (Fig. 324),
(3) rotation of shoulder into flexion from lateral position (Fig. 325),
(4) horizontal adduction bringing the elbow in medially (Fig. 326),
(5) flexion of the shoulder by pushing the elbow upward (Fig. 327),
(6) extension of the shoulder by bringing the elbow down (Fig. 328).

Fig. 323 Seated G-2–1

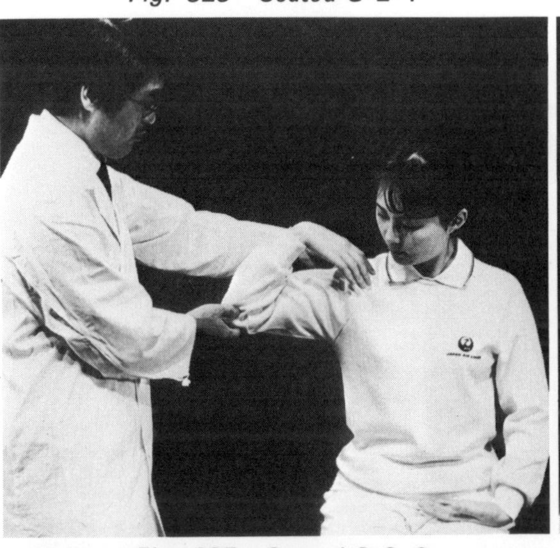

Fig. 324 Seated G-2–2

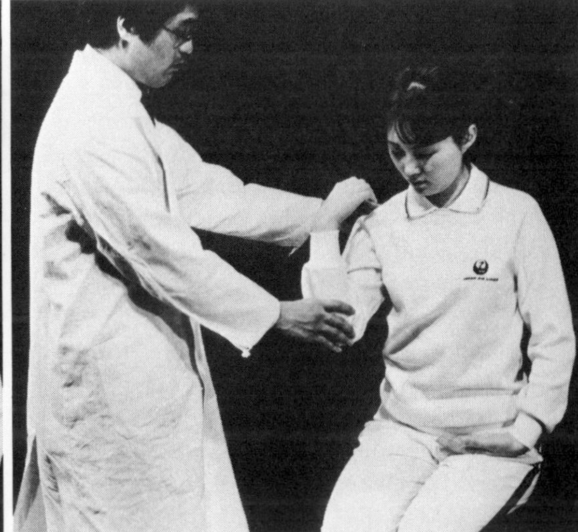

Fig. 325 Seated G-2–3

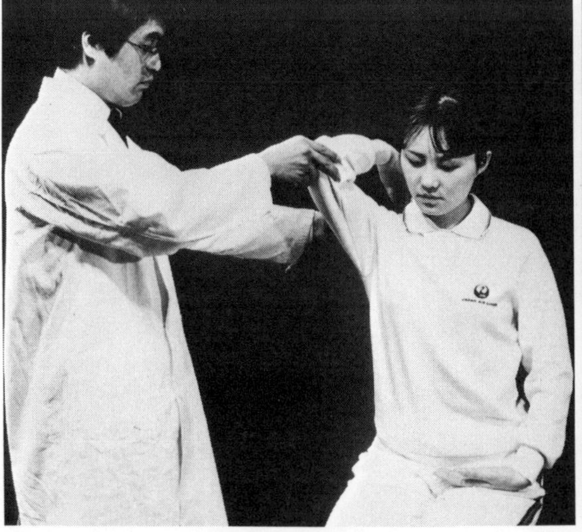

Fig. 326 Seated G-2–4

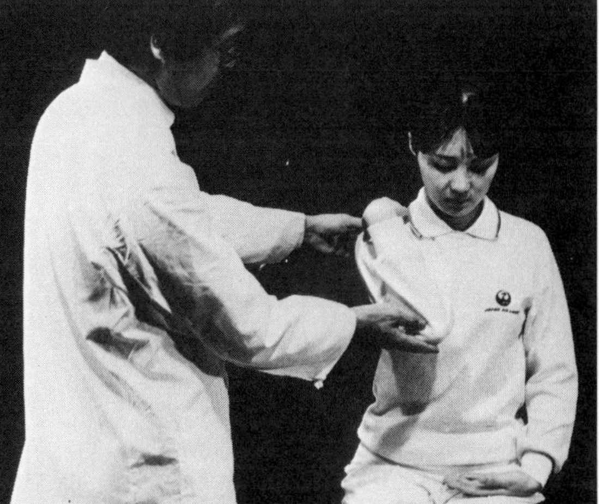

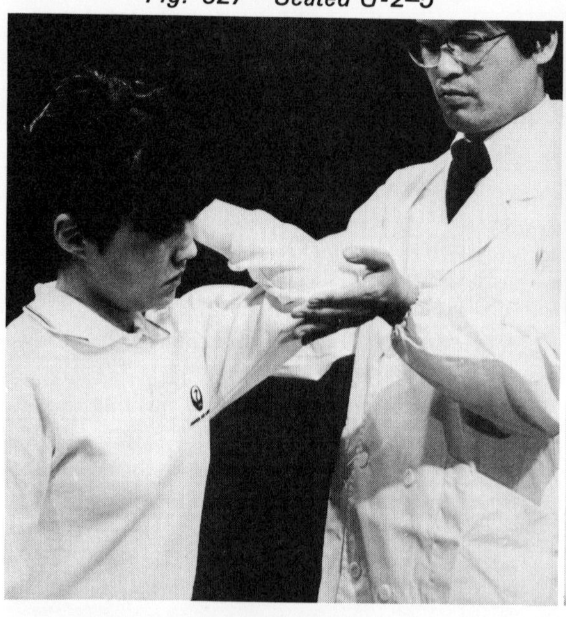

Fig. 327 Seated G-2–5

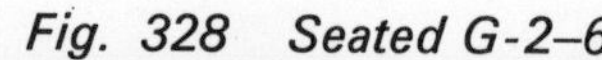

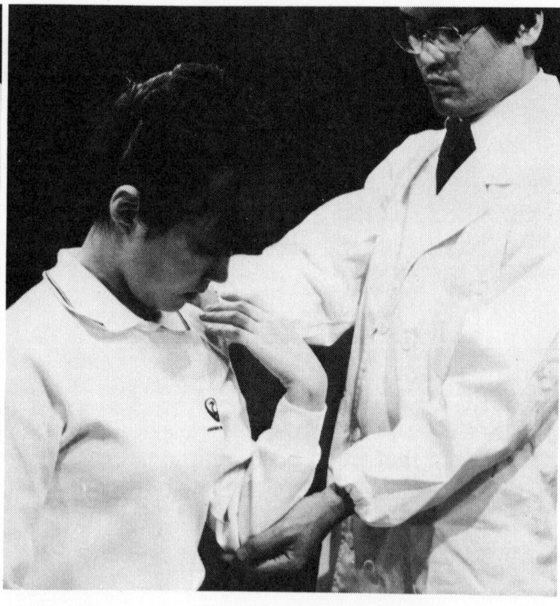

Fig. 328 Seated G-2–6

Sōtai I: In the same posture as during the mobility examination, the patient first raises her right elbow flexed, directly in front. She then lowers her elbow back down to her side describing a sagittal arc. As the patient lowers her arm, the therapist applies resistance with one hand placed under her elbow (Figs. 329 to 331). They hold tension at a suitable position for a few seconds and then release together. This procedure is repeated two or three times.

Sōtai II: The patient first raises her right elbow flexed, straight out to her side. From that posture, pivoting at the shoulder, the patient moves her elbow downward to her left

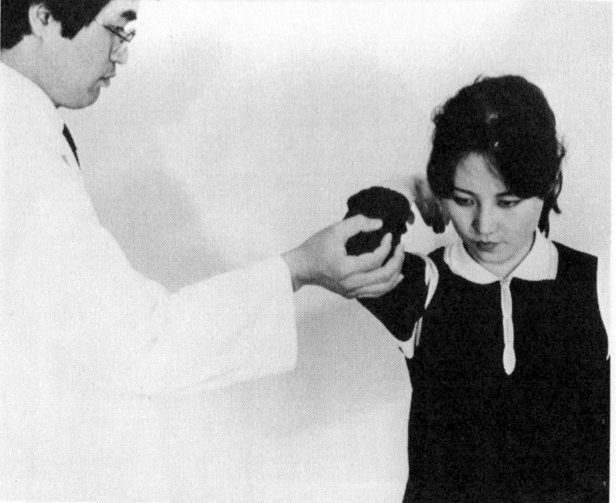

Fig. 329 Seated G-2–7

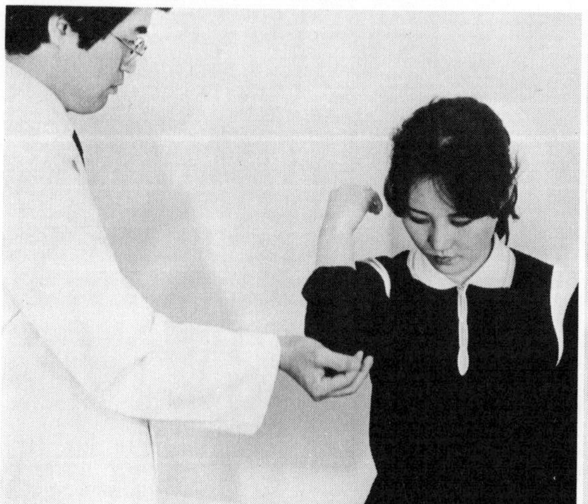

Fig. 330 Seated G-2–8

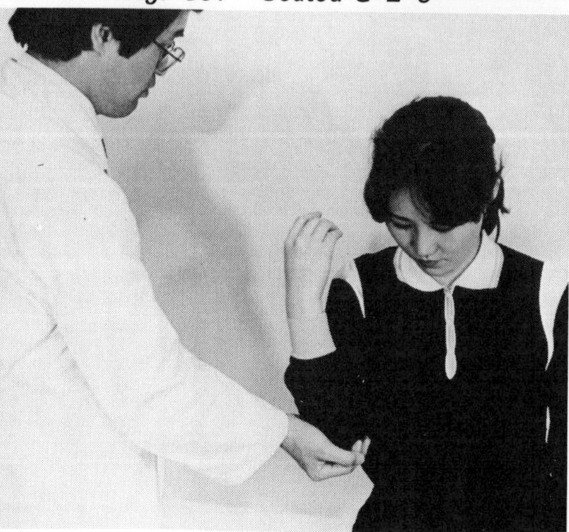

Fig. 331 Seated G-2–9

Fig. 332
Seated G-2–10

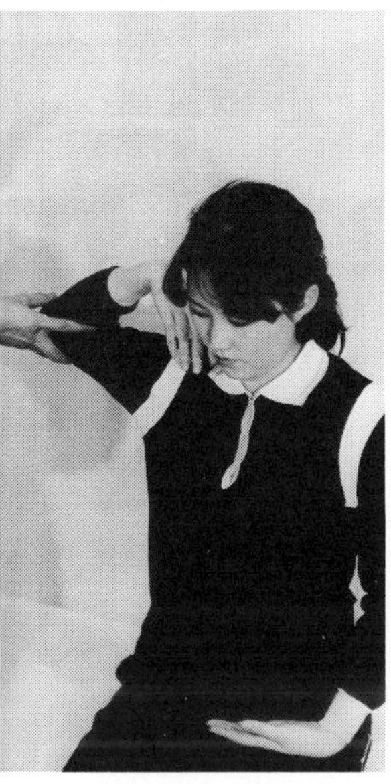

Fig. 333 Seated G-2–11

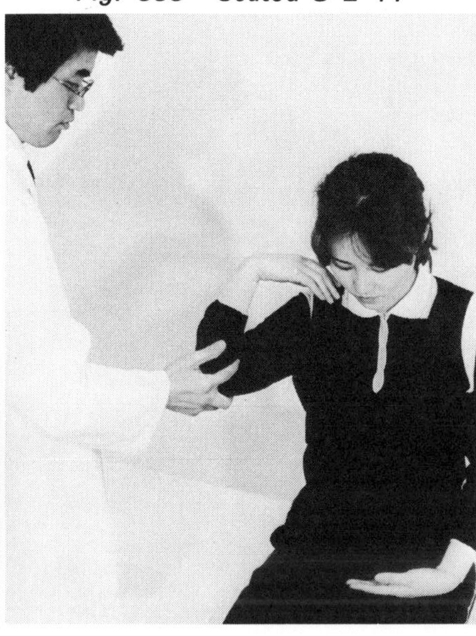

Fig. 334 Seated G-2–12

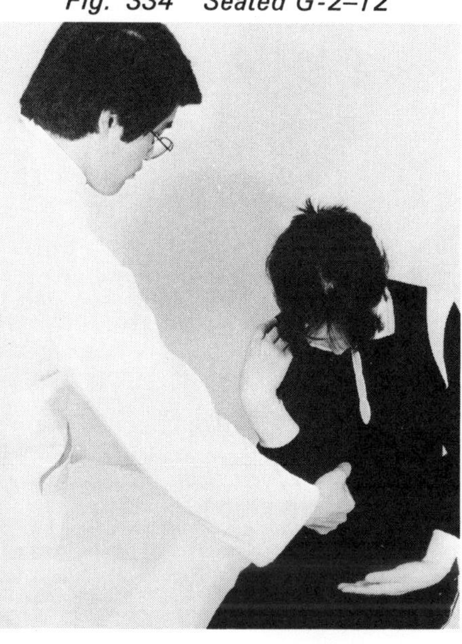

describing a diagonal arc. The therapist gives resistance to her arm movement by placing a hand under her right elbow (Figs. 332 to 334). They hold tension at a suitable position and release after a pause, and then repeat the procedure.

Sōtai III: First the patient raises her right elbow flexed, out to her side. She lowers her elbow diagonally forward and down, The therapist places one hand upon her right shoulder and his other hand under her elbow and gives resistance (Figs. 335 to 337). They maintain tension for three to five seconds at a suitable position and release together, and then the procedure is repeated.

Fig. 335
Seated G-2–13

Fig. 336 Seated G-2–14

Fig. 337 Seated G-2–15

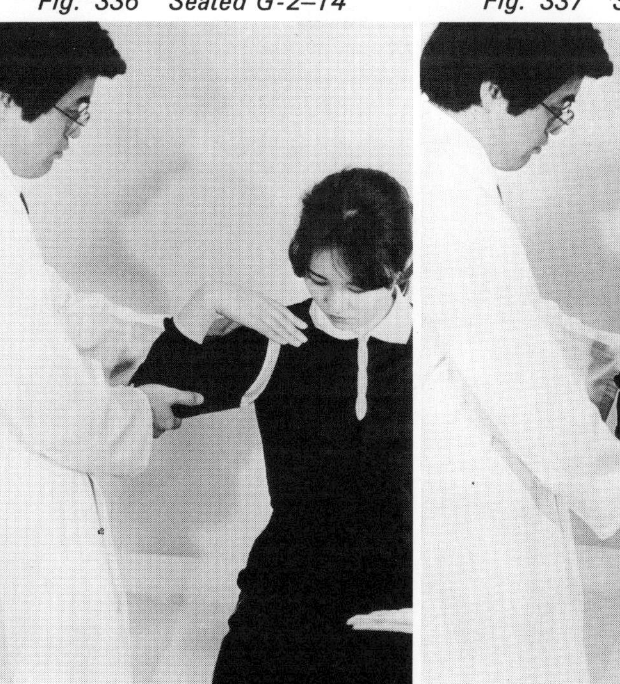

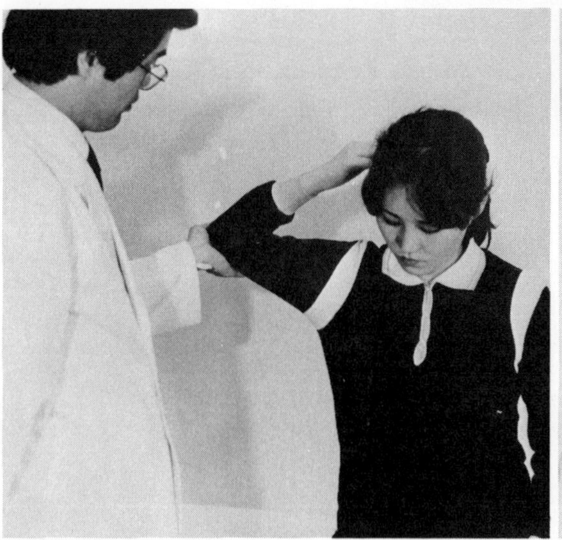

Fig. 338 Seated G-2–16

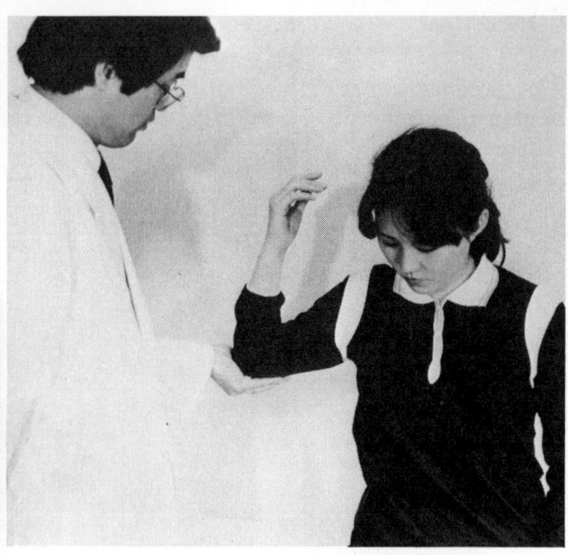

Fig. 339 Seated G-2–17

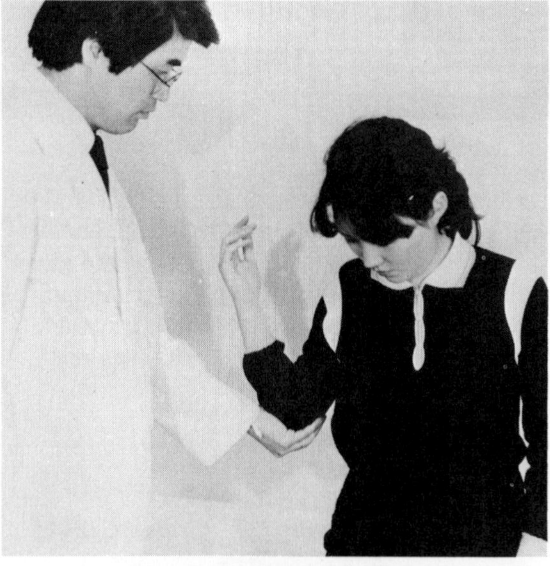

Fig. 340 Seated G-2–18

Sōtai IV: The patient first raises her right elbow flexed, out to her side. She then lowers it laterally straight down to her side. The therapist gives resistance to this movement (Figs. 338 to 340). When a suitable position is reached, tension is held briefly and then released siumultaneously, and then the procedure is repeated.

Seated H-1

Dōshin: In the seated position, the patient extends her right or left arm anterolaterally with the palm turned upward. Holding the patient's extended arm at the elbow and wrist, the therapist flexes and extends her elbow joint,

Fig. 341 Seated H-1–1

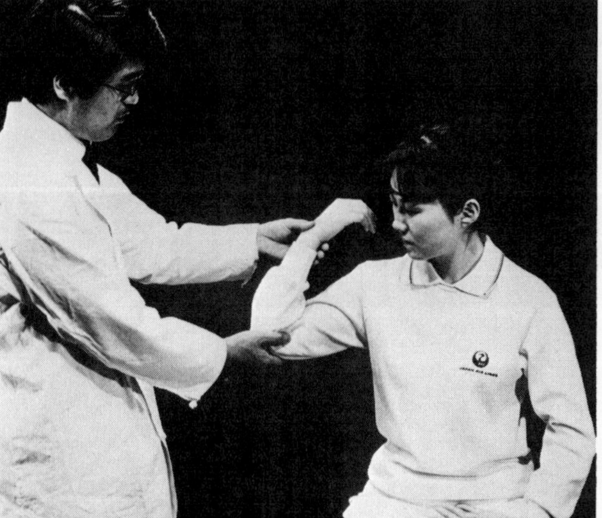

Fig. 342 Seated H-1–2

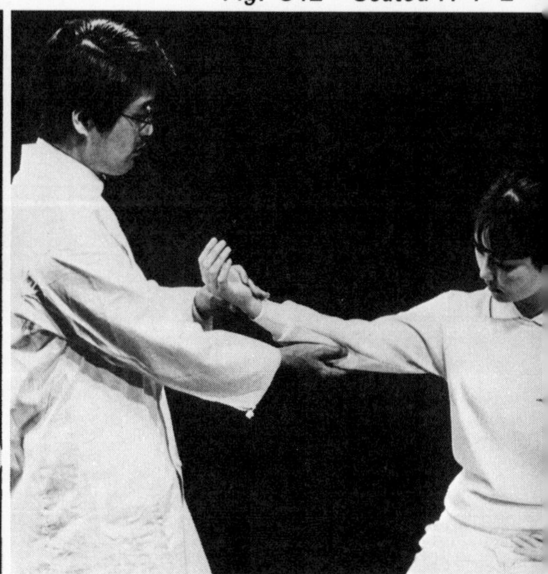

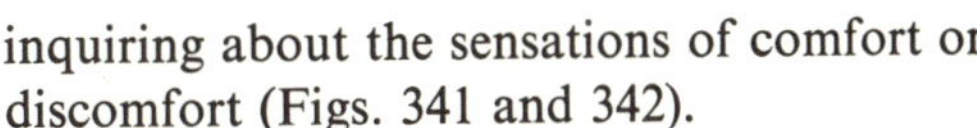

inquiring about the sensations of comfort or discomfort (Figs. 341 and 342).

Sōtai I: The patient first flexes her right arm at the elbow, touching her fingertips to her shoulder. She then extends her flexed arm. Holding her elbow and wrist (Figs. 343 and 344), the therapist gives resistance to her arm extension movement. They hold tension at a suitable position for a few seconds and then release together. This procedure is repeated two or three times.

Fig. 343 Seated H-1–3

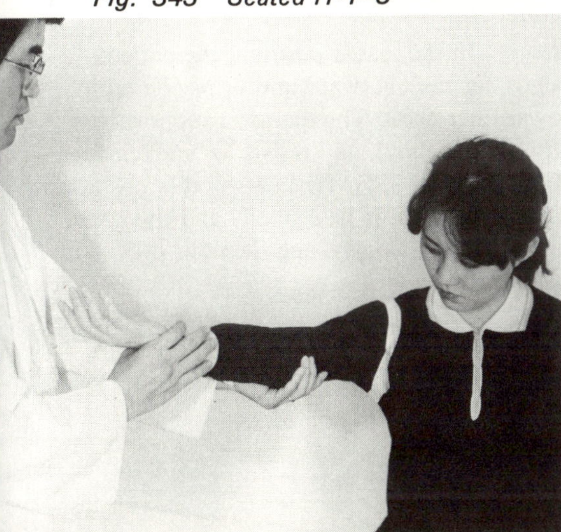

Fig. 344 Seated H-1–4

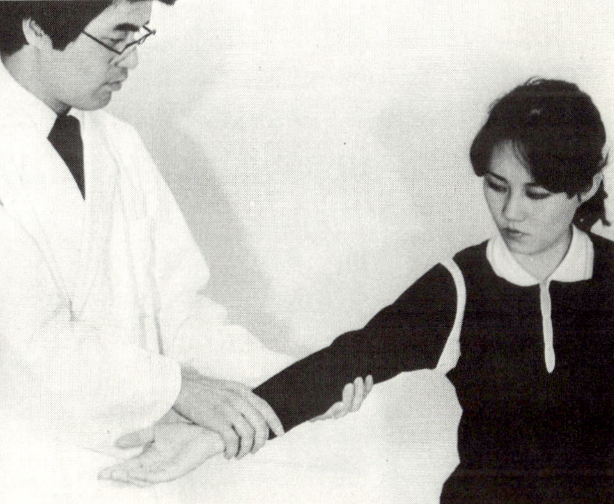

Fig. 345 Seated H-1–5

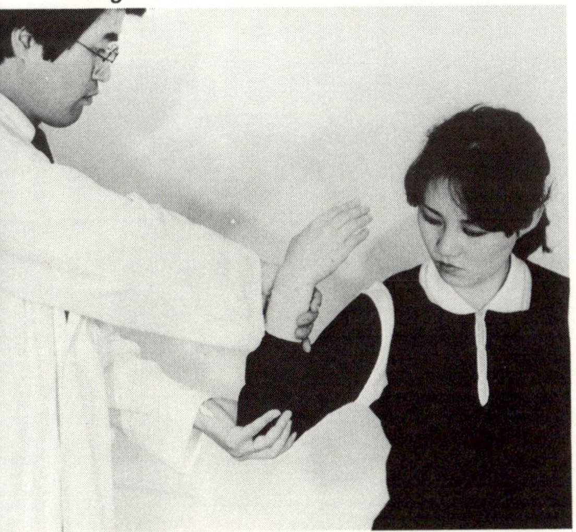

Fig. 346 Seated H-1–6

Sōtai II: The patient first extends her right arm anterolaterally. She then attempts to flex this arm at the elbow and bring her fingertips to her shoulder. By holding her elbow and wrist, the therapist gives resistance to this movement (Figs. 345 and 346). They hold tension at a suitable place and then release this after holding briefly, and then repeat the procedure.

Fig. 347 Seated I-1–1

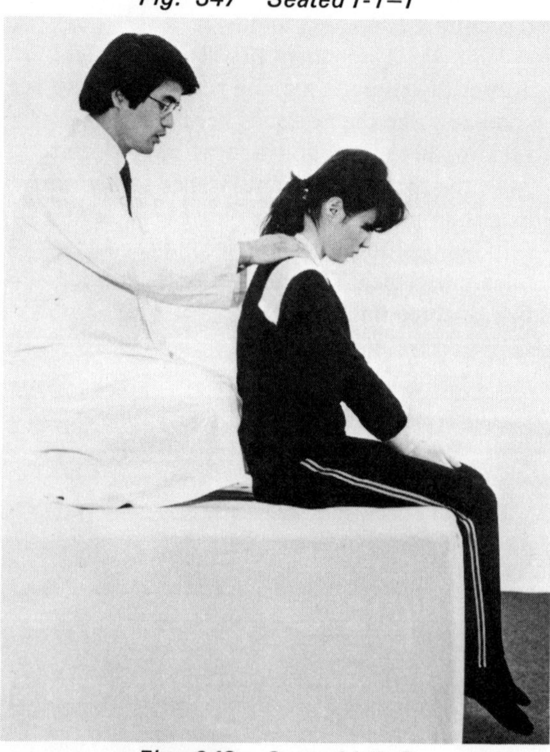

Seated I-1

Sōtai: The paitent holds her palms together in the seated position and reaches for the floor by leaning her torso forward in deep anterior flexion. The therapist holds her shoulders from behind to resist the movement of her torso (Figs. 347 to 349). They hold tension at a suitable position for a few seconds and then release together. The procedure is repeated two or three times.

Seated I-2

Sōtai: In the seated position, the patient bends her neck forward and brings her chin toward her chest. The therapist supports her chin from behind, and resists her movement (Figs. 350 and 351). When a suitable position is reached, tension is held briefly and then released simultaneously, and then this procedure is repeated.

Fig. 348 Seated I-1–2

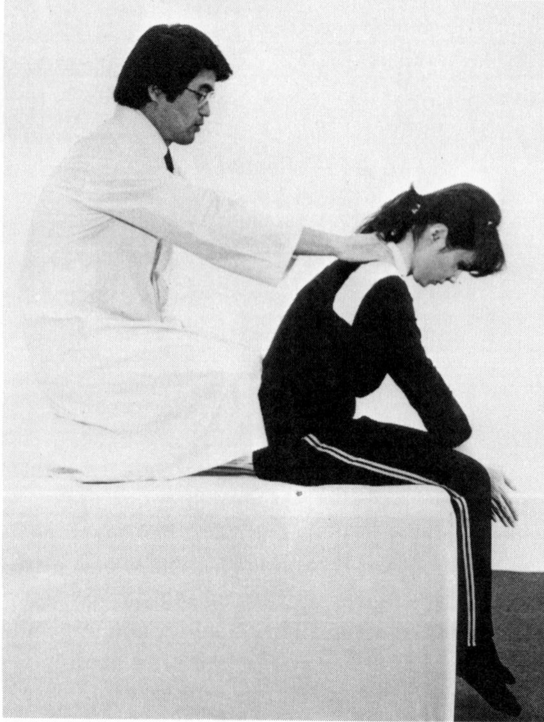

Fig. 349 Seated I-1–3

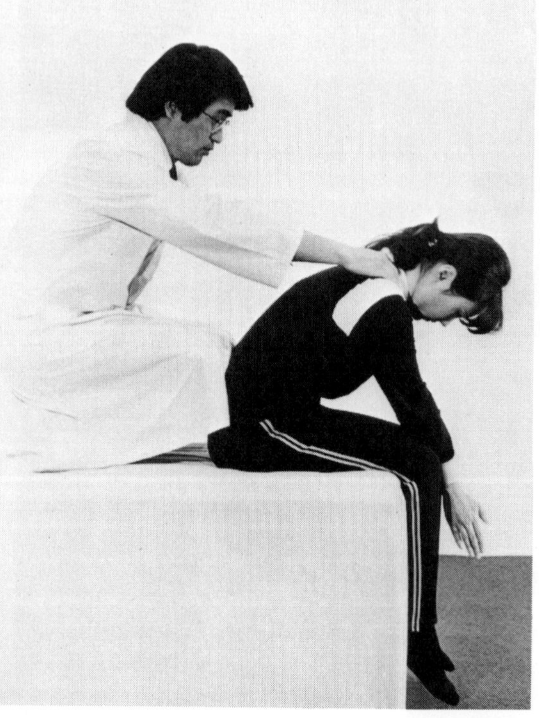

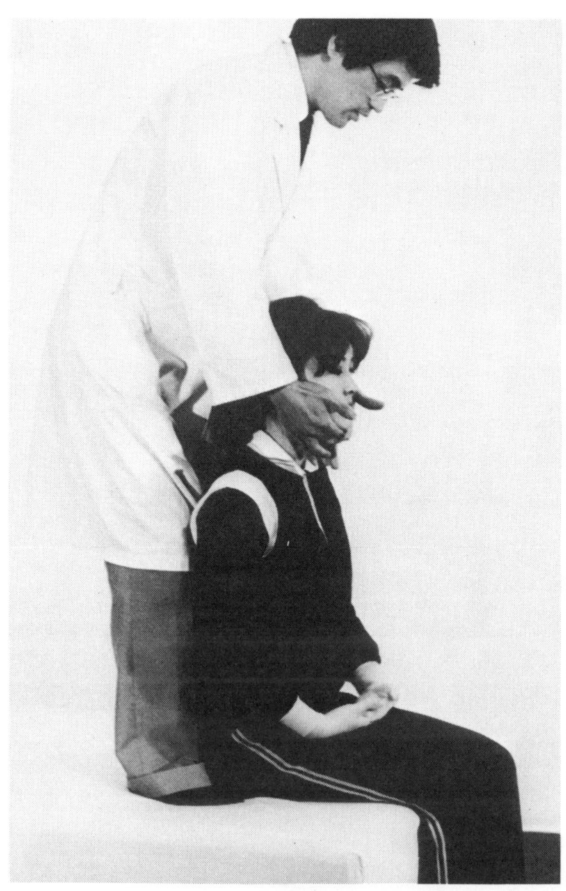

Fig. 350 Seated I-2–1

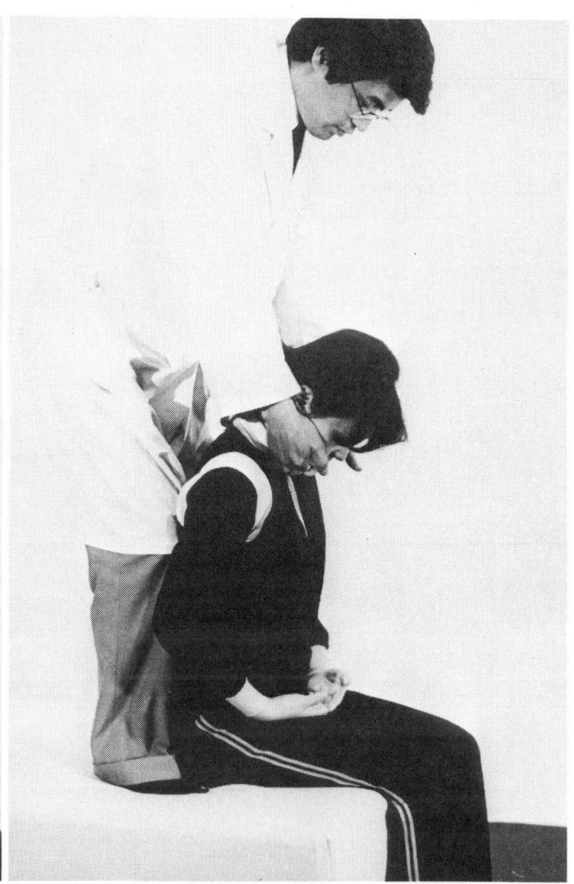

Fig. 351 Seated I-2–2

Seated I-3

Sōtai: From the basic seated position, the patient extends her neck, bending it back fully. Placing his hands on her neck, the therapist gives resistance to her movement (Figs. 352 and 353). They hold tension at a suitable position and release after a pause, and then repeat the procedure.

Fig. 352 Seated I-3–1

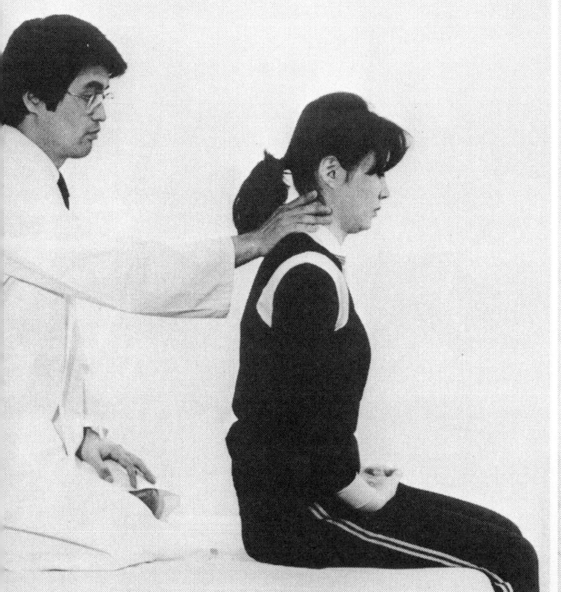

Fig. 353 Seated I-3–2

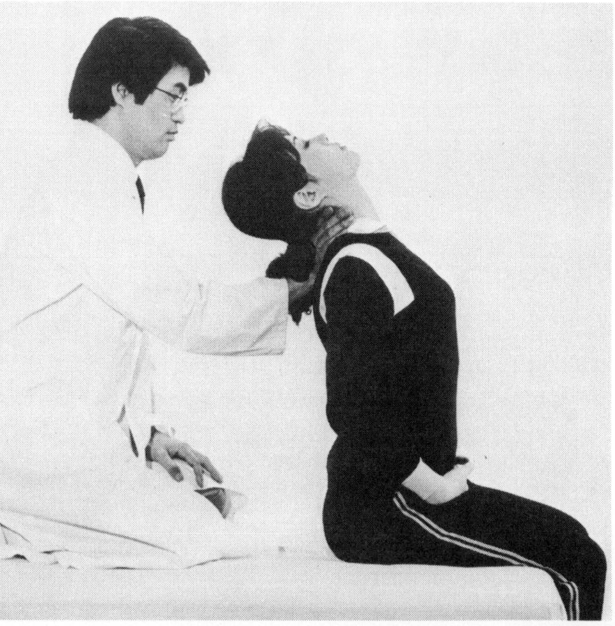

Fig. 354 Seated I-4–1

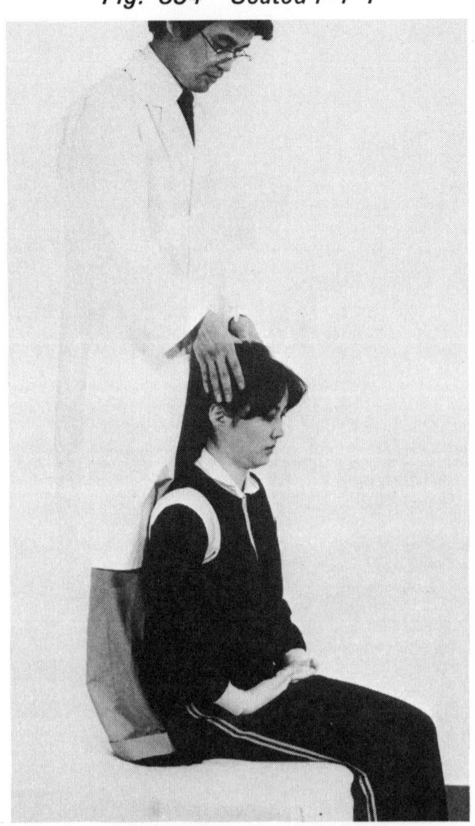

Fig. 355 Seated I-4–2

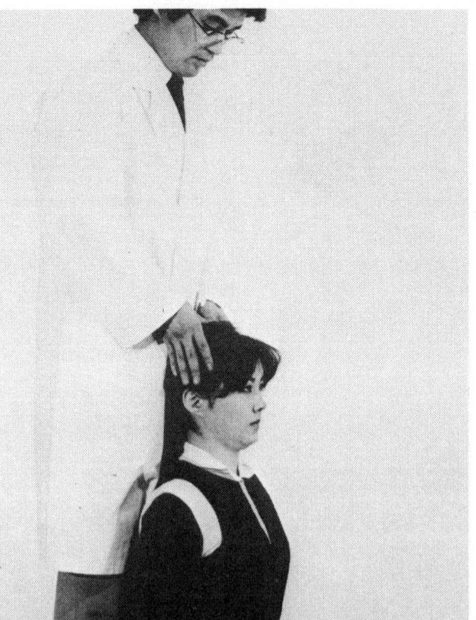

Fig. 356 Seated I-5–1

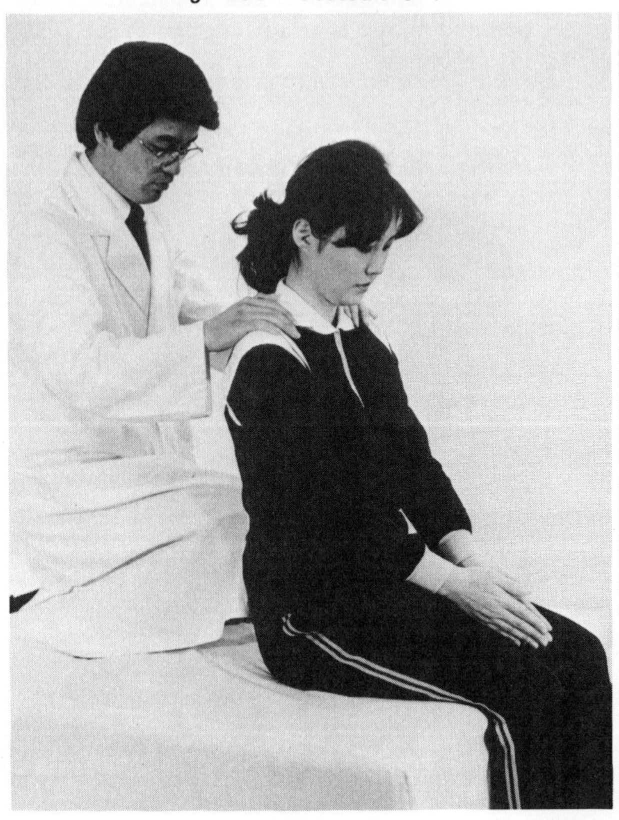

Fig. 357 Seated I-5–2

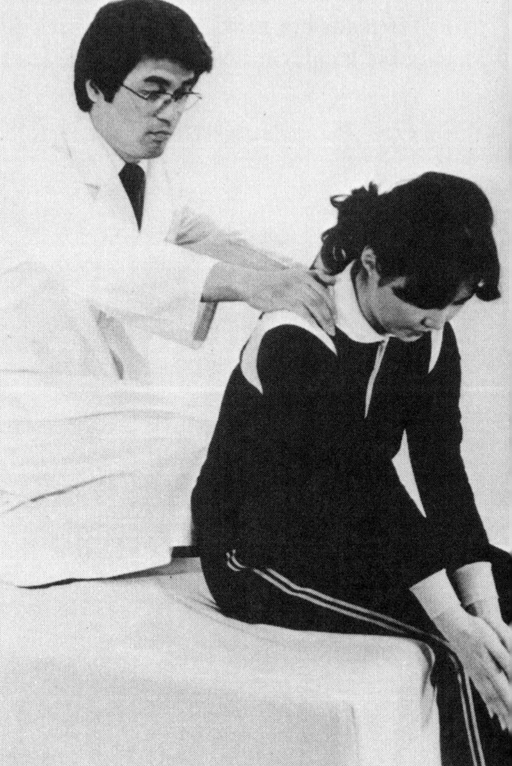

Seated I-4

Sōtai: In the seated position, the patient draws her chin in and extends her spine so as to elevate her head. Applying pressure on her parietal region, the therapist gives resistance to the spinal extension movement (Figs. 354 and 355). They hold opposing pressure for three to five seconds in a suitable position and release together after a pause. The procedure is repeated two or three times.

Seated I-5

Sōtai: In the seated position, the patient holds her palms together. She then moves her hands forward and down at a diagonal, flexing her trunk forward and bringing her forehead down toward her right knee. The therapist holds the shoulders of the patient from behind while pushing lightly on her lumbar region with his knees, providing gentle resistance to her movement (Figs. 356 to 358). They hold tension at a suitable position and release after a pause. The procedure is repeated two or three times.

Fig. 358 Seated I-5–3

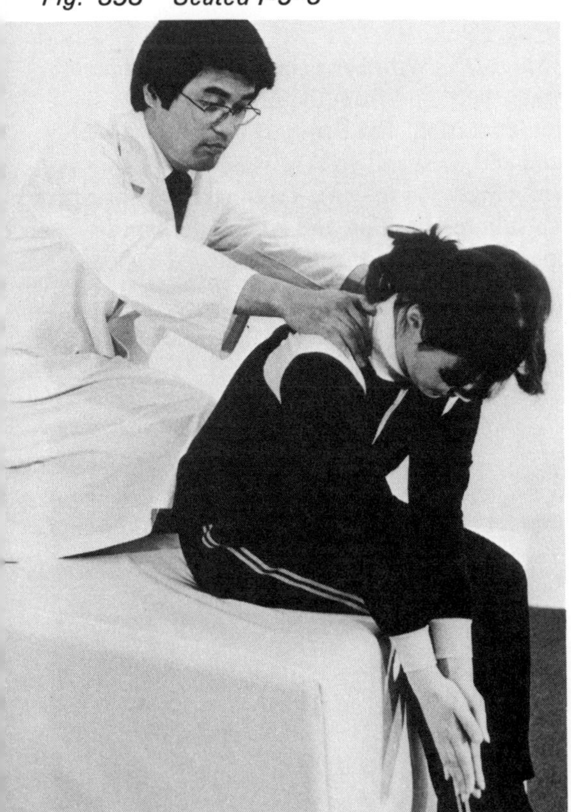

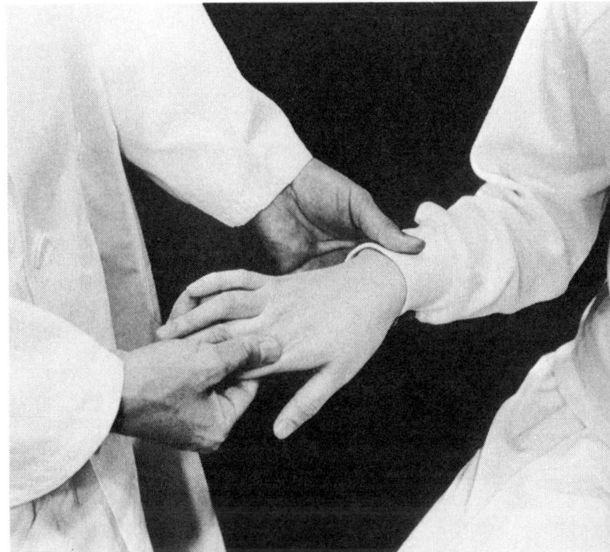

Fig. 359 Seated J-1–1

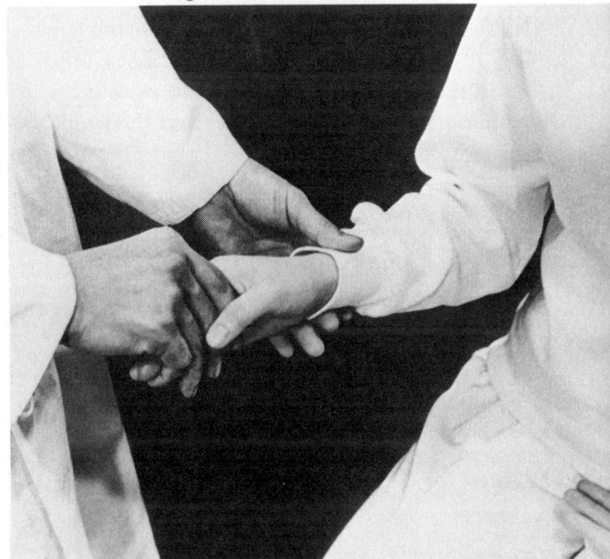

Fig. 360 Seated J-1–2

Seated J-1

Dōshin: The therapist holds the seated patient's right or left hand. He then rotates her lower arm into the pronated position and then the supinated position asking the patient about sensations of comfort and discomfort (Figs. 359 and 360).

Fig. 361 Seated J-1–3

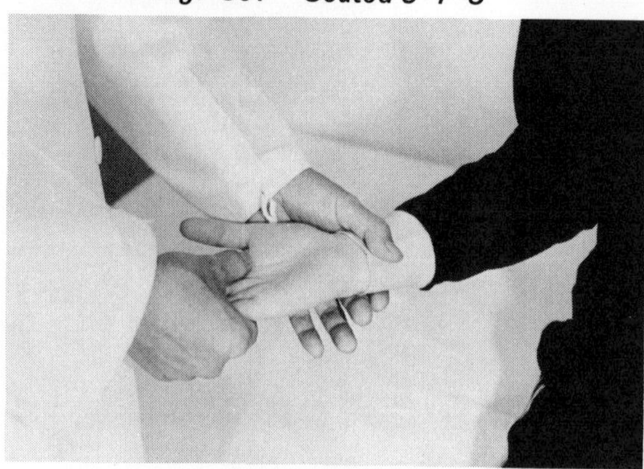

Fig. 362 Seated J-1–4

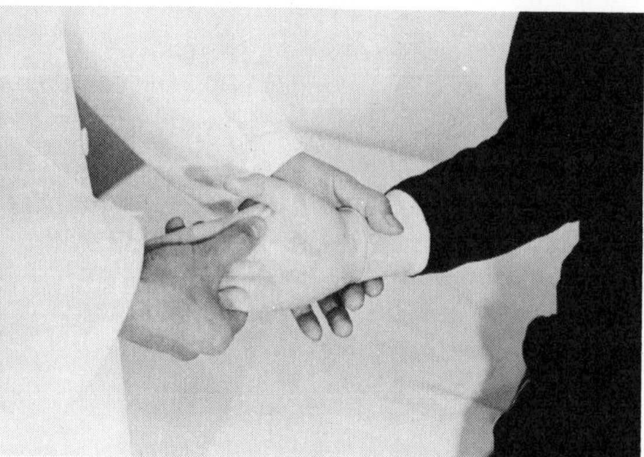

Fig. 363 Seated J-1–5

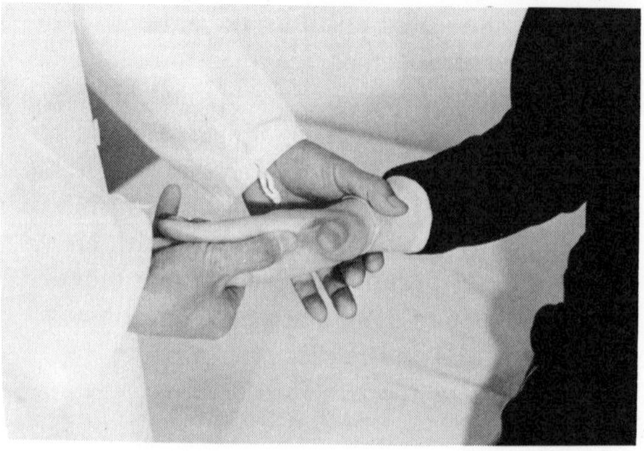

Sōtai I: With her palm open, the patient rotates her right hand from the supinated to the pronated position. The therapist holds her right hand and wrist, and gives ressistance to this movement (Figs. 361 to 363). They hold tension at a suitable position and release together after holding it briefly, and then repeat the procedure.

Fig. 364 Seated J-1–6

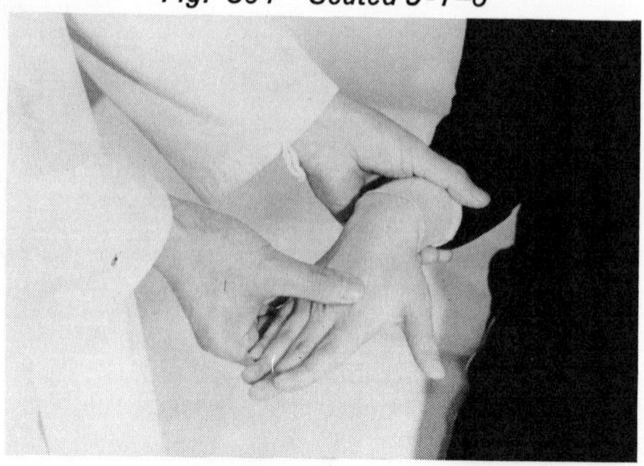

Sōtai II: With her palm open, the patient rotates her hand from the pronated to the supinate position. The therapist holds the patient's hand and wrist and gives resistance to this movement (Figs. 364 to 366). Tension is held briefly at a suitable position and is released simultaneously. This procedure is repeated two or three times.

Fig. 365 Seated J-1–7

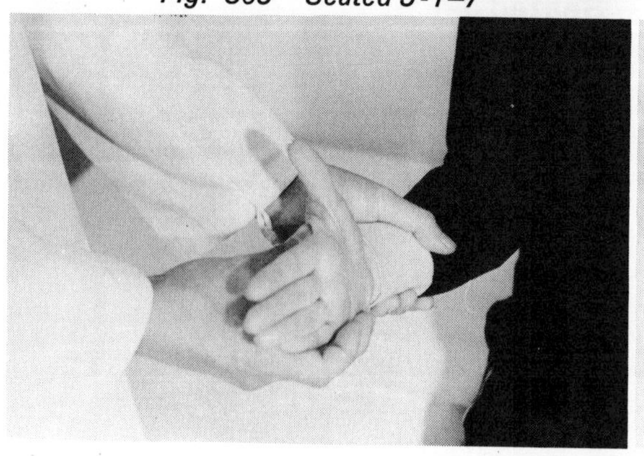

Fig. 366 Seated J-1–8

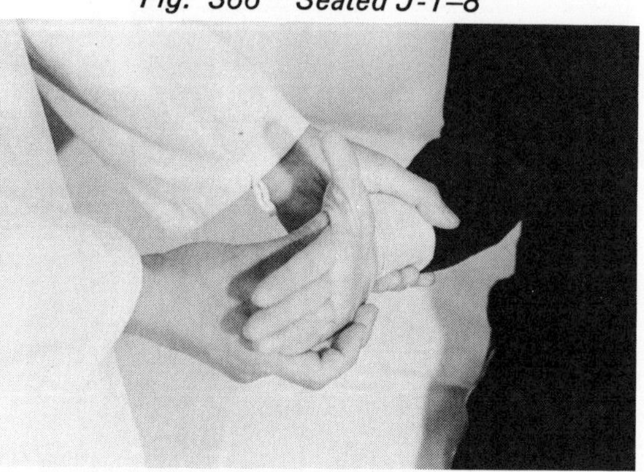

Seated J-2

Dōshin: Holding the seated patient's hand, the therapist flexes her wrist medially (radial deviation) and then laterally (ulnar deviation), inquiring about sensations of comfort or discomfort (Figs. 367 and 368).

Fig. 367 Seated J-2–1

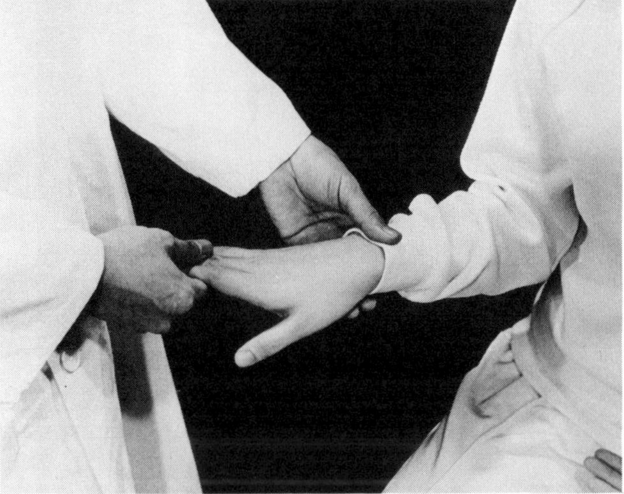

Fig. 368 Seated J-2–2

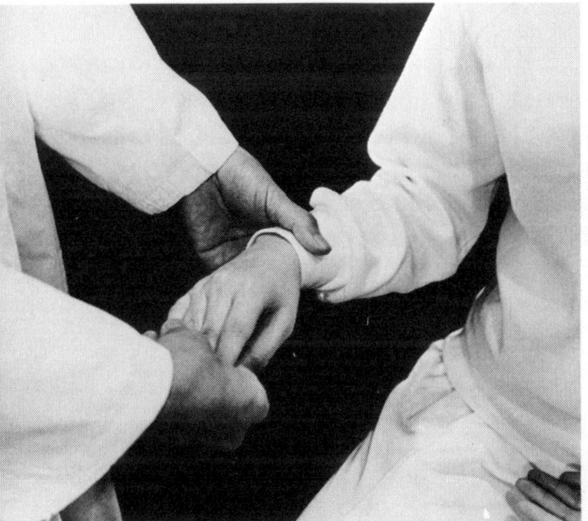

Fig. 369 Seated J-2–3

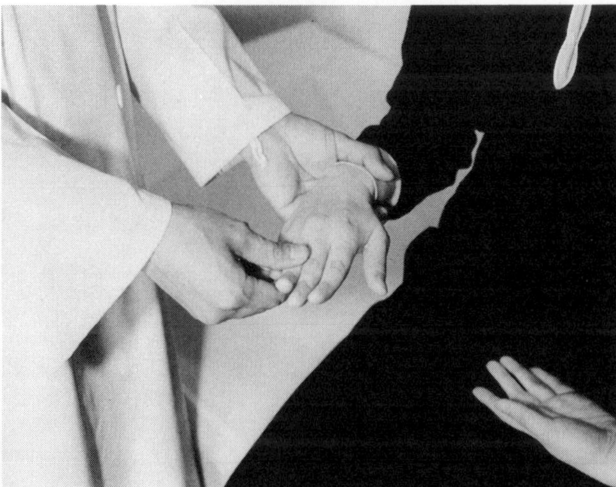

Fig. 370 Seated J-2–4

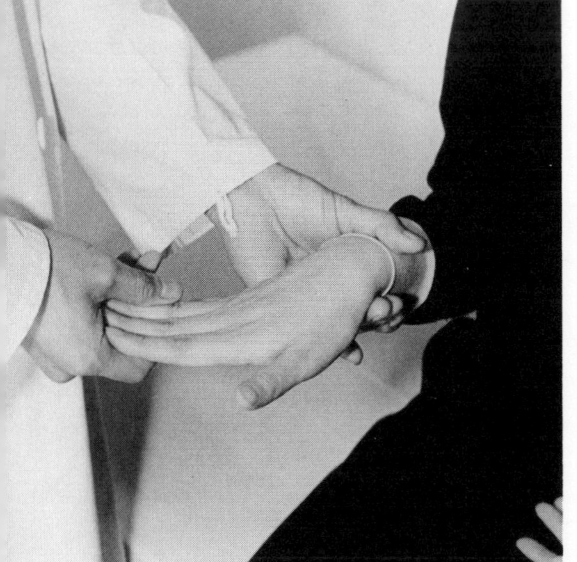

Sōtai I: The patient flexes her wrist in the ulnar direction from the radial deviation position. Holding her fingers and wrist, the therapist gives resistance to this movement (Figs. 369 and 370). They hold opposing pressure at a suitable position and release together after a few seconds. The procedure is repeated two or three times.

Fig. 371 Seated J-2–5

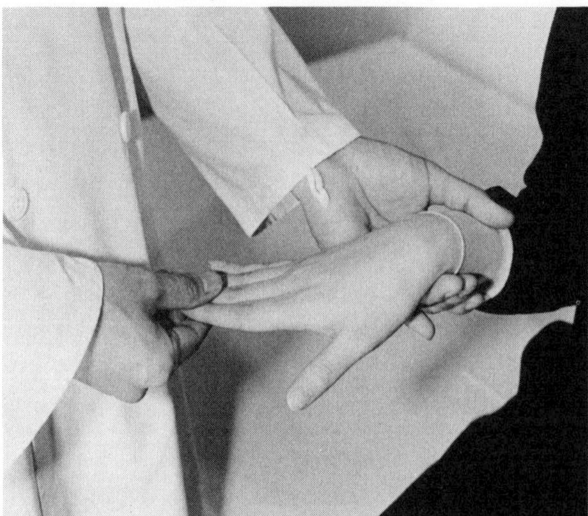

Fig. 372 Seated J-2–6

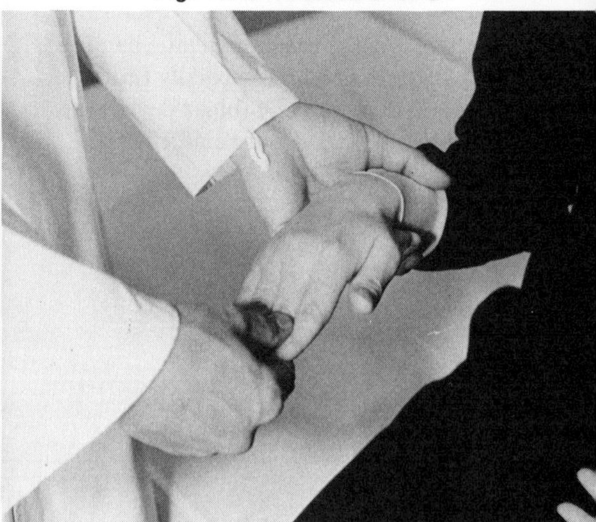

Fig. 373 Seated J-3–1

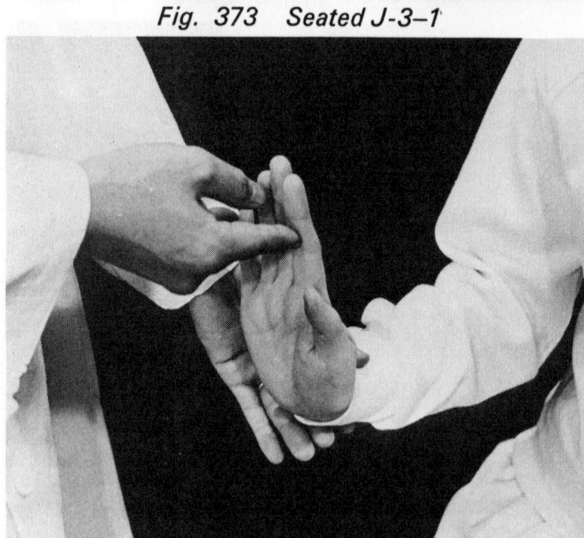

Sōtai II: This Sōtai movement is just the reverse of the above procedure, and the patient flexes her wrist in the opposite direction from ulnar deviation into radial deviation. The therapist grips her fingers and wrist as shown and provides resistance (Figs. 371 and 372). Tension is briefly held in a suitable position before being released.

Seated J-3

Dōshin: The therapist holds the right or left hand of the seated patient in the manner illustrated in Figure 373, and flexes her wrist toward the back of the hand (extension), and then toward the palm (flexion) inquiring about sensations of comfort and discomfort (Fig. 374).

Fig. 374 Seated J-3–2

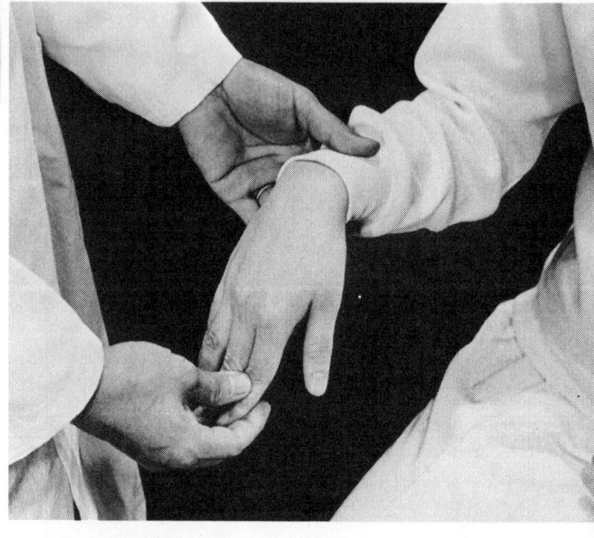

Fig. 375 Seated J-3–3

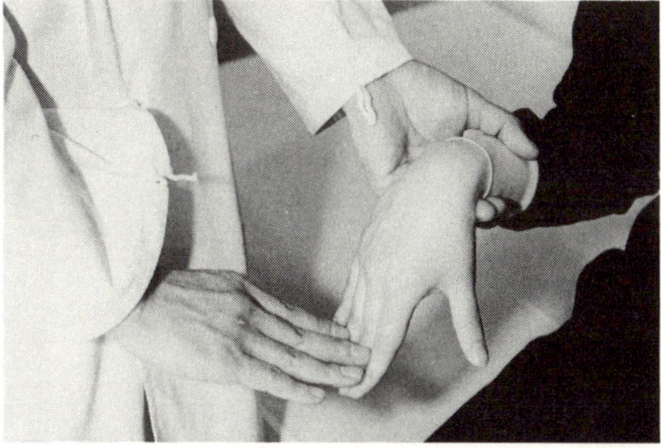

Fig. 376 Seated J-3–4

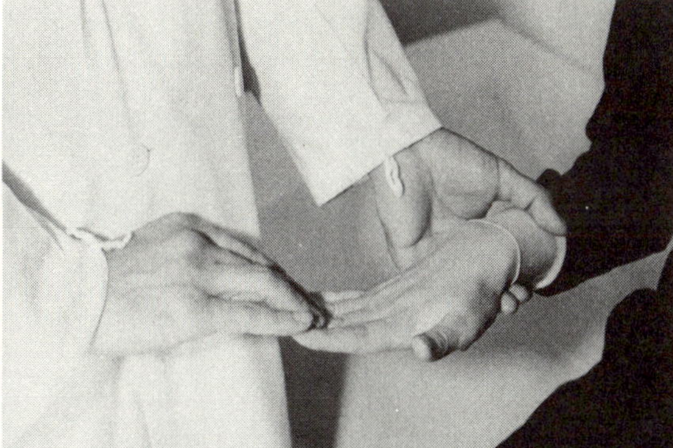

Fig. 377 Seated J-3–5

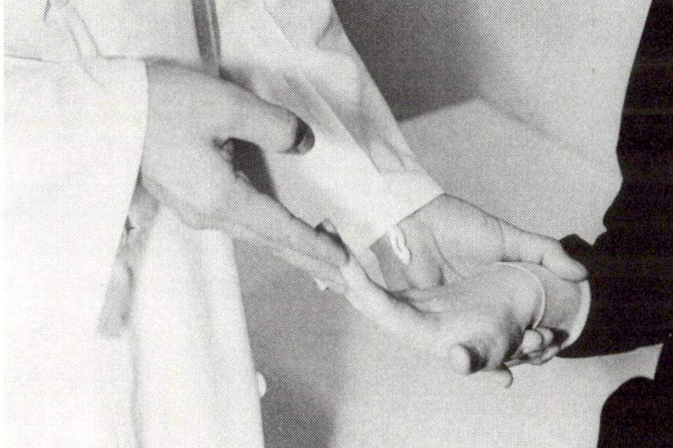

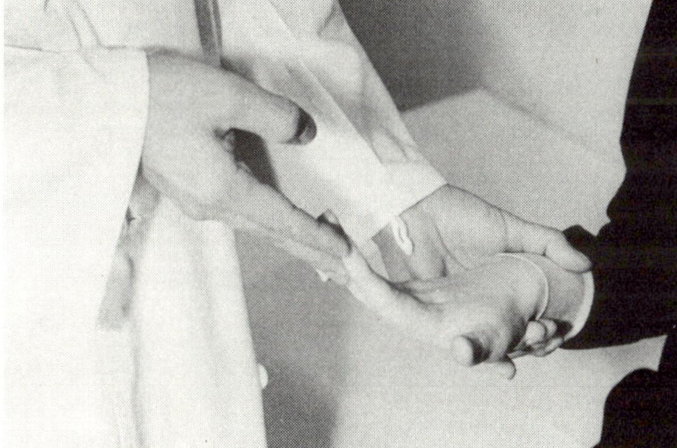

Fig. 378 Seated J-3–6

Fig. 379 Seated J-3–7

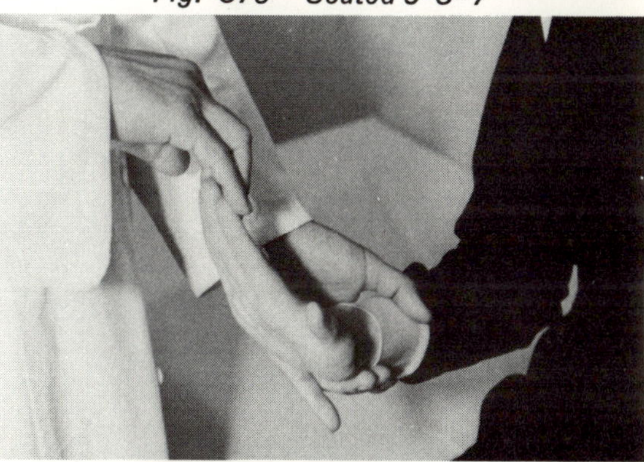

Sōtai I: The patient extends her wrist joint by moving her hand through an arc beginning in palmer flexion and ending in dorsal extension. Holding her wrist and fingertips, the therapist applies resistance (Figs. 375 to 377). They hold tension at a suitable position and then release simultaneously. The procedure is repeated two or three times.

Sōtai II: The patient flexes her wrist joint by moving her hand from dorsal extension into palmar flexion. The therapist gives resistance by holding the patient's fingers and wrist (Figs. 378 to 380). They maintain opposing pressure briefly at a suitable position before releasing simultaneously. The procedure is repeated two or three times.

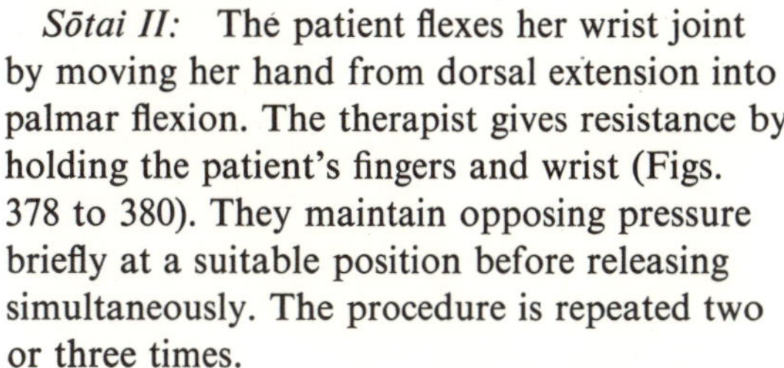

Fig. 380 Seated J-3–8

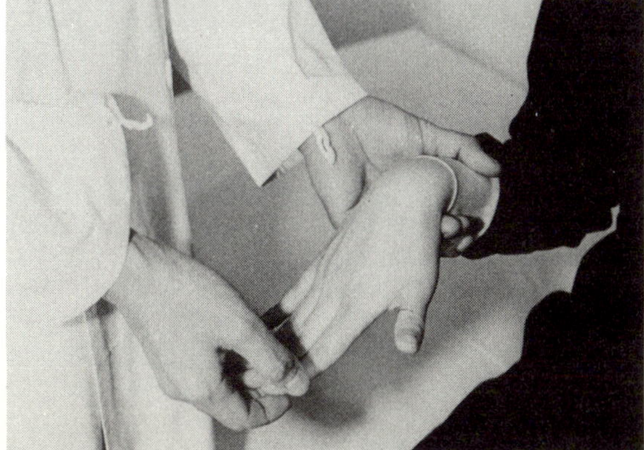

3. PROPER POSITION AND HAND PLACEMENT FOR THERAPIST

Sōtai, or slow movement of the body in the comfortable direction during exhalation, viewed from the standpoint of its kinetics or dynamics, can be explained as an integration of subtle biomechanics by slow movement. Even though Sōtai consists of slow movements of the body without use of much force, this does not mean the therapist can assume any position in relation to the patient, or that his hands can be used without care in their placement. Even the slightest variation in the dynamics of the movement brings into play corresponding kinesiological principles. It is difficult to correct distortions in physical structure when these principles are disregarded. And furthermore, when the therapist places himself in relation to the patient without regard for these principles, he may end up with distortions himself. This could in effect reverse the roles of the therapist and patient by the therapist receiving distortions. Ideally, when Sōtai is performed, distortions in the therapist's body will also be corrected. Therefore, guidelines are given below for the positioning of the theapist in relation to the patient, and where exactly to hold the patient during Sōtai movements.

Position of Therapist in Relation to Patient

For Sōtai techniques Supine A through M, the therapist standing either at the head or feet of the patient, lines himself up with the longitudinal median line of the patient (Fig. 1). Resistance can be offered against the patient's movement in this position and Sōtai movements of flex-

Fig. 1

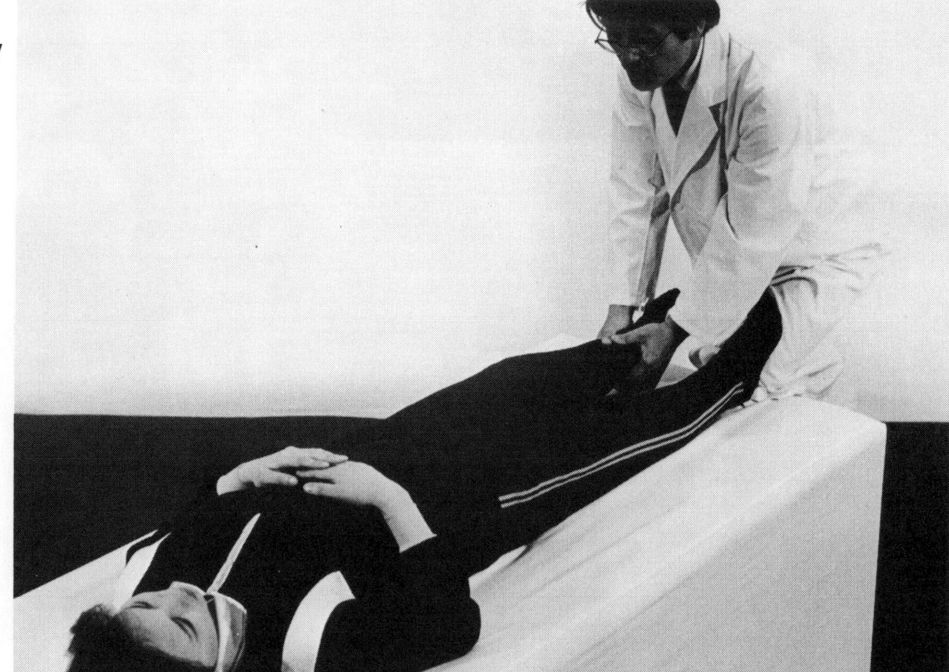

ion, extension, contraction, or rotation can be performed on either anterior, posterior, or lateral parts. In technique Supine N, the therapist resists arm rotation movement, standing to the side of the patient.

In Sōtai techniques Prone A-2 and D, the therapist places himself in line with the patient's median line (Fig. 2). In technique Prone B, it is easier to perform the Sōtai standing to the side of the patient. The Sōtai movement and method of applying resistance is identical to that of technique Prone A.

When performing Sōtai with the patient in the seated position, the therapist is most often directly in front or behind the patient. In some techniques, however, the therapist stands off to the side. Figures 3, 4, and 5 are some examples of this. As shown for technique Prone B-1, assisting the patient from the side allows the therapist to avoid awkwardness and it makes the technique easier to perform.

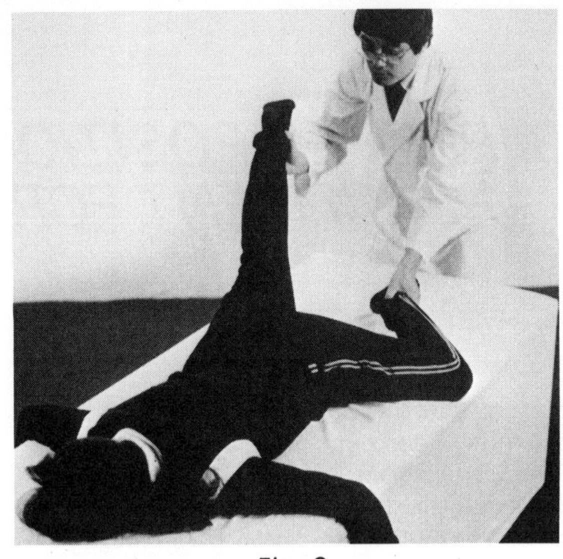

Fig. 2

Fig. 3

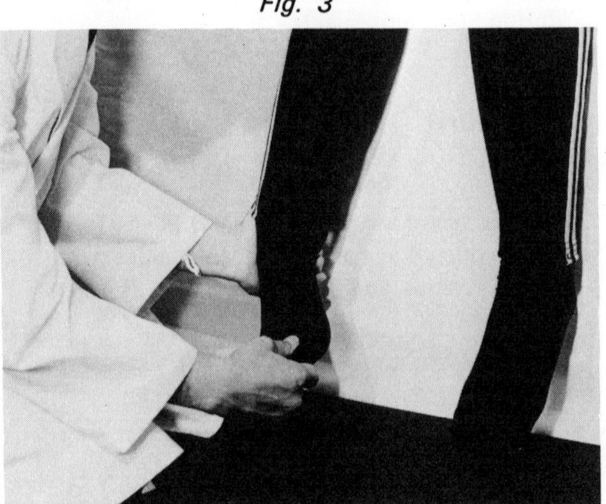

Fig. 4

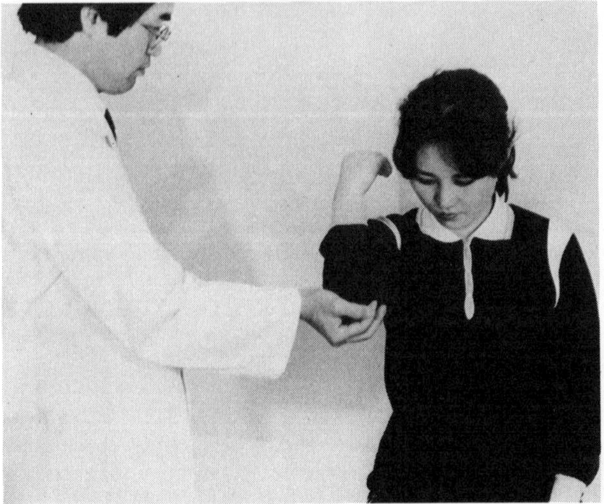

Fig. 5

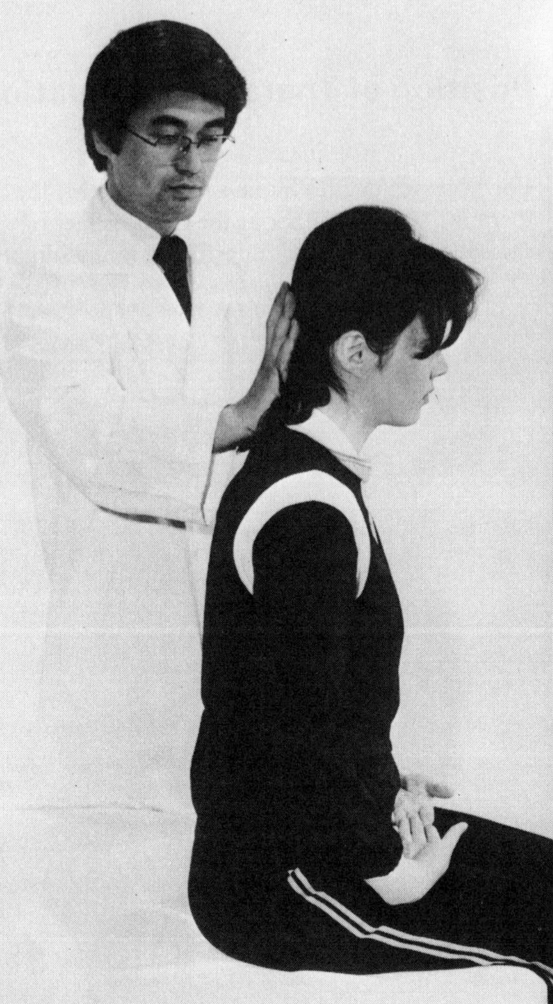

Hand Placement of Therapist

Fig. 6

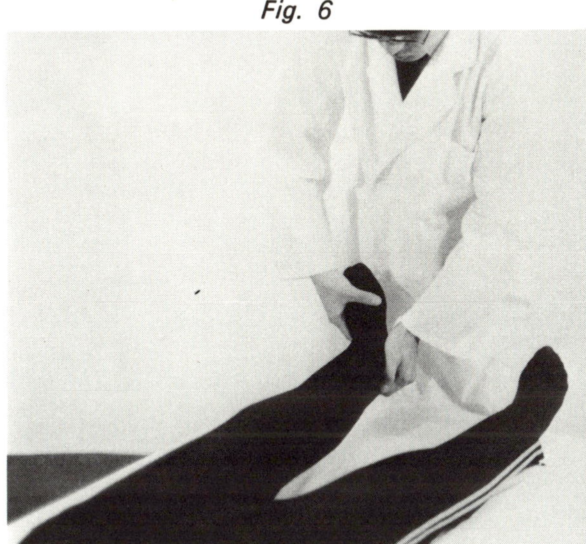

Fig. 7

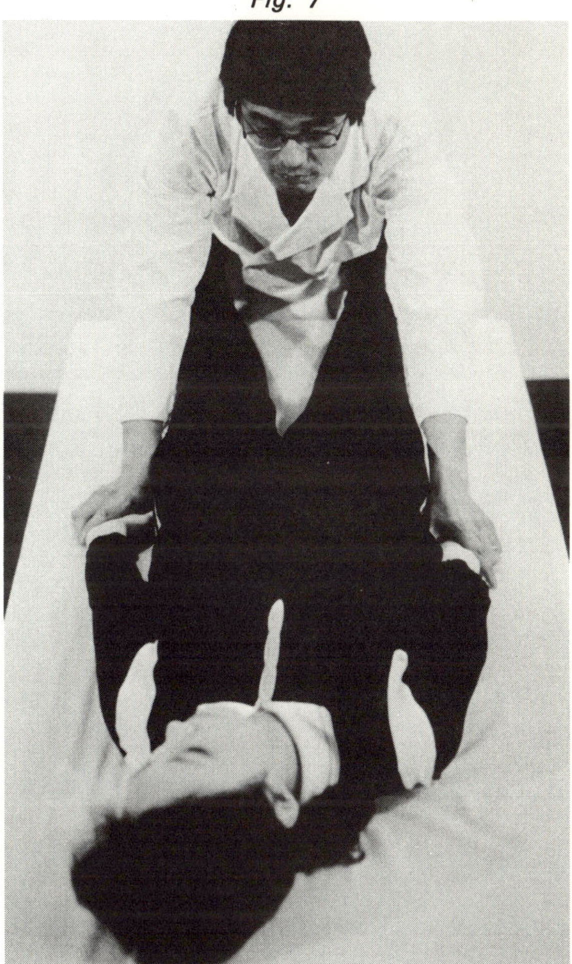

Where the therapist must place his hands during each Sōtai movement is given with the explanation of the Sōtai techniques. The precise manner in which to place the hands on the patients are explained below.

In all Sōtai techniques except Supine G, L, and M, apply resistance at a distal point from the center of movement and hold firmly by matching the contours of that part with the hands (Figs. 6 through 9). The therapist must not grip too strongly, but instead must firmly "place" his hands on the part to be held.

Fig. 8

Fig. 9

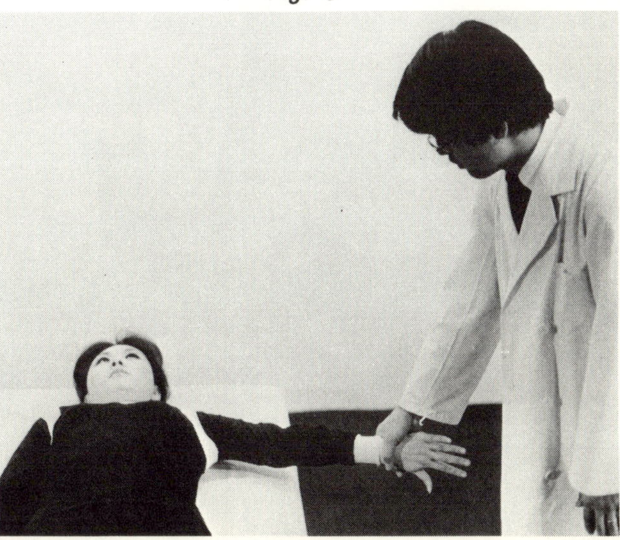

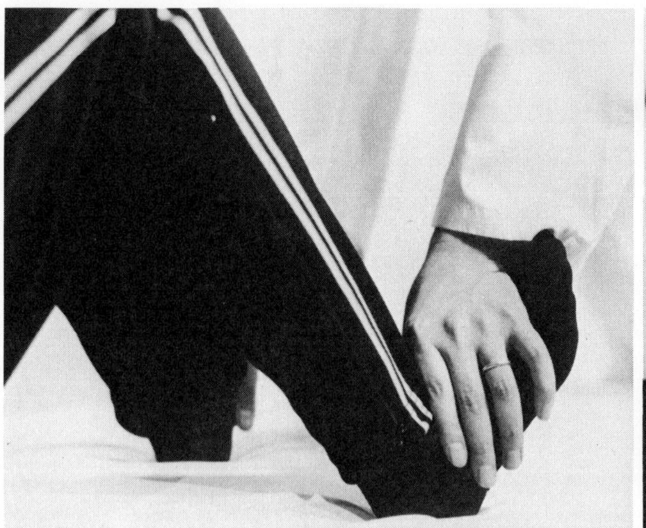

Fig. 10

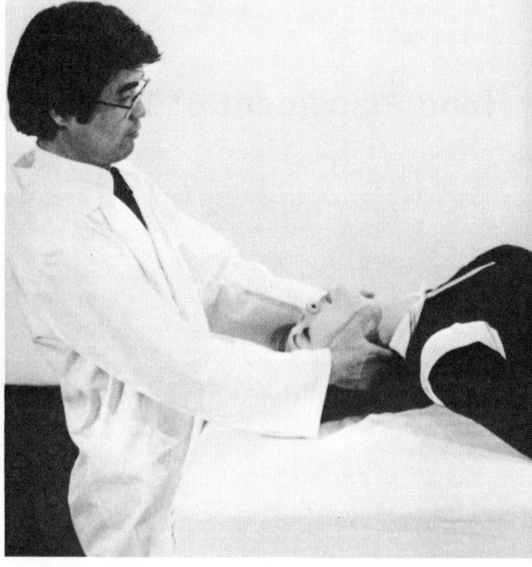

Fig. 11

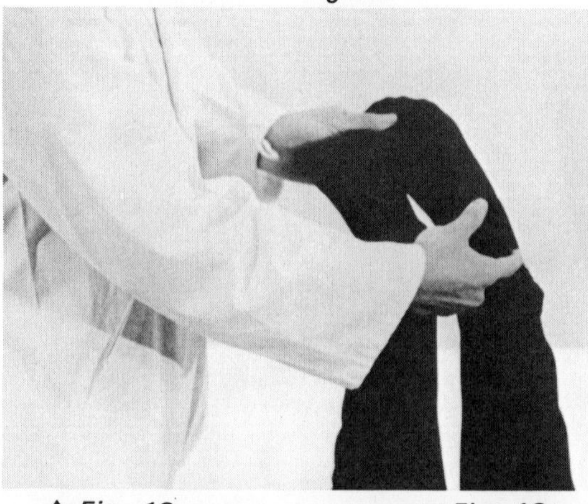

▲*Fig. 12*

In technique Supine G, L, and M, the point of resistance is proximal to the center of movement, and the hands are firmly fitted to match the contours of the part held (Figs. 10 and 11). It is important not to grip too strongly, but to keep the hands firmly in place.

In techniques Prone A-2 through D, the hands are placed on points of resistance distal to the center of movement (Figs. 12 to 14).

The placement of the therapist's hands varies even with the same movement by whether the

▼*Fig. 13*

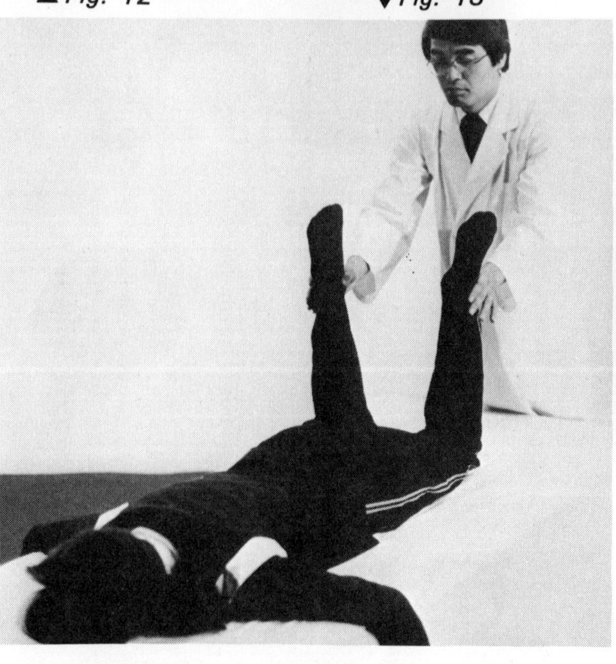

Fig. 14

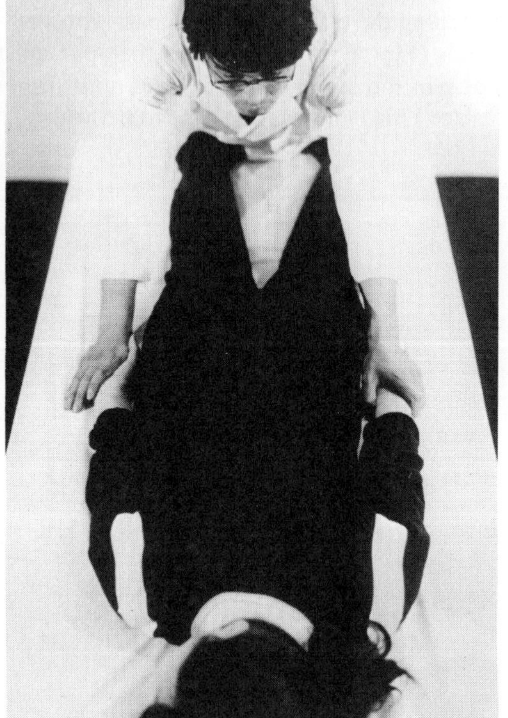

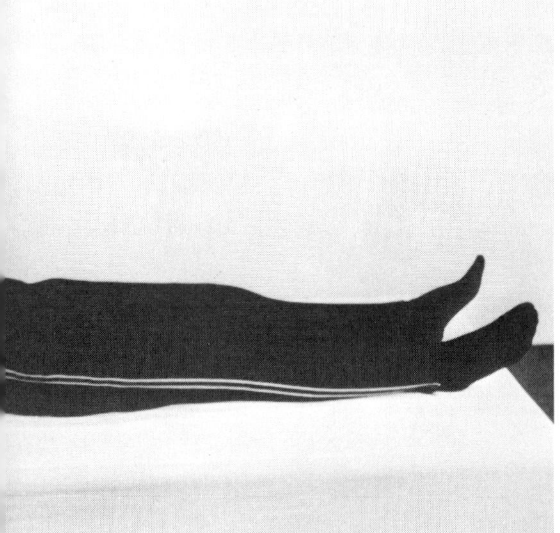

knees of the patient are together (Figs. 15 and 16) or held apart about shoulder width (Figs. 17 and 18). The trick in making Sōtai effortless and easy is to find the most suitable point of resistance (or support) for a particular movement.

Fig. 15

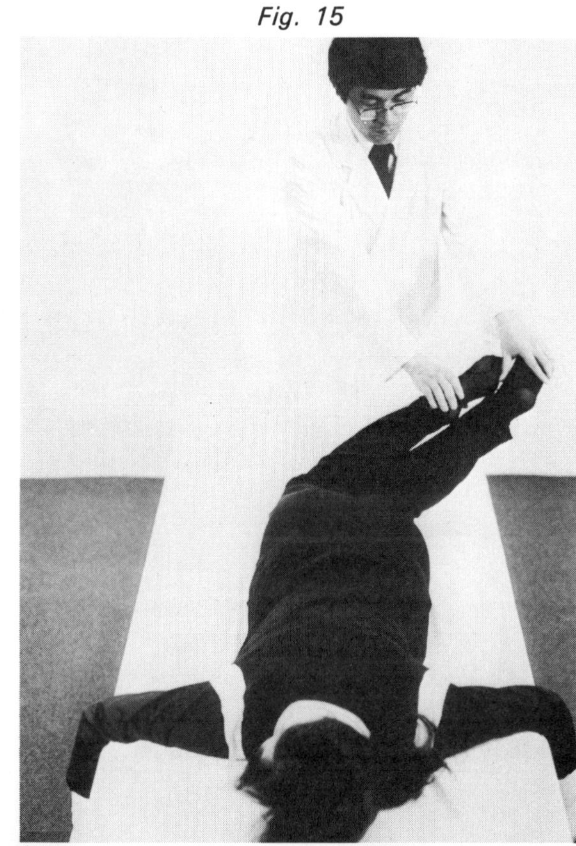

Fig. 16

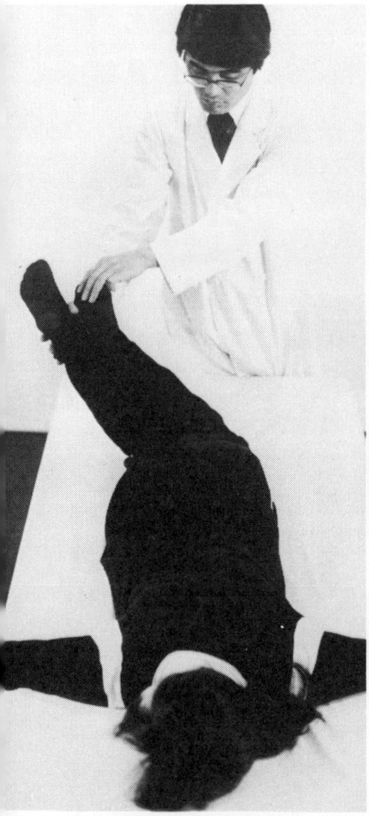

Fig. 17

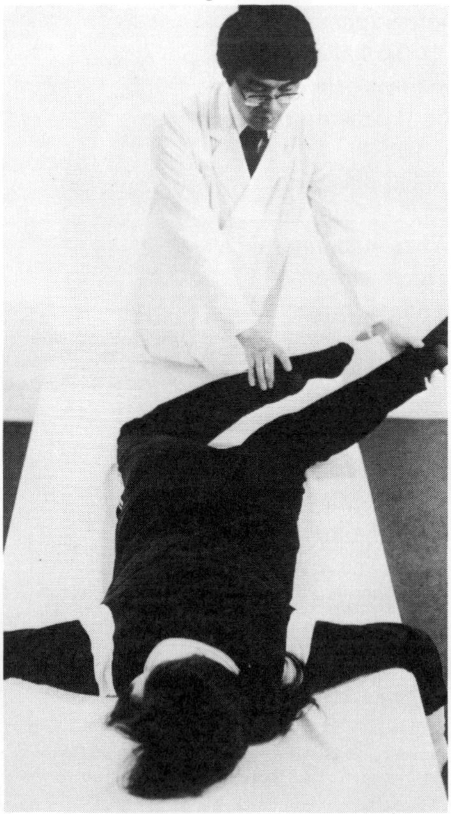

Fig. 18

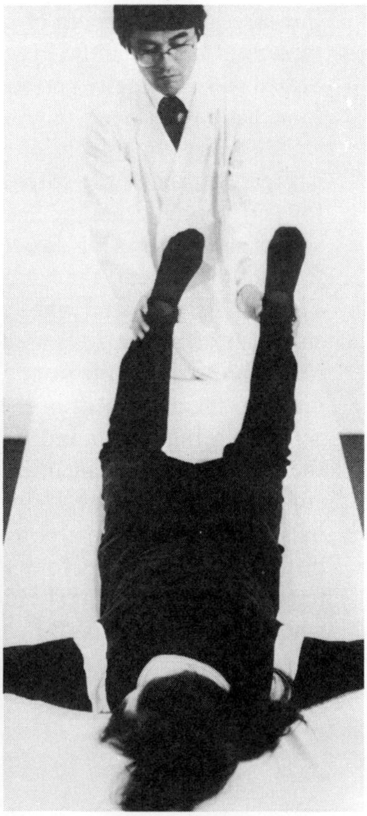

Fig. 19

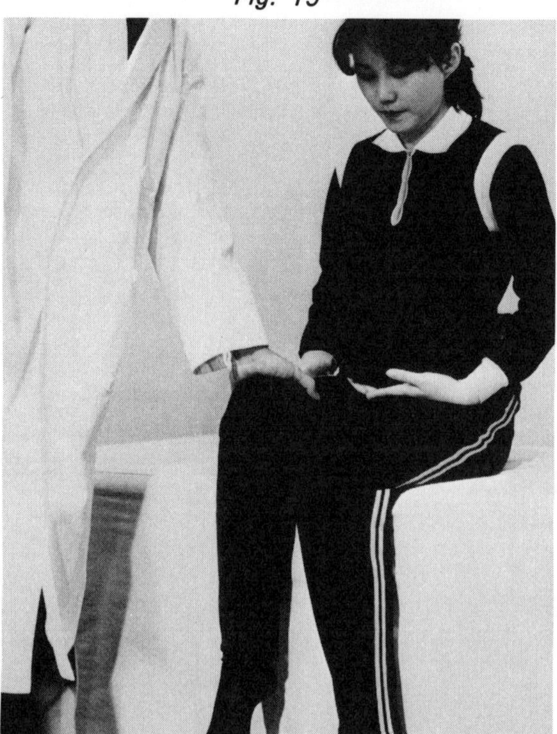

Fig. 20

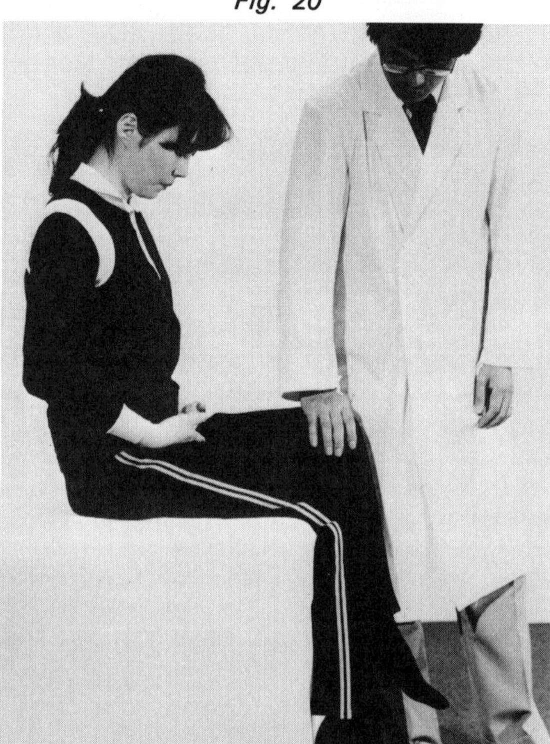

Fig. 21

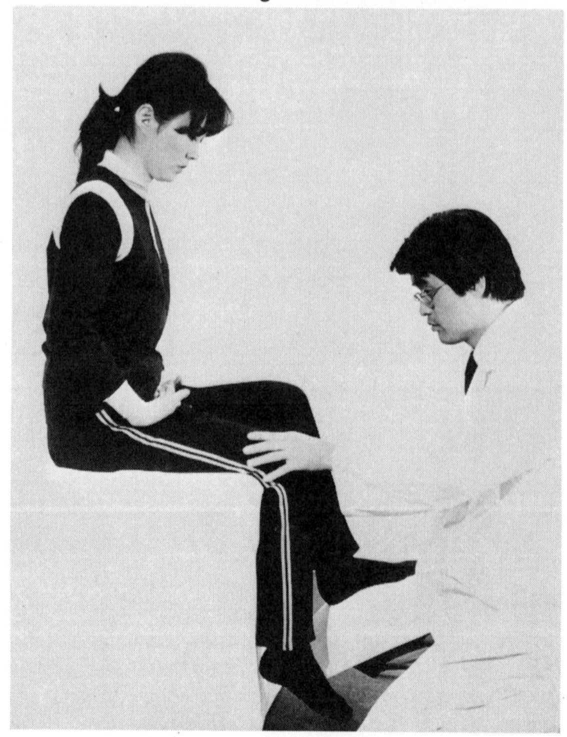

The therapist is standing off to the side in this case for the purpose of photographing the placement of his hands (Fig. 19). Technique Seated A-1 is actually performed using this same hand placement, only with the therapist standing directly in front of the patient.

Figure 20 shows the correct hand placement for performing technique Seated A-1 from the side of the patient (Fig. 20). (When standing in front of the patient, the hand placement of Figure 19 is used, and when standing to the side, that of Figure 20 is used.)

Figure 21 shows the same Seated A-1 technique so the movement of the patient is the same as in Figures 19 and 20. However, once the principle of movement in linkage is understood, it becomes clear where to place the hands for best results, and whether the therapist must use his knees for support. The difference in this technique becomes apparent when it is compared with Figure 19.

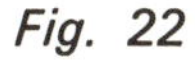

Fig. 22

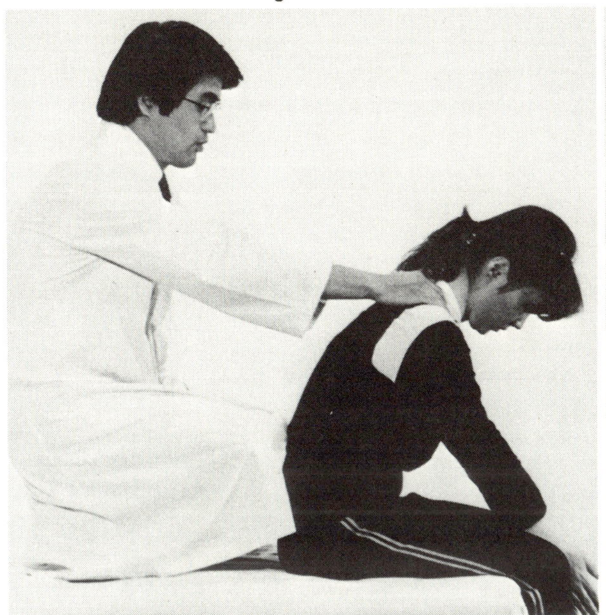

Fig. 23

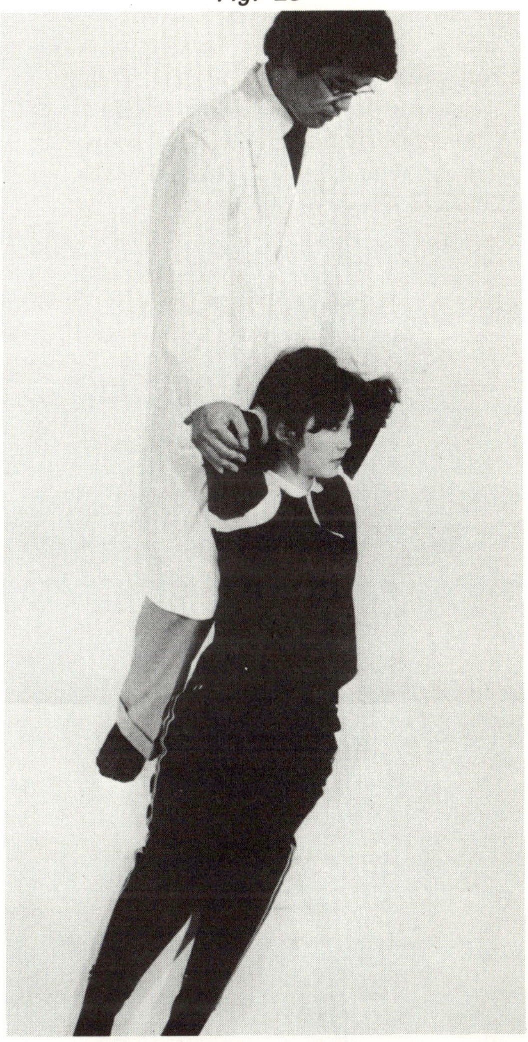

Figure 23 shows another example of using the therapist's knees. In this movement, the patient tends to get in an unstable position, so the therapist's use of his knees stabilizes the patient. This even makes the movement appear more stable.

When the hand placement conforms with the principles of motion, it will naturally result in the correct positioning and good form (Figs. 24 and 25).

Fig. 24

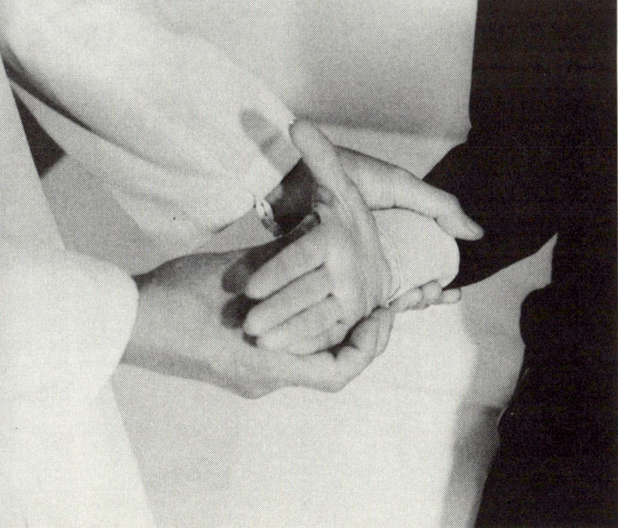

Fig. 25

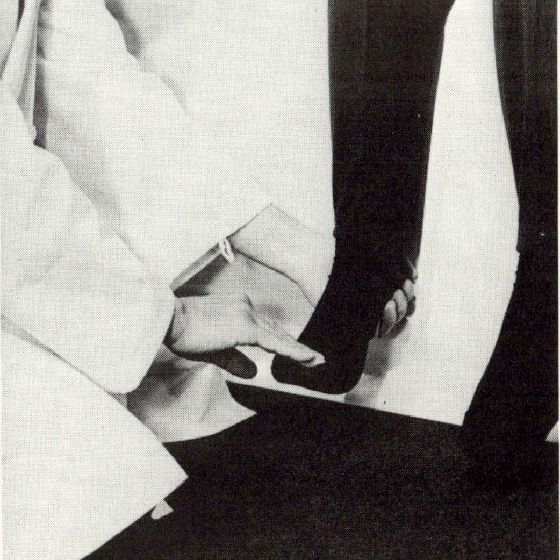

The placement of the therapist's hands for the same Sōtai technique is different between standing to the side of the patient and standing directly behind (Figs. 26 and 27).

When performing techniques Seated I-2 and -3, the movement is smoother and more stable when the hand is placed proximal to the center of movement.

By comparing Figures 27 and 28, it is apparent how these two forms can be clearly distinguished into that of greater and lesser stability. In Figure 27, the therapist's hand is near the cervical spine and his elbow is close to the patient. Figure 28 on the other hand, gives an appearance of instability.

Fig. 26

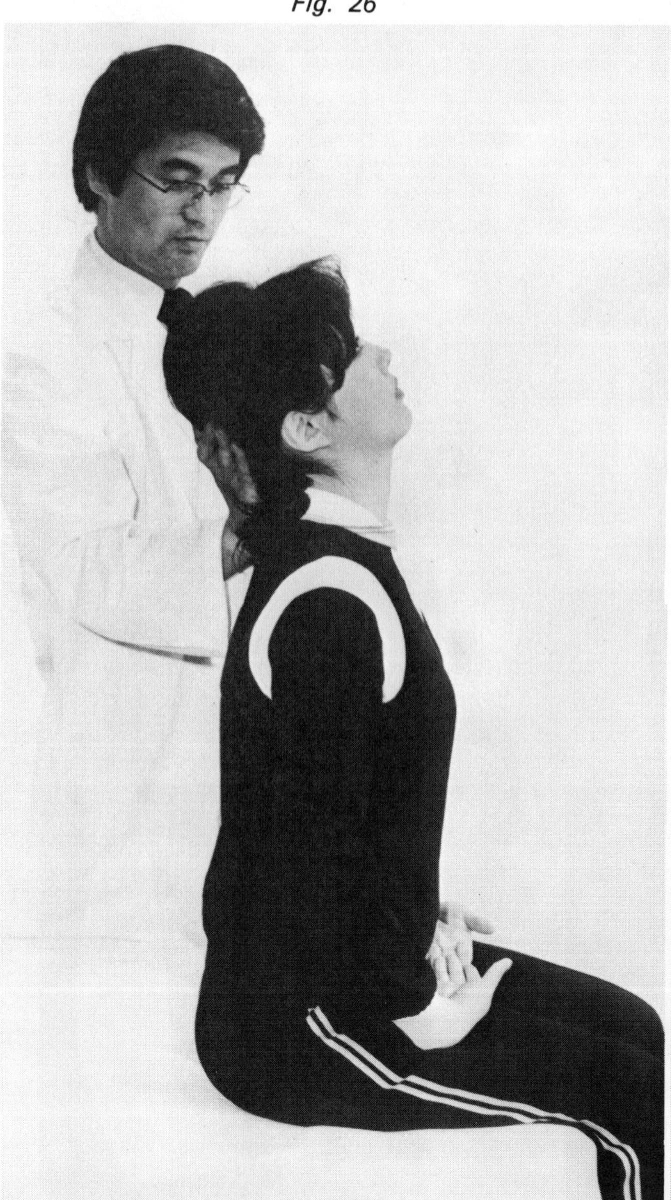

Fig. 27

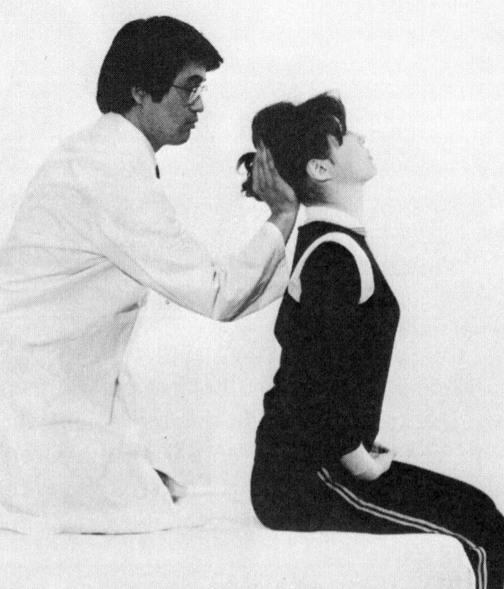

Fig. 28

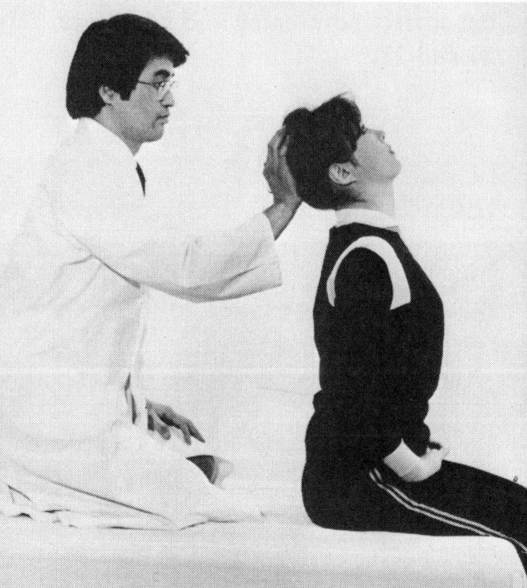

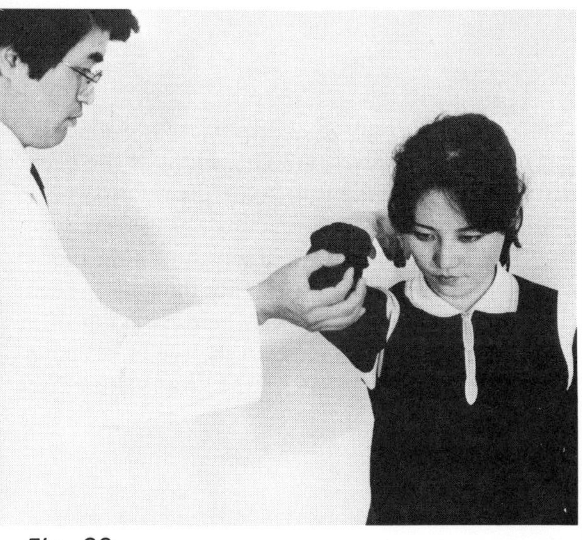

Fig. 29

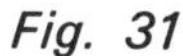

Fig. 30

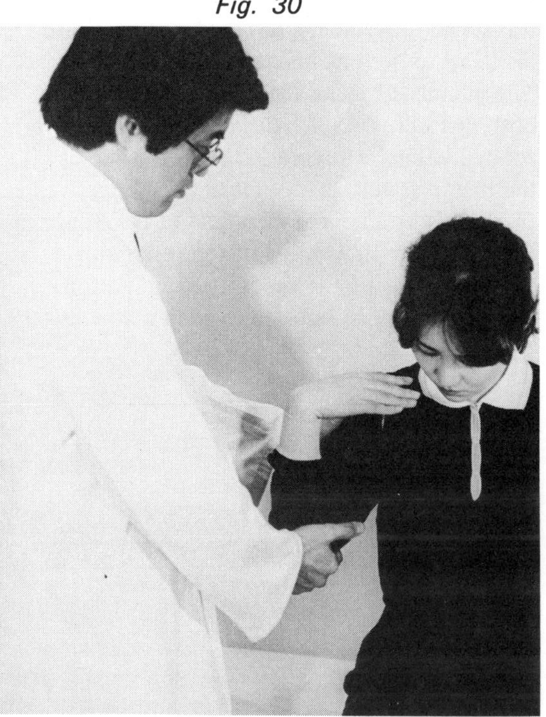

Fig. 31

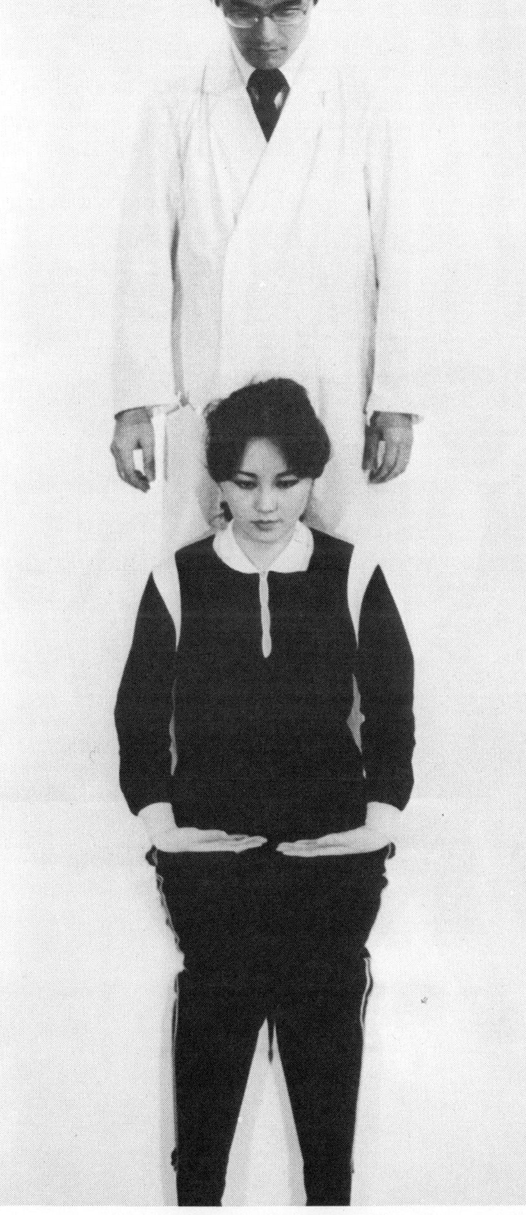

It is better in some cases for the sake of stability, that the therapist place both hands on the patient rather than just one (Figs. 29 and 30). Furthermore, even the same technique can be performed with greater ease and stability, depending on the movement, when both hands are used for support. The greatest stability can be achieved by the therapist keeping his elbow either at his side or next to the patient. When the therapist's elbow is right between the patient and him, the movement will become more difficult for the patient, and also the therapist will tire easier.

The Sōtai techniques of Seated D, E, F and I are done in the basic stance with the therapist standing behind the patient (Fig. 31). In this case, first the therapist must see if the patient is tense in anticipation. (The object of the Sōtai technique can be better attained when the patient's palms are made to face upward. When the palms are placed down, the movement can become strained and ineffective, and thus the aim of the treatment could be defeated.)

In technique Seated D-1 and 2 (rotation and transverse movement), the therapist uses both his knees as well as his hands (Figs. 32 and 33). The manner of using the knees is the same in both D-1 and D-2. When the patient's torso is rotated left as in Figure 32, the left knee of the therapist acts as a point of resistance. The therapist's knees serve as points of resistance in the transverse movement of the torso also.

Note: During the mobility examination, the left knee must be used in such a way as to facilitate the rotation or transverse movement. The knees, however, are not placed at the back or side of the patient to *cause* the rotation or transverse movement.

There are many ways in which to hold the patient, but in some cases only the fingers need be used (Fig. 34). In cases where the point of resistance is chosen close to the center of movement, holding lightly with the fingers does the job.

Fig. 32 *Fig. 33* *Fig. 34*

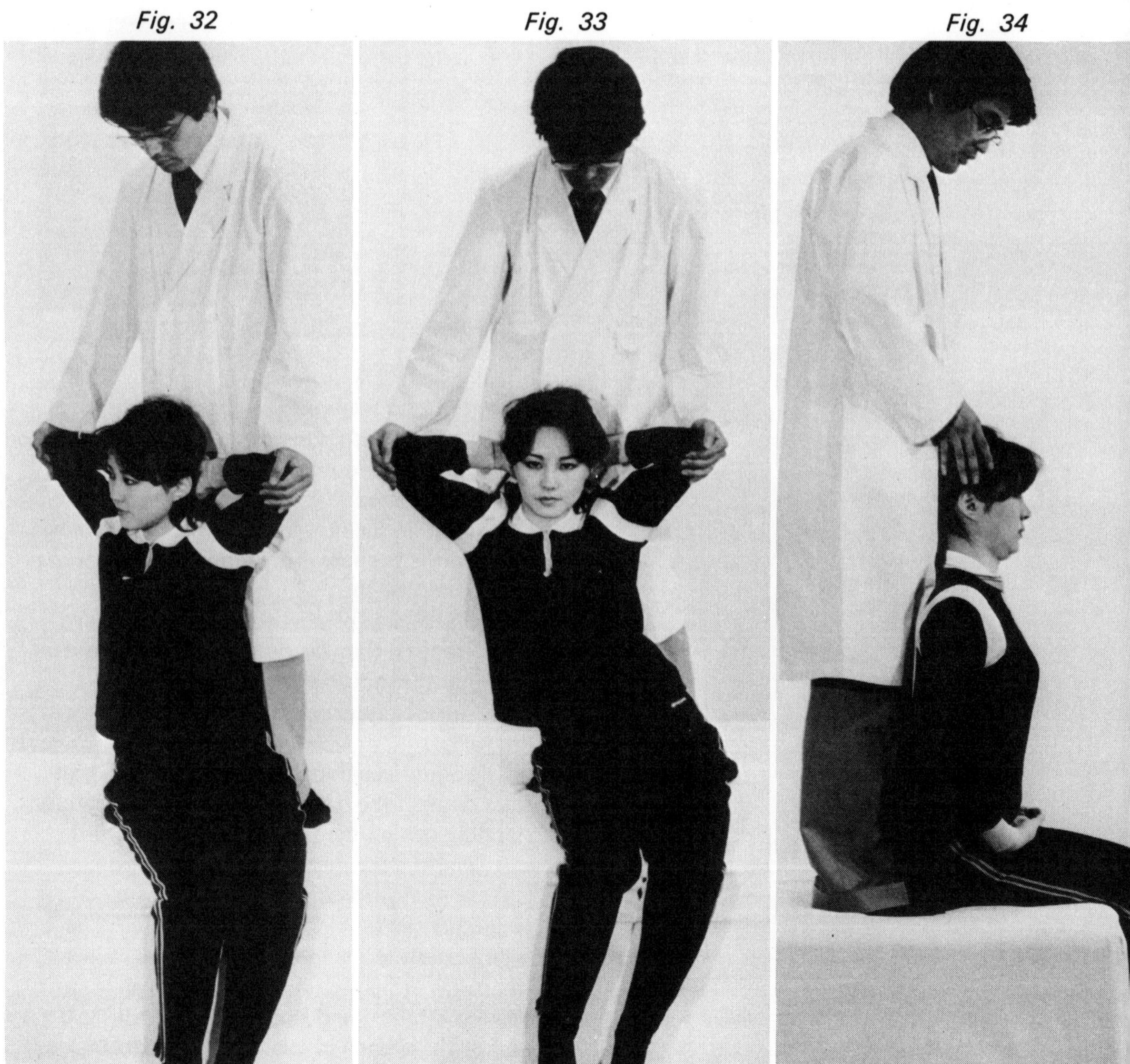

4. CHECKPOINTS FOR MORPHOLOGICAL OBSERVATION

The human body is formed by the mutual linkage of its respective parts—the head, the torso, and the upper and lower limbs. Therefore when the balance and proportion of the body is offset (the balance in just one part, or the balance between one part and the rest of the body), this change is first expressed as a change in physical sensation and movement. At the same time, this imbalance also extends to other parts of the body to produce changes in the form and function.

As a general example of morphology relating organic function; when the right shoulder is stiff a tendency toward stomach problems may be indicated, while stiffness in the left shoulder could indicate liver dysfunctions. It is also possible to say that the right soulder being higher than the left is an indication of a healthy appetite. The object of morphological observation is to interpret these variations in physical form.

It is essential that the patient be examined from head to toe in all postures including the standing, sitting, Seiza, supine, and prone postures. When one masters this art, the diagnosis of illnesses through morphological observation alone becomes a possibility. Morphological observation is simple because merely the disturbance in physical proportion and balance are examined. Once the technique of interpreting physical form is learned, one becomes capable of judging the state of his own health as well as that of his family and friends. This is therefore an invaluable technique for the prevention of disease. After a morphological examination is performed, the results serve to indicate the appropriate Sōtai technique and exercises for the patient. The morphological observations also serve as a guideline which demonstrates the improvements brought about as a result of the Sōtai Therapy.

Anterior Aspect (Standing, Seated, and Seiza Postures)

1) Tortility and inclination of neck
2) Tortility and difference in height between right and left shoulders
2) Tortility and curvature of arms; tortility of wrists
4) Difference in the level and position of the nipples
5) Tension and stiffness in pectoral and abdominal muscles
6) Tortility and difference in height between the right and left iliac spine
7) Difference between right and left patellas (anterior-posterior positioning and orientation)
8) Orientation of feet (average angle created by the opening between the feet is 60°)
9) Tortility and inclination of entire body
10) Manner of crossing legs in the seated position
11) Color and luster of skin

Fig. 1 *Fig. 2* *Fig. 3*

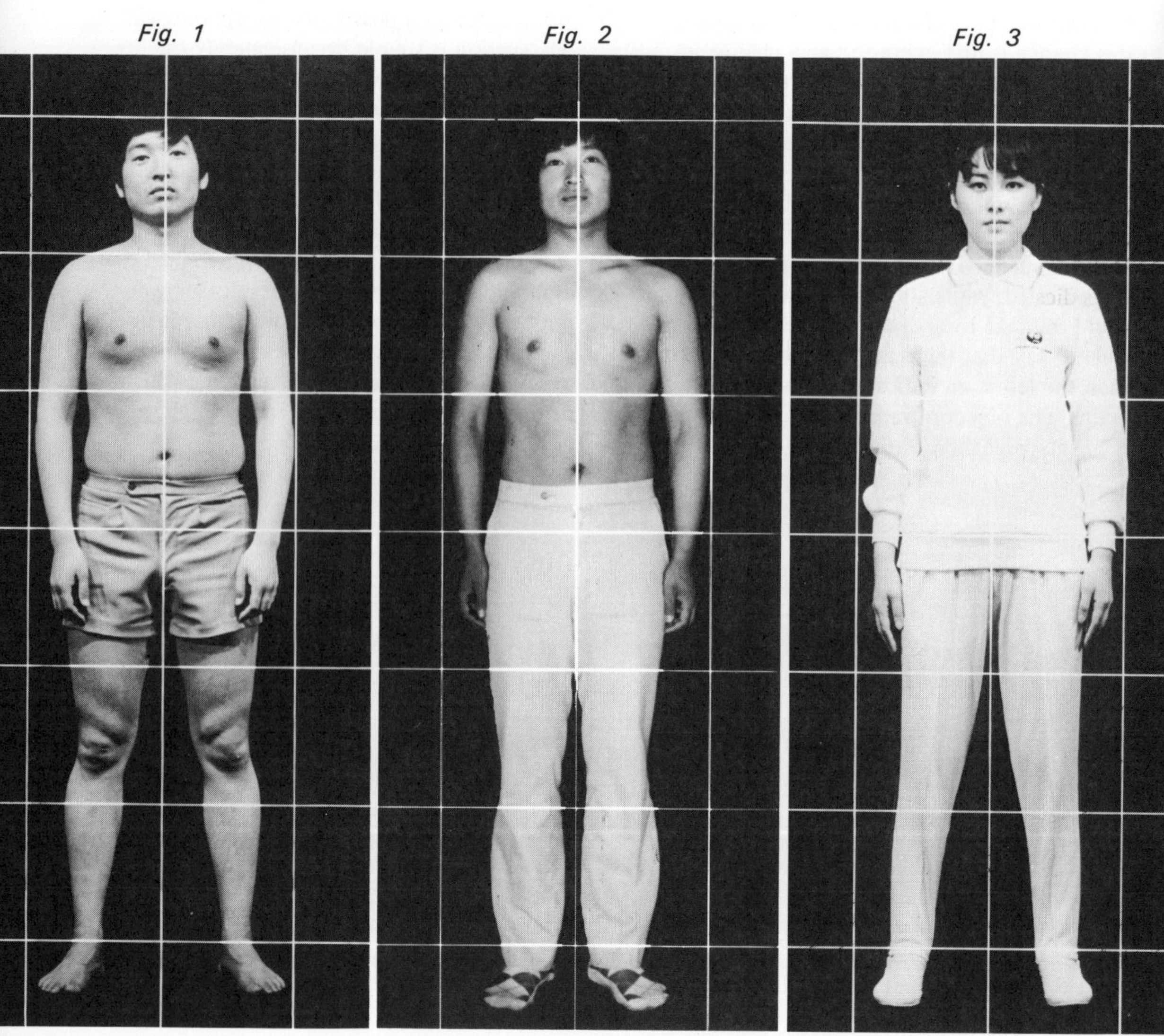

A comparison can be made between the most recent photograph of this individual and that two years earlier (Figs. 1 and 2). When every aspect is examined in detail, one can see that there has been considerable change. This man came into contact with Sōtai Therapy after incurring a lumbar injury on a trampoline. The first photograph was taken immediately after this injury.

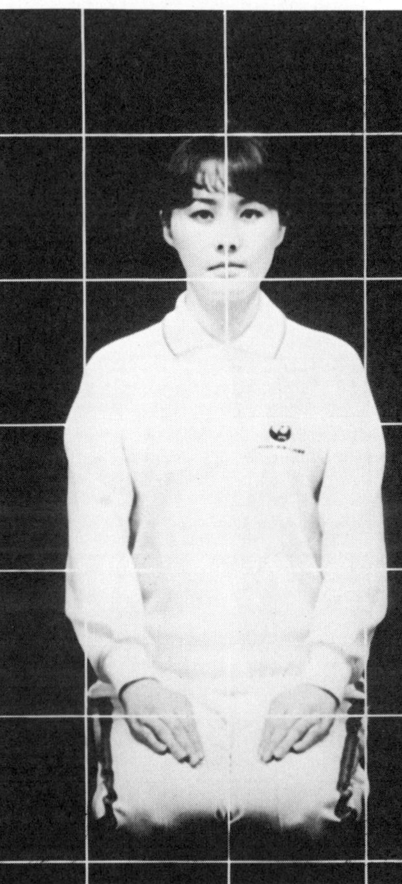

Fig. 6

Fig. 4

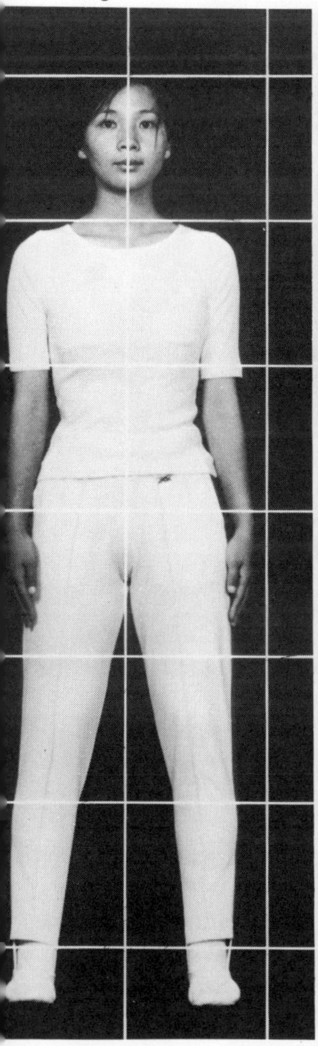

Fig. 5

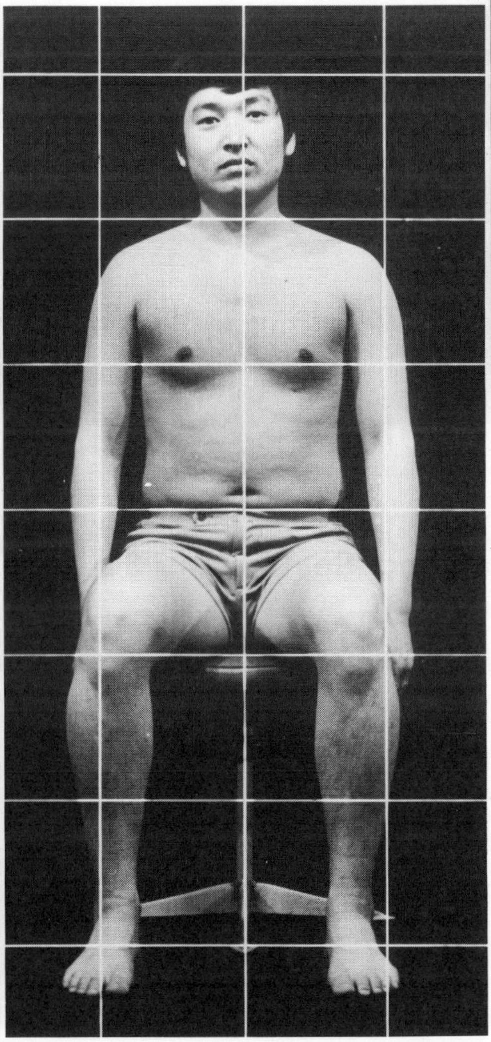

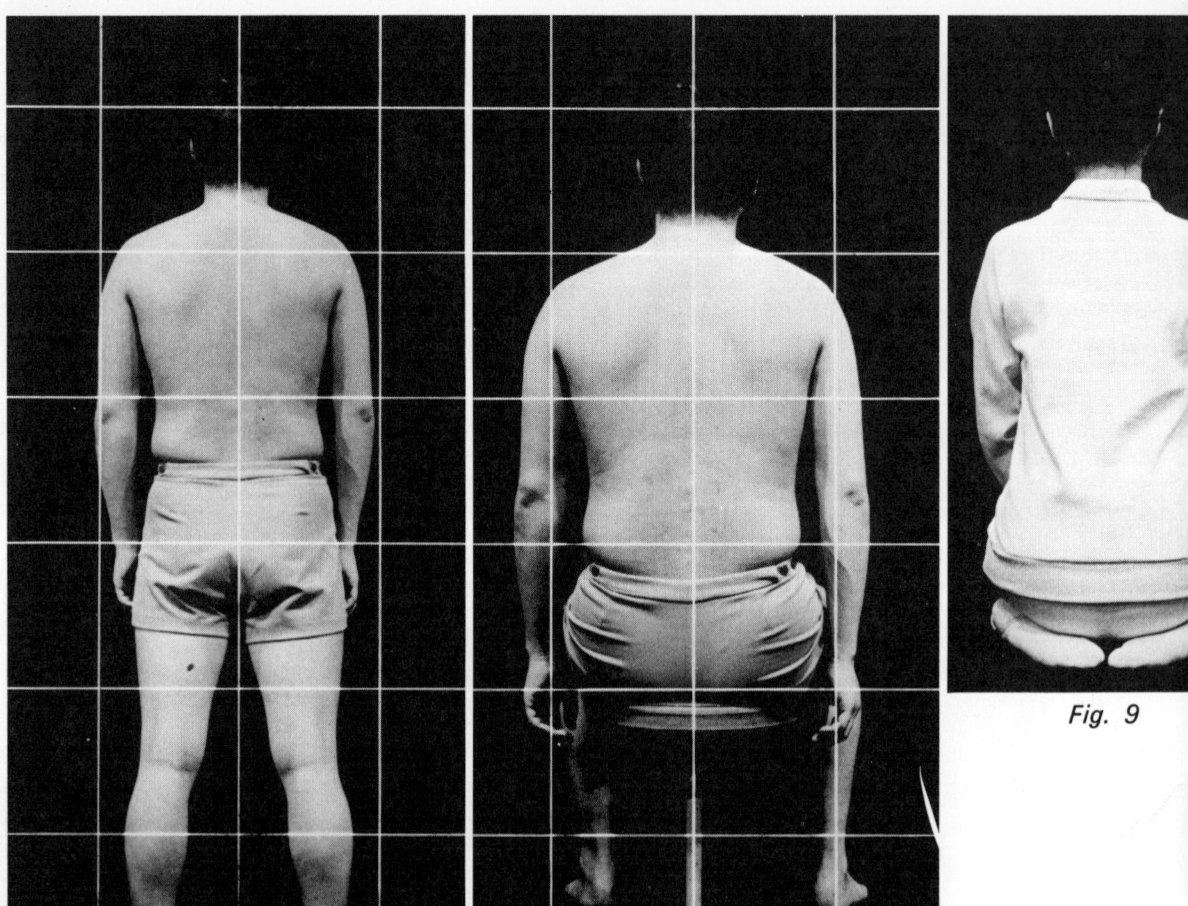

Fig. 7

Fig. 8

Fig. 9

Posterior Aspect (Standing, Seated, and Seiza Postures)

1) Tortility and inclination of neck; induration in the nape
2) Difference in height between right and left scapulae
3) Tortility and curvature of spine
4) Protrusion, tension, and stiffness in dorsal muscles
5) Tortility and curvature of arms; tortility of wrists; difference in space between arm and trunk
6) Difference in height of the right and left elbows, and difference in orientation
7) Difference between right and left gluteus muscles
8) Variation of form between right and left legs
9) Difference in position between right and left heels
10) Opening between the thighs (seated and Seiza postures)
11) State of physiological curvature of the spine
12) Manner in which the buttocks rest upon the plantar arches in the Seiza position
13) Color and luster of skin

Fig. 10

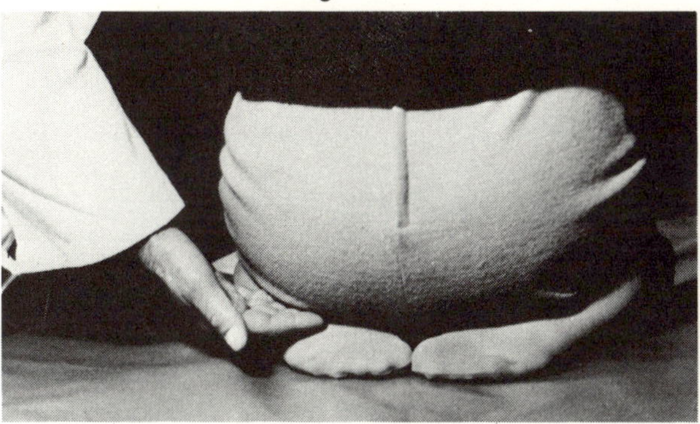

In the Seiza posture, the big toes of the right and left feet should lightly touch one another. The hips should settle fully upon the plantar arches so that there is no gap and fingers cannot be placed between the buttocks and soles.

Fig. 11

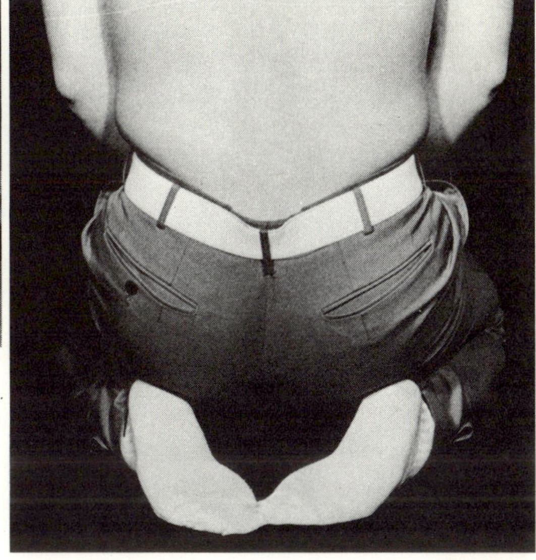

When the first toes of both feet are in light contact and a hand can be easily placed in the space between the hips and the plantar arches, there exist abnormalities in the overall physical structure (by Japanese standards).

Fig. 12 *Fig. 13*

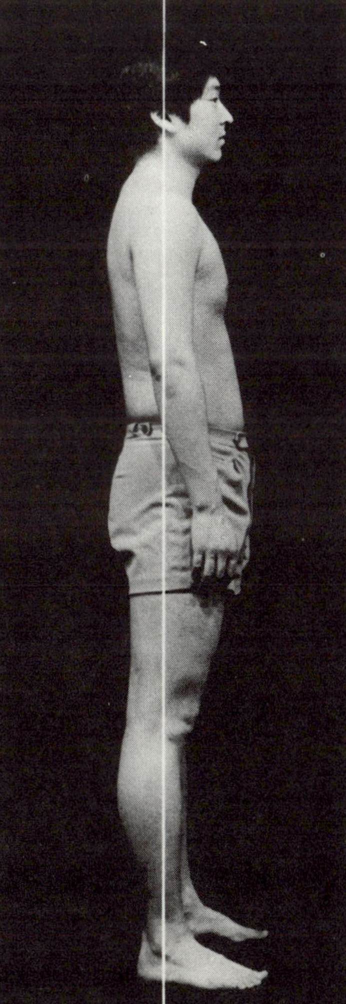

Lateral Aspect (Standing and Seated Postures)

1) Stability and straightness of standing posture
2) Comparison of the position of the head
3) Difference between right and left shoulders
4) Comparison of dorsal and ventral morphology
5) Tortility of arms; tortility and orientation of fingers
6) Morphology of lower abdomen
7) Color and luster of skin

A vertical line through the center of gravity should pass through the auricular opening, the anterior side of the sacrum (promontory of sacrum), anterior to the center of the knee joint, and slightly anterior to the lateral malleolus (ankle).

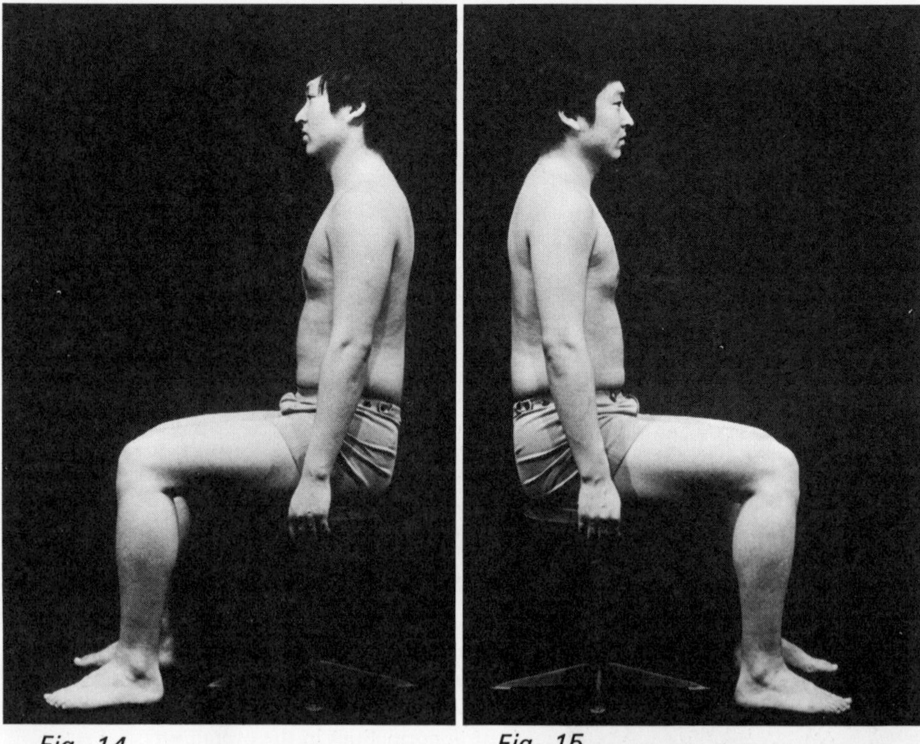

Fig. 14

Fig. 15

Fig. 17

Fig. 16

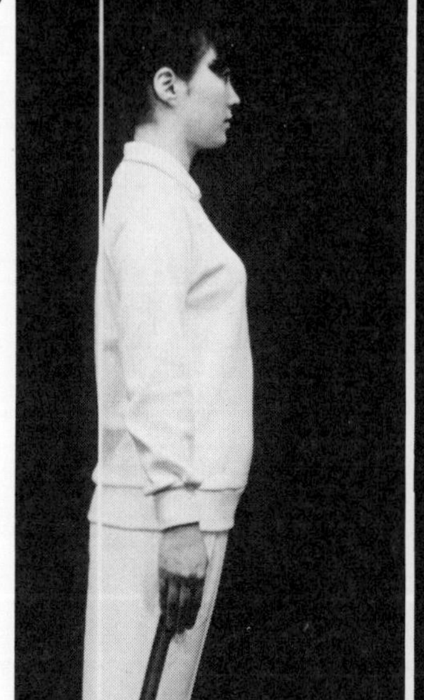

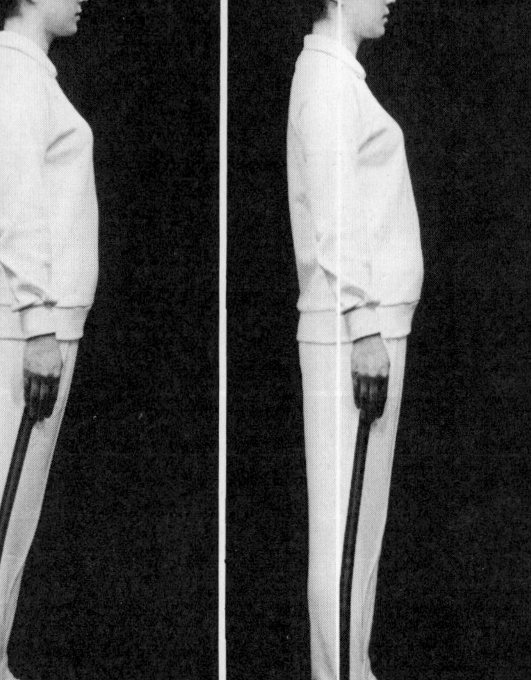

Fig. 16: Standing posture with center of gravity shifted slightly forward (army posture).

Fig. 17: Comfortable posture for the person (comfortable posture).

Supine and Prone Postures (Viewed from Either Side and from Head)

1) Comparison of right and left lateral views
2) Tortility and inclination of neck
3) Difference between right and left halves of chest
4) Difference between right and left ilia
5) Tension and stiffness in muscles of legs
6) Tortility and curvature in spine
7) Tension and stiffness, or protrusion of the back muscles
8) Tension and stiffness, or protrusion of the gluteus muscles
9) Color and luster of skin

Fig. 18

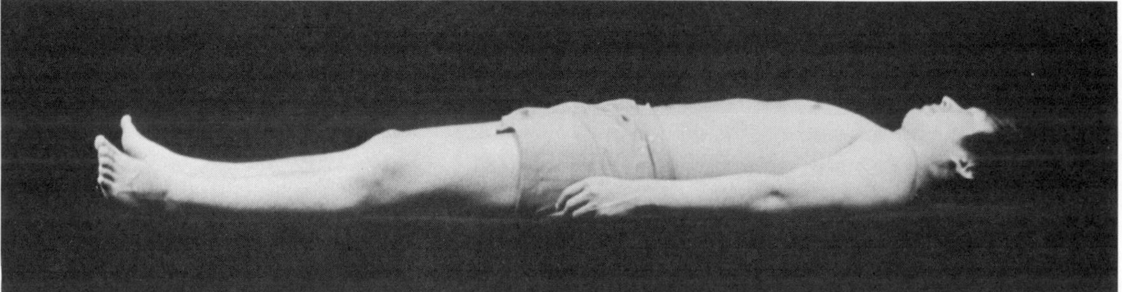

Fig. 19

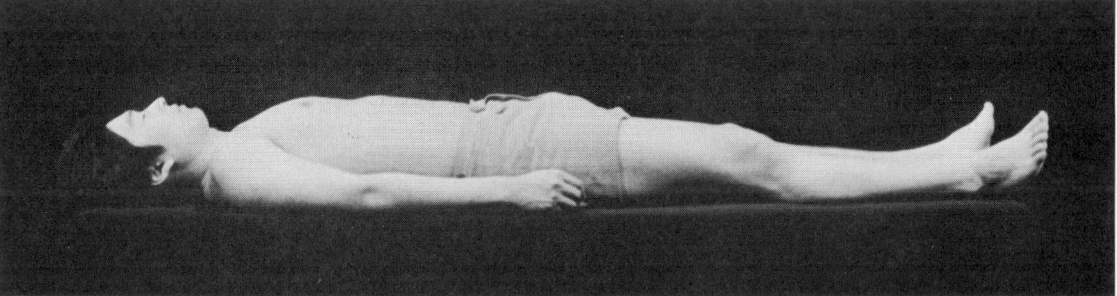

Fig. 20

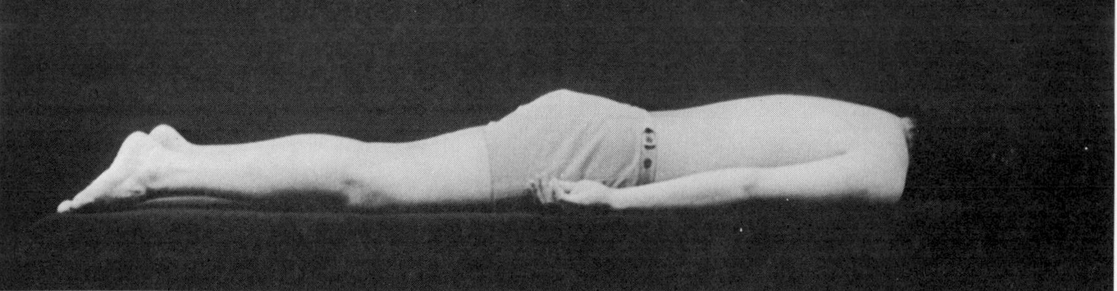

Fig. 21

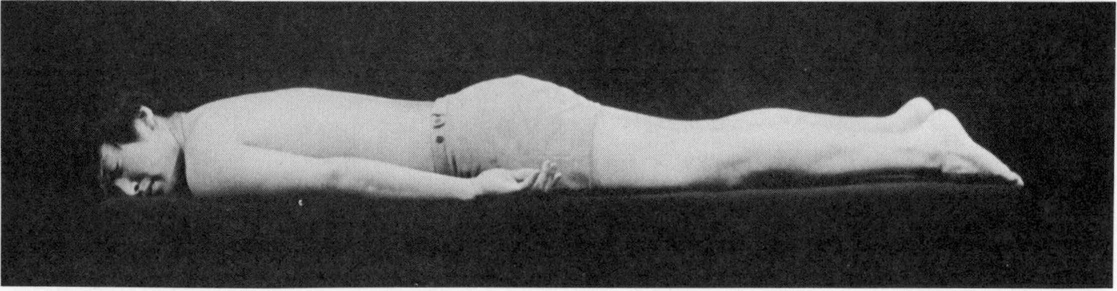

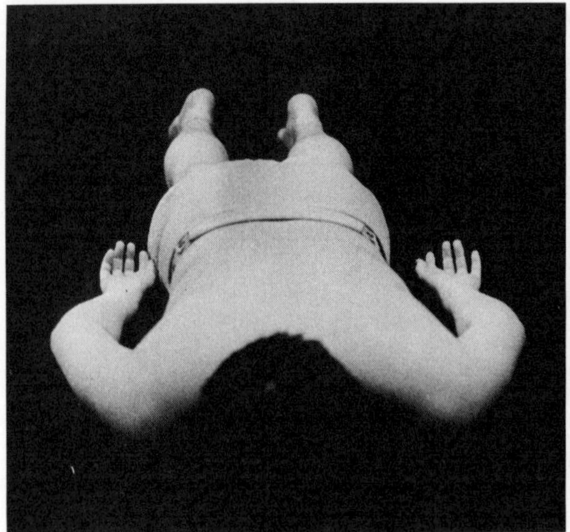

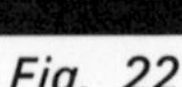

Fig. 22

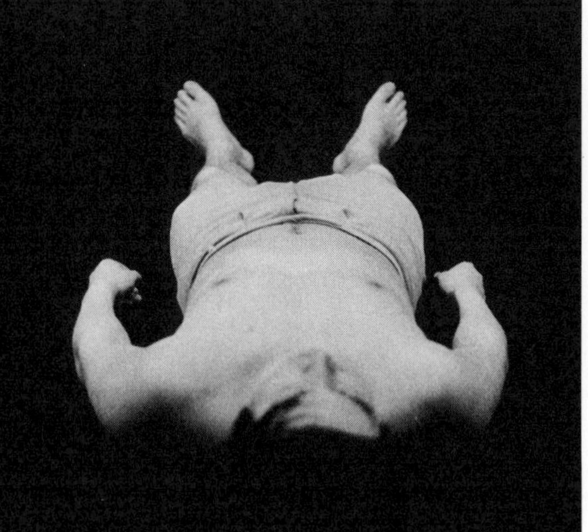

Fig. 23

Supine and Prone Postures (Longitudinal View from Feet)

1) Alignment of the body
2) Condition of the feet (corns, callouses, indurations; tortility curvature, and indurations in the toes)
3) Angle of feet opening
4) Differnce in the length of the legs, and the amount of tortility and curvature
5) Difference between right and left knees
6) Differences in position and orientation of right and left patellas
7) Tortility of ankles
8) Color and luster of skin

Fig. 24

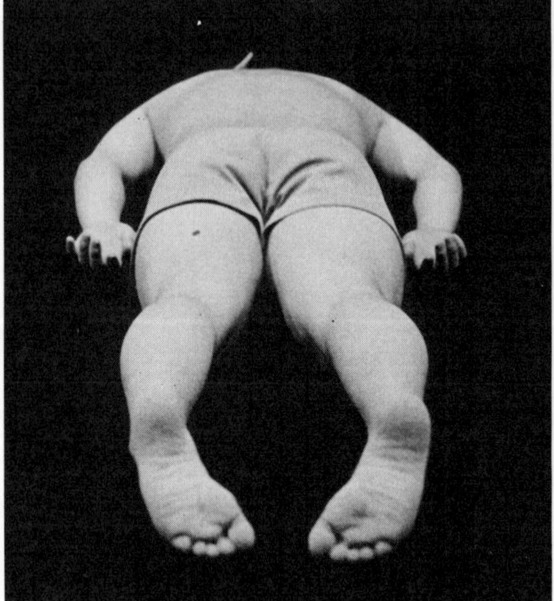

Fig. 25

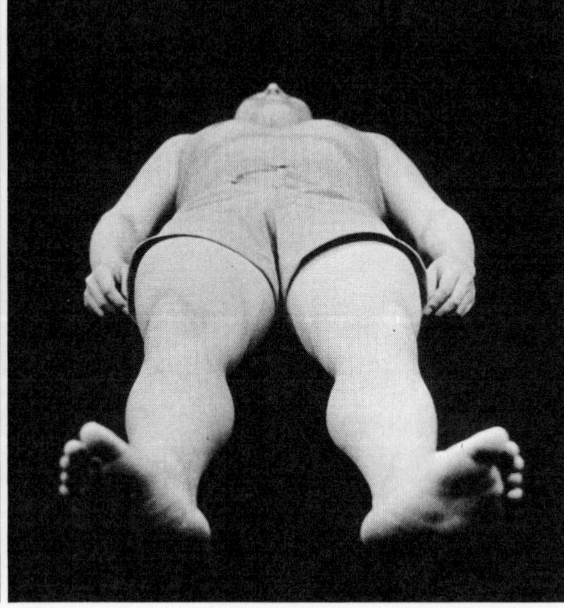

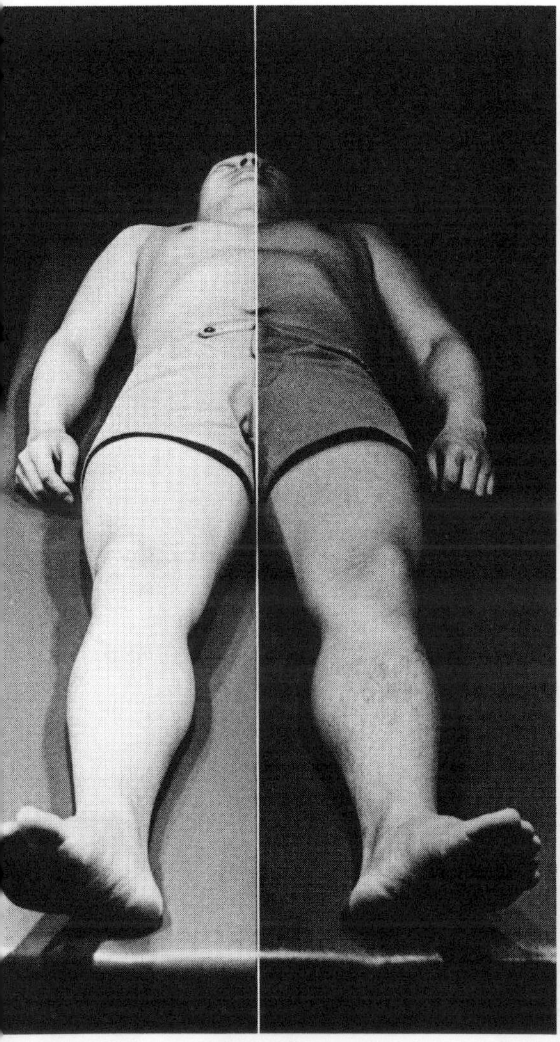

Fig. 26

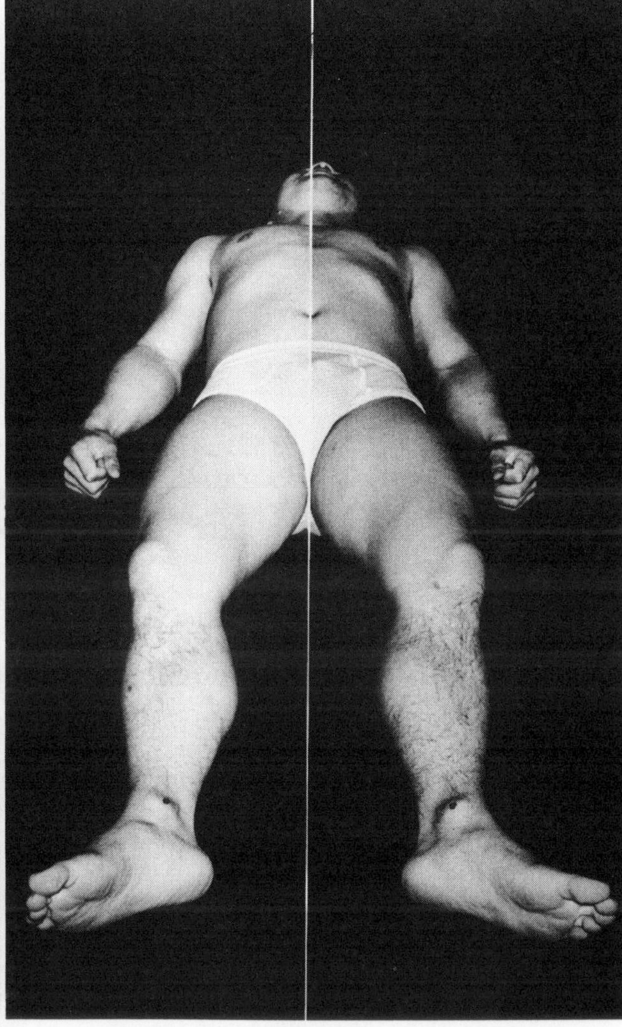

Fig. 27

To accentuate the morphological features and to aid in the interpretation of the differences between the right and left halves of the body, one side of the photographs have been shaded to provide contrast. The photographs are examples of two males between who distinct differences can be seen in morphology.

	Fig. 26	Fig. 27
A) Leg length difference	right longer	left longer
B) Right and left patellas	facing outward	normal position
C) State of extension	inclined left	inclined right
D) Chest	right higher	left higher
E) Feet opening angle	fully open	normal

Fig. 28

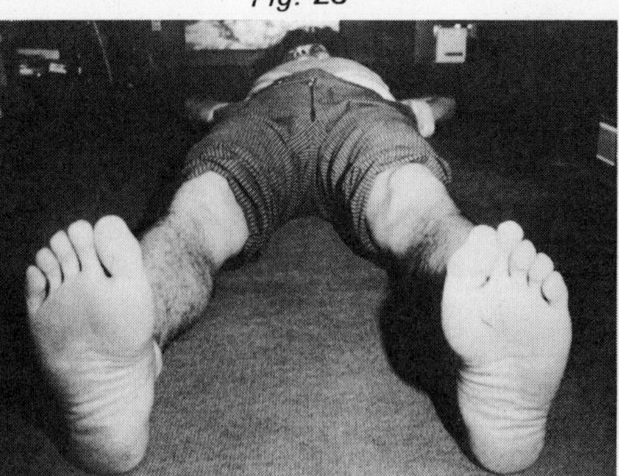

Fig. 29

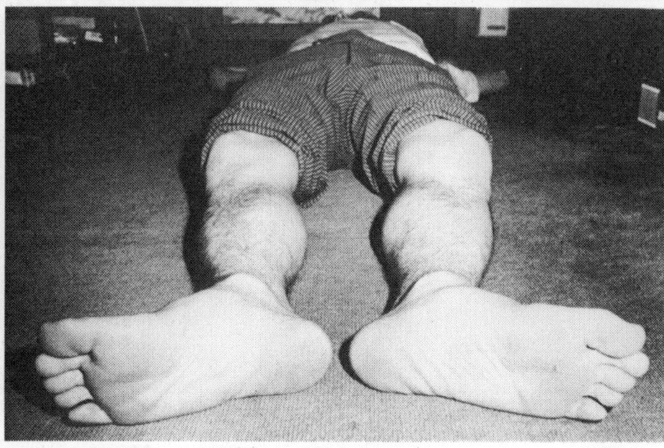

The feet of this patient open to 180 degrees when relaxed in the supine position. Even when his feet are rotated together toward the center, they do not turn farther than vertical. This is an example of unusual plantar morphology.

Observation of Scapulae Positions in Standing Forward Flexion Posture and Three Variations of the Prone Position

In patients who suffer from lumbago and stiffness of the neck and shoulders, there usually exist a difference in height between the right and left scapulae. Figure 30 shows this height difference being measured with a scoliometer. A measured value of more than 4° is considered abnormal. The scoliometer in the figure indicates a value of 5°.

When observing the scapulae with the subject in the prone position, the head may be positioned in three different ways: facing right as shown in Figure 31, facing downward as shown in Figure 32 and facing left as shown in Figure 33. It is important to take into account the difference between the numerical values for the side to which the subject can turn with ease and that of the side to which it is more difficult to turn. (*Note:* Approximately 70 percent of the people turned their heads to their left in the prone position.)

Close and careful observation is essential for people with scoliosis, cervical distortions, lumbago, or abnormalities in the lower limbs. (Fig.

Fig. 30

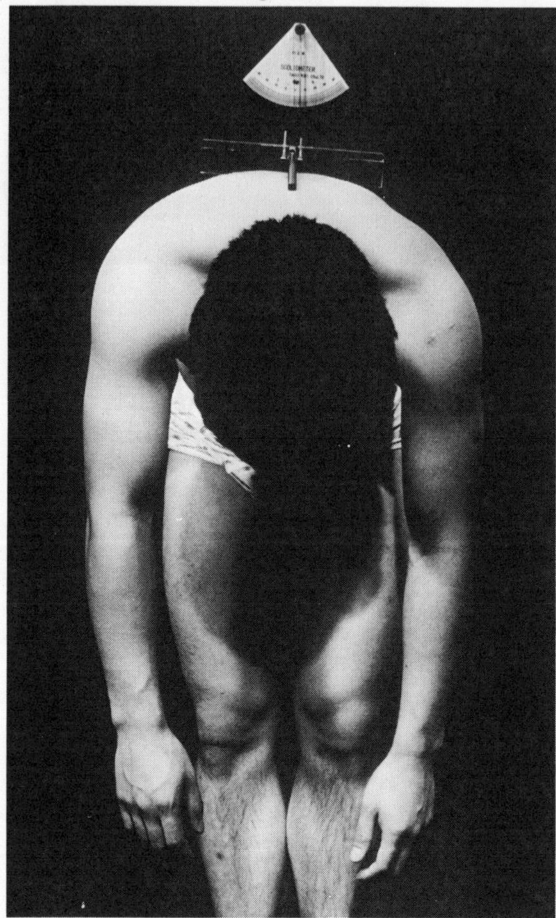

31: R2°, Fig. 32: R1.5°, Fig. 33: R1°)

Recently, much attention has been aroused over the frequent occurence of scoliosis in young people. There is one noteworthy report in recent literature related with this.

The angular values measured with a scoliometer were divided into the following categories: 0°–2.5°, 2.6°–3.5°, 3.6°–4.5° and over 4.5°. Subjects in each angle value category were tested for physical performance. The results indicated that those individuals in the 3.6°–4.5° and over 4.5° categories were inferior in physical performance.

Consequently, 0°–2.5° was designated as normal, and those in the 2.6°–3.5° range were labeled "Type I." Type I persons are still within the normal range, but should pay closer attention in their daily life to posture. Individuals in the 3.6°–4.5° range, labeled "Type II,"should take positive action to correct their posture and improve their physical condition. Those persons in the over 4.5° category should receive various physical examinations.

A cause and effect relationship was observed between the presence of scoliosis and vital capacity, lung capacity ratio, as well as the function of the back muscles.

Kōshu Eisei Jōhō (Public Health Journal),
April 1979

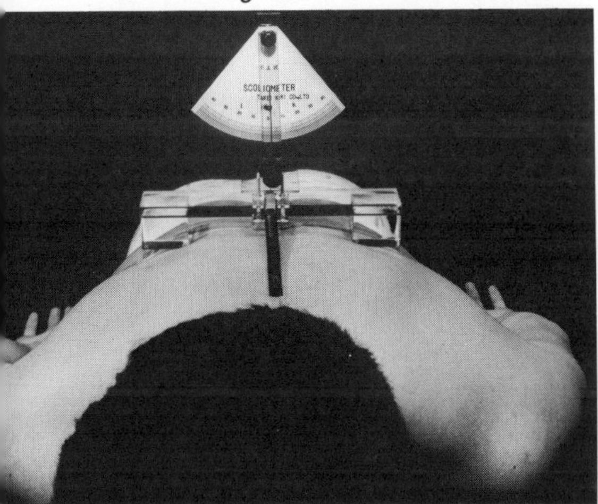

Fig. 31

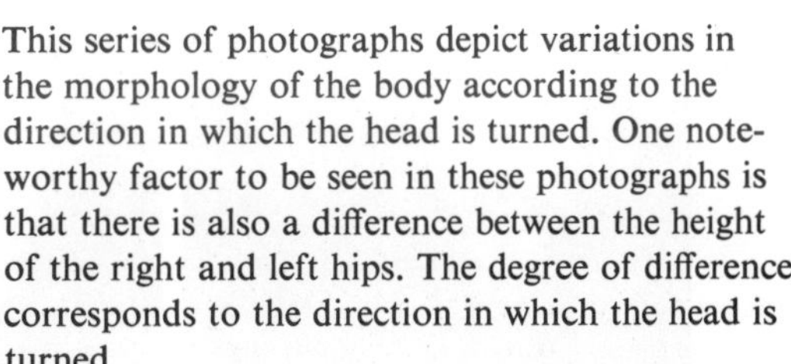
This series of photographs depict variations in the morphology of the body according to the direction in which the head is turned. One noteworthy factor to be seen in these photographs is that there is also a difference between the height of the right and left hips. The degree of difference corresponds to the direction in which the head is turned.

Data from Kawakami Lab.

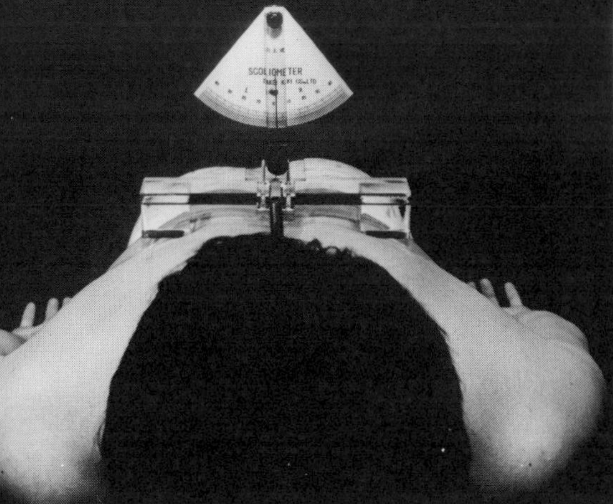

Fig. 32

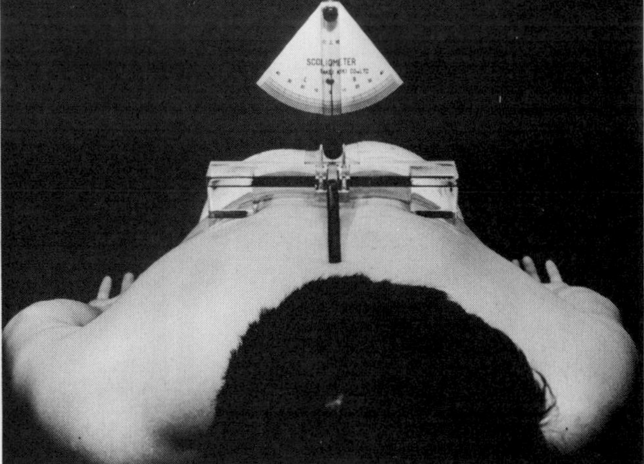

Fig. 33

Physical Distortion and Its Transition Viewed by X-ray (1)

Figures 1 through 33 present various aspects of superficial morphology, but with x-ray the observation of internal distortions and their transition over time is possible. Although a great many radiographs are taken daily, the number of medical personal studying these radiographs from a broad morphological perspective are few. Even when radiographs are examined closely, the observation of morphological features is usually limited to localized areas.

Dr. Hiroshi Suzuki of the Suzuki Orthopedics Hospital in the city of Toyohashi routinely studies radiographs of the entire body from a broad morphological perspective, by imposing a center of gravity line onto the radiograph. Dr. Suzuki's studies are a valuable contribution in research of physical therapy.

In the designing of artificial joints of the leg, one method used to determine the necessary strengths is to study the amount of muscular force acting upon the joints when the patient

This is an example of good functional structure. In order to exaggerate the changes brought about when the subject changes from a two legged stance to a one legged stance, the female subject holds weights, respectively equal to 20 percent and 40 percent of her body weight. The vertical white

Fig. 34 A B C

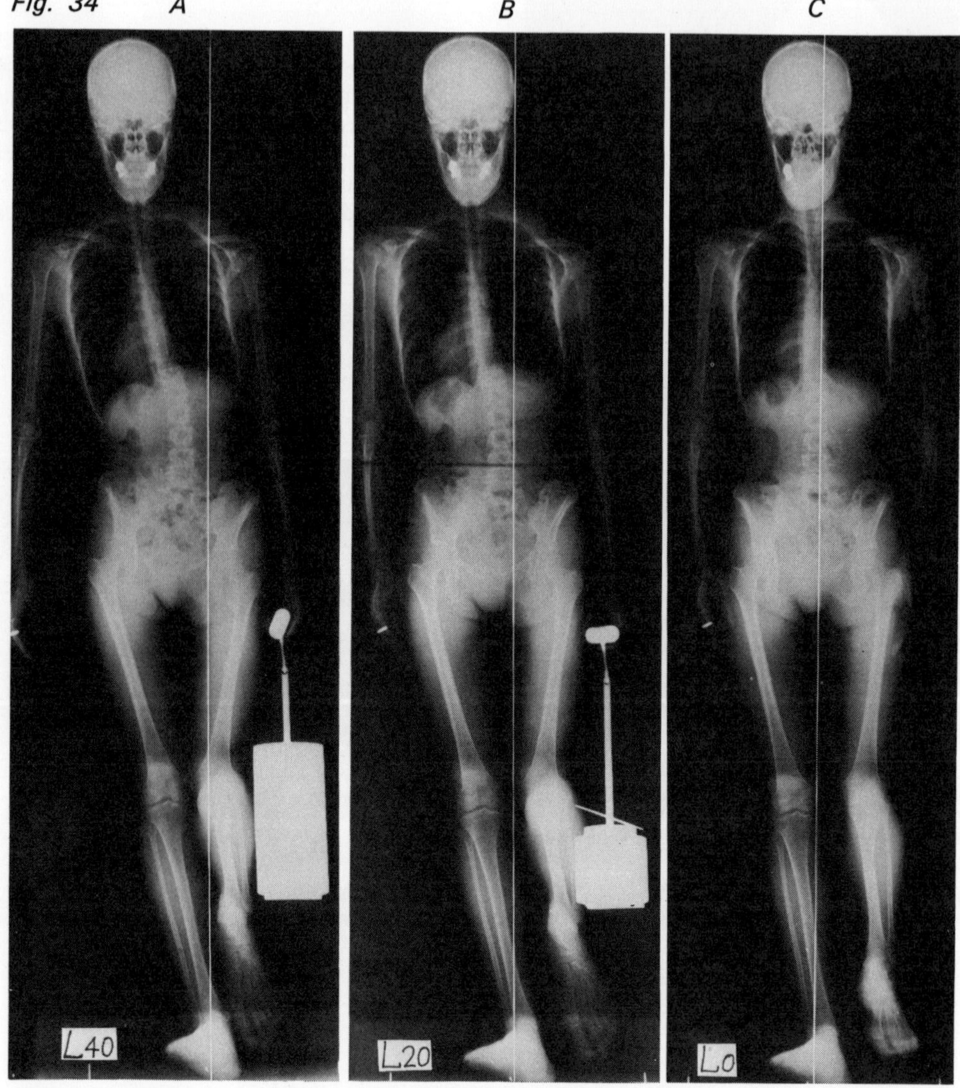

stands on one leg. Some 60 full length radiographs with a center of gravity line have been studied, and also the joints of the hip, knee, and ankle are considered individually.

Going a step beyond the external morphological observation, radiographs reveal changes in minute detail of the skeletal structure. The features which are externally visible will not be discussed here, but it can be seen that there is a close relationship between form (posture), function (quality of one legged stance and quantity of force on joint) and the shifting of the center of gravity (change in stance).

Compared to the figure showing statisfactory function of the leg, the inclination of the torso is greater and the posture is more awkward in the figure showing poor function of the leg. In addition, the amount of the shift in the center of gravity is greater and the shift tends to occur more suddenly. Since the center of gravity line passes close to the fulcrum of the joints in the leg, it may be said that strong muscular forces are not coming to bear on these joints.

line passes through the center of gravity. Carrying a weight on one side produces a slightly unnatural one legged stance. When the weight is increased, the unnatural postural compensation also increases in order to maintain balance.

Fig. 35 *A* *B* *C* *D*

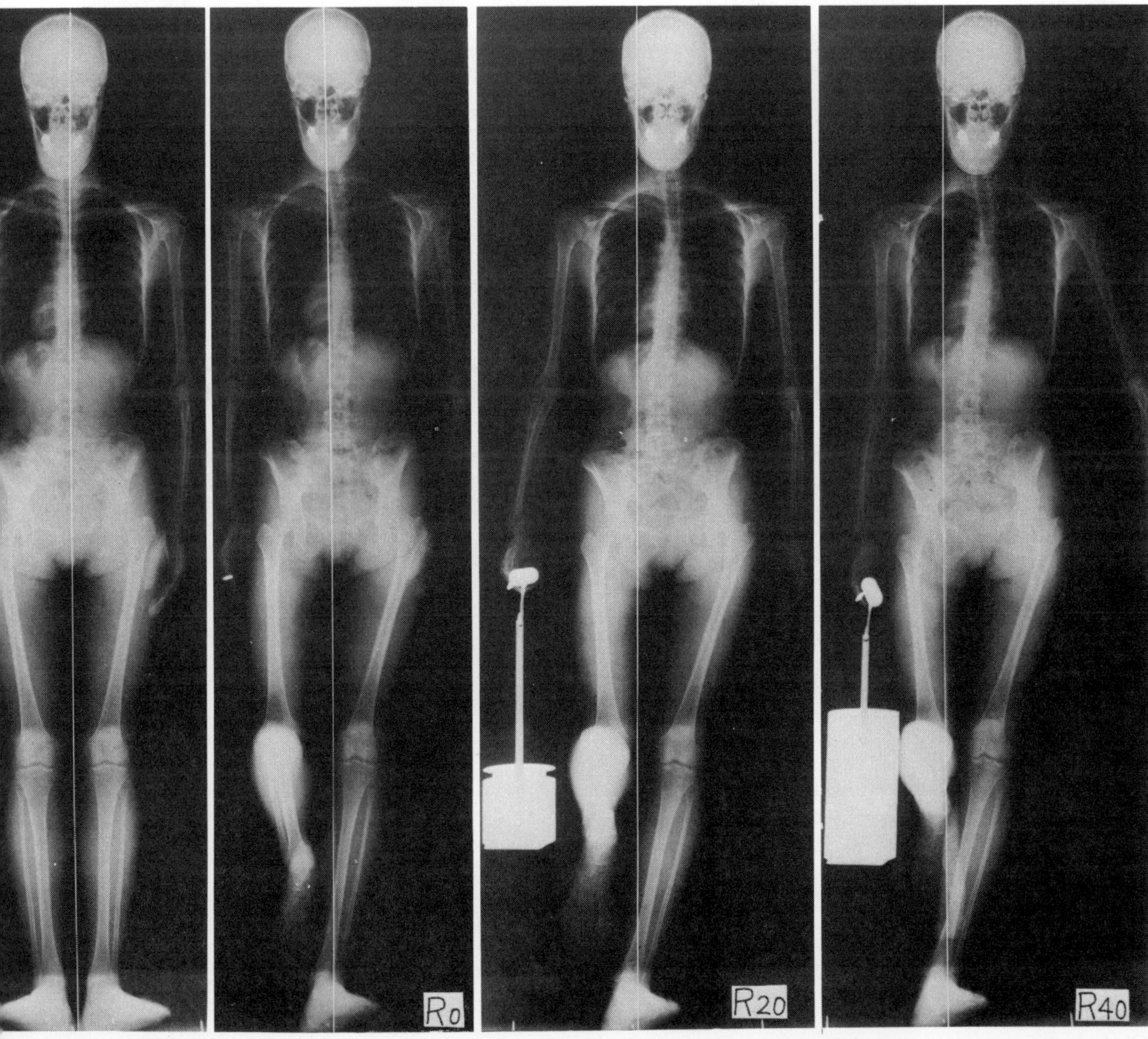

Physical Distortion and Its Transition Viewed by X-ray (2)

Figures 36, 37, and 38 are examples of poor functioning. The figures were taken three months, seven months, and one year after the patient underwent surgery for fractures in the femur and tibia.

Fig. 36 A B C

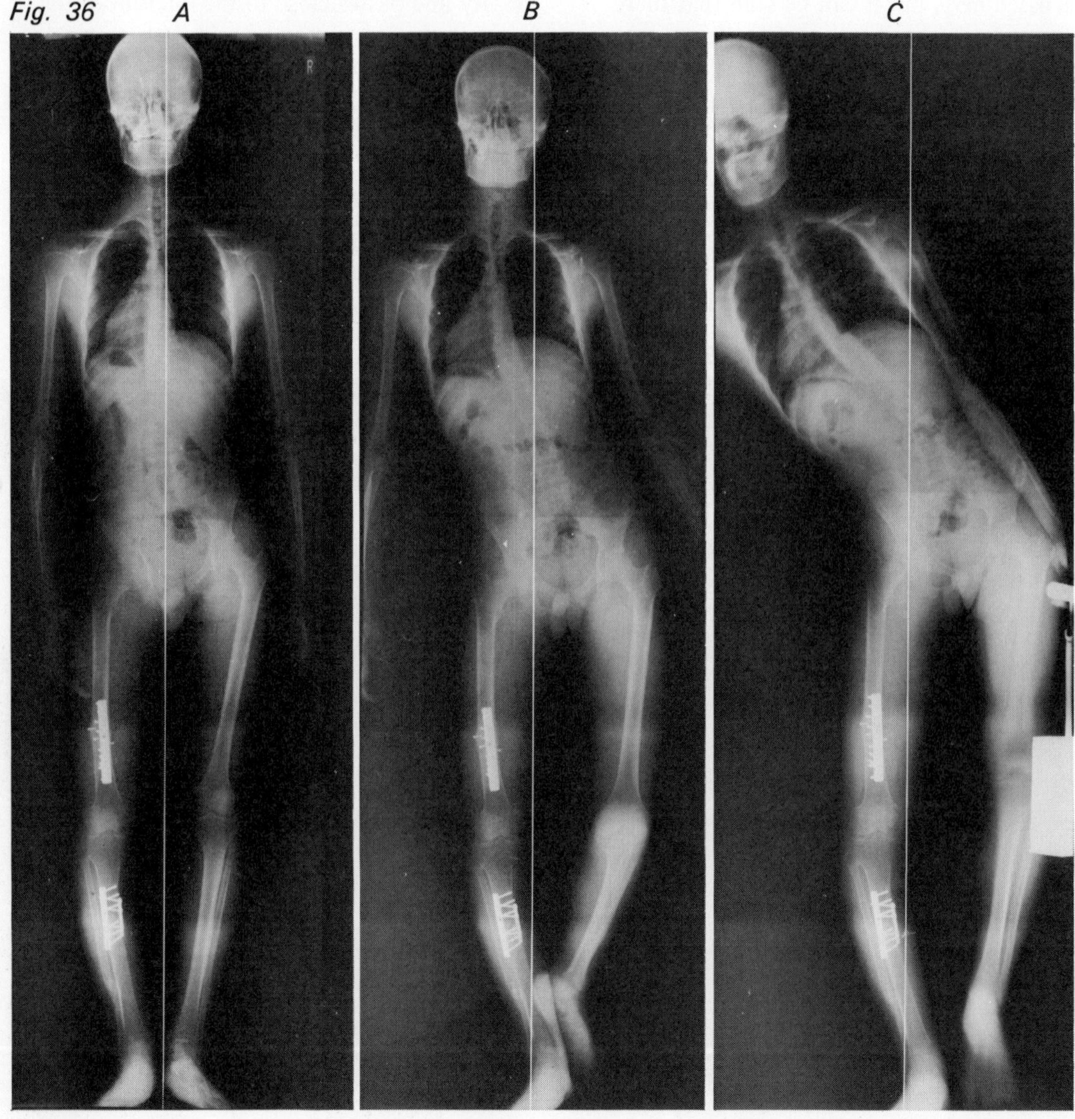

Awkwardness of the posture is pronounced (three months after surgery).

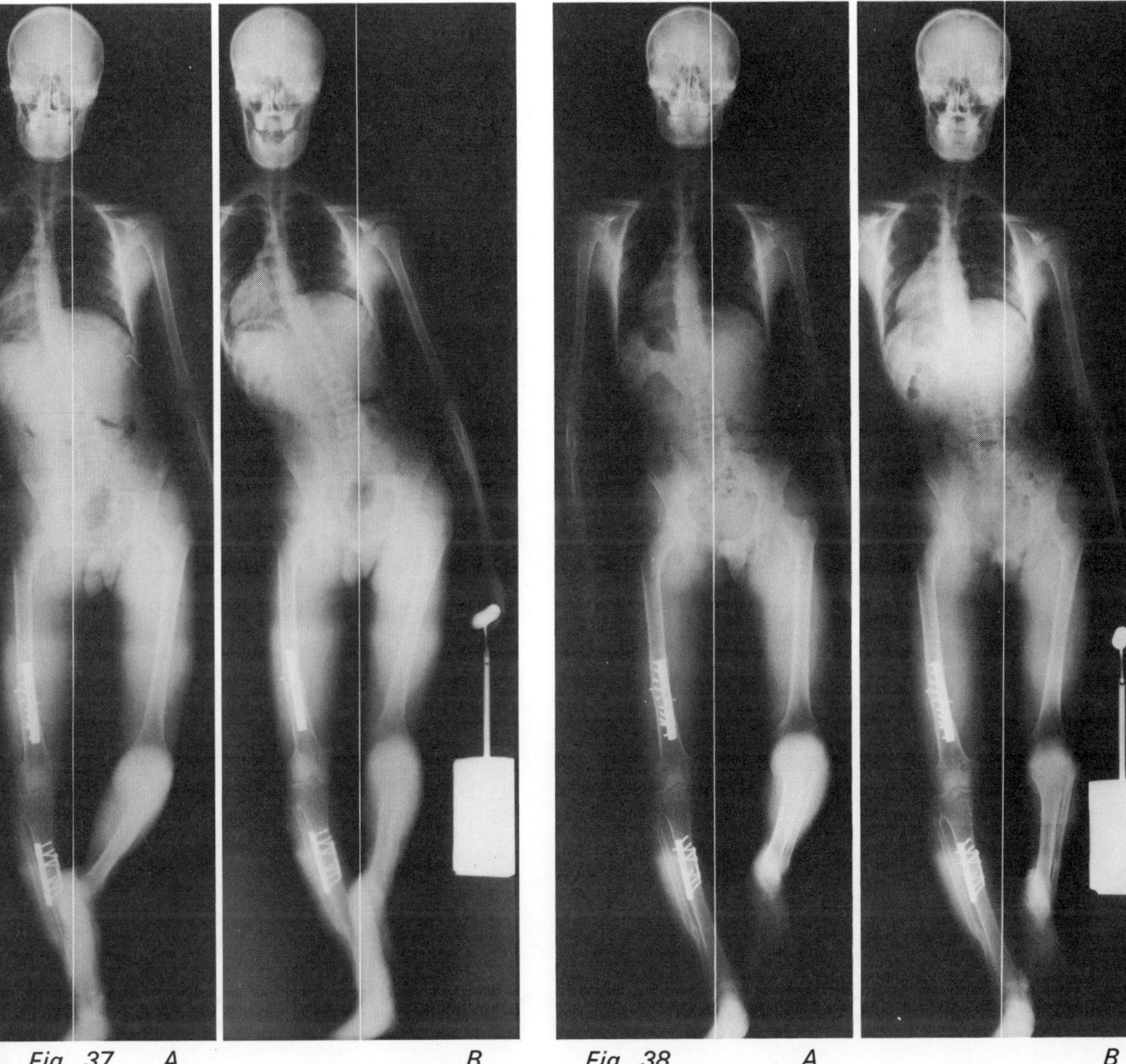

Fig. 37 A B

Fig. 38 A B

Awkwardness has been reduced partially (seven months after surgery).

Awkwardness of posture is further reduced. Improvement becomes evident when this photograph is compared to Figure 34-A. The recovery of a more natural posture is represented by the increase in the distance between the center of gravity line and the hip and knee joints of the leg supporting the weight. This allows the joints to support greater muscular forces and thereby increases stability.

Source: Suzuki Orthopedics Hospital

5. KINESIOLOGICAL LINKAGE AND RESPONSE OF BODY

In our day to day activities, our body makes a great variety of movements within the physiological limits of its joints. These movements made for various purposes, for the most part, are performed without special awareness of it. (In rehabilitation training or similar therapy, movements are practiced so that patients can perform them without need for special attention or effort.) There are times, however, when we move our body with specific awareness. Normally automatic movements come to a person's attention when there is acute pain or soreness (discomfort), as well as when there are impediments due to aging. Regardless of the situation, there are ways to make the movements necessary in carrying out daily activities easier, and these methods can be learned quite easily. As one example, a person can find the best position in which to hold the right arm that will make turning the head the easiest.

In this chapter an experiment using a water tank studying the body's responese to flexion and rotation of the neck, with attention to the shifting of weight, is detailed.

Kinesiological Effects of Neck Movements

The model in the water tank is using her back and toes as points of support (Fig. 1). The mechanism was set up so that when her knees were pushed forward 3 centimeters or more, her hips floated slightly upward. Also, applying more than 5 kilograms of force to either side of the center support axis caused a rotation. (5 kilograms of weight to the right causes inclination of subject to the right.) Vertical center lines have been added on the figures to serve as an index of movement and inclination.

When slowly turning her head to either side, the subject's hips move contralateral to the direction of neck rotation (Figs. 2 and 3). The difference in the degree of hip movement between rotation to the right and to the left is not significant. (About five seconds taken to complete neck rotation, the same hereafter.).

Similarly, when the neck is slowly flexed to the right and left sides, there is hip movement contralateral to the head movement (Figs. 4 and 5). The right and left differences in this case is also not significant. (About three seconds taken to complete neck flexion movement, the same hereafter.)

Fig. 1

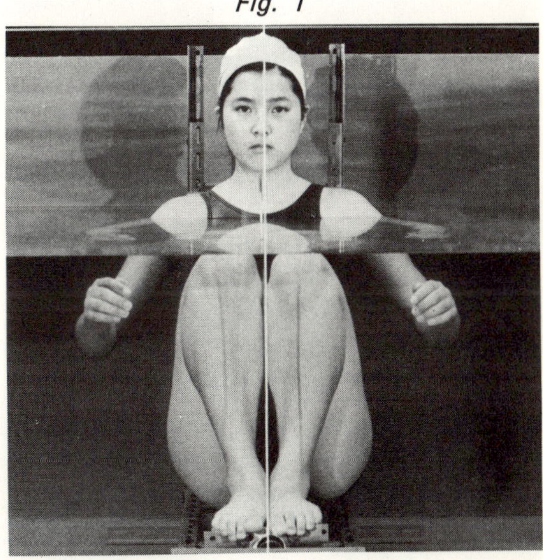

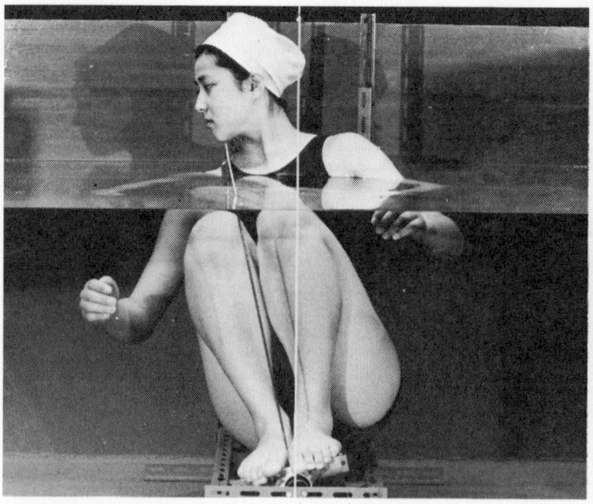

Fig. 2

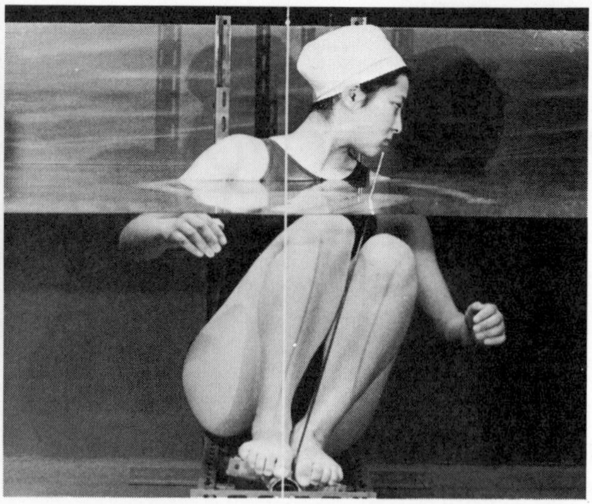

Fig. 3

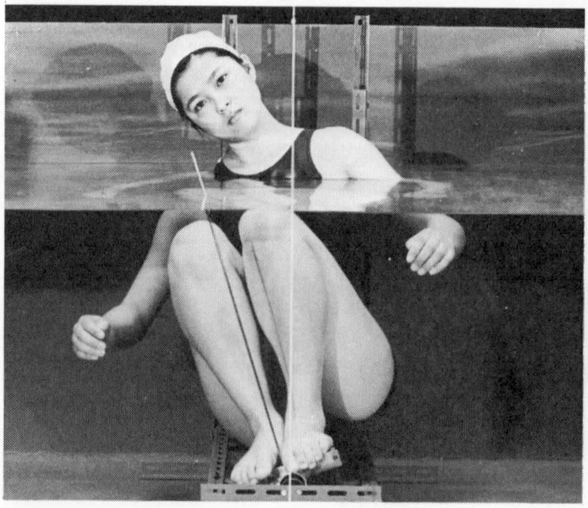

Fig. 4

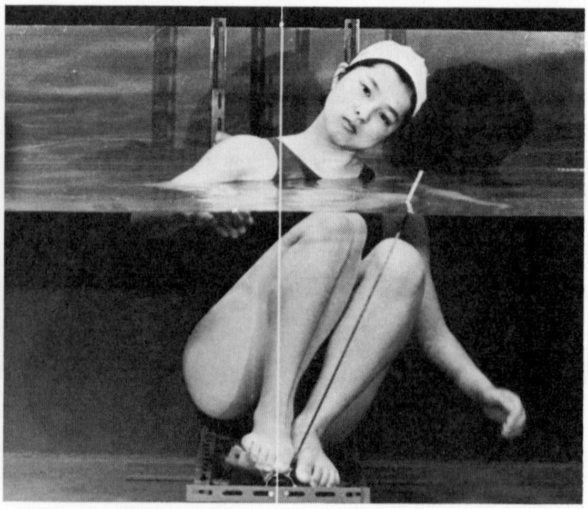

Fig. 5

When the right foot is used as the support point during bilateral neck rotation, hip movement is more pronounced during right rotation than during left rotation (Figs. 6 and 7). Also, the head is displaced farther from the center line when the rotation is toward the right, and the neck movement appears easier.

When the right foot is used as the support point during slow bilateral neck flexion, hip movement appears greater during left flexion than during right flexion (Figs. 8 and 9). Displacement of the head from the center line is also greater during left flexion.

Neck rotation using the left foot as the sup-

Fig. 6

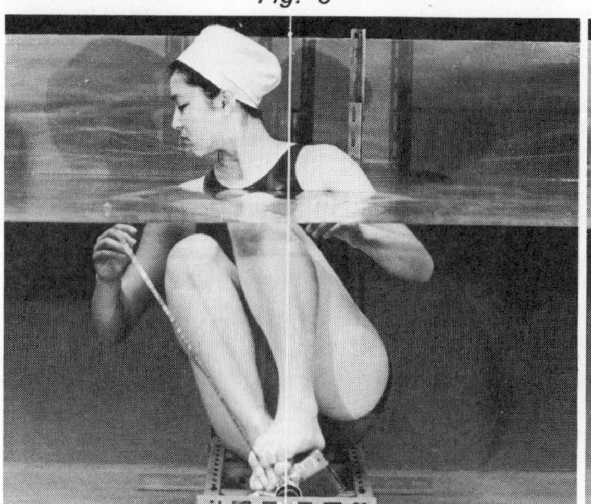

Fig. 7

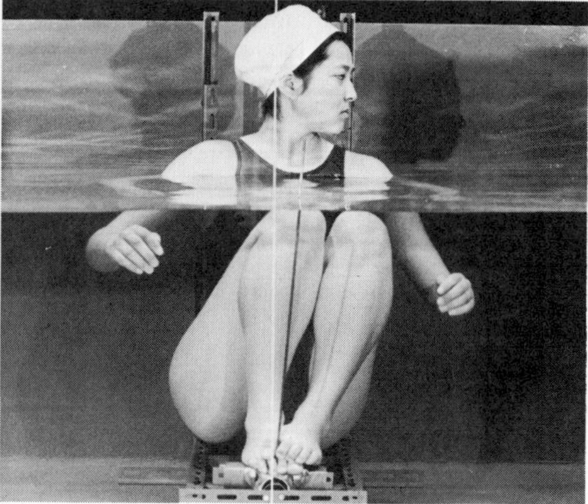

port point shows that both hip movement and head displacement are greater during rotation to the left than to the right (Figs. 10 and 11).

For neck flexion with the left foot as the support point, hip movement and head displacement are greater during right flexion (Figs. 12 and 13).

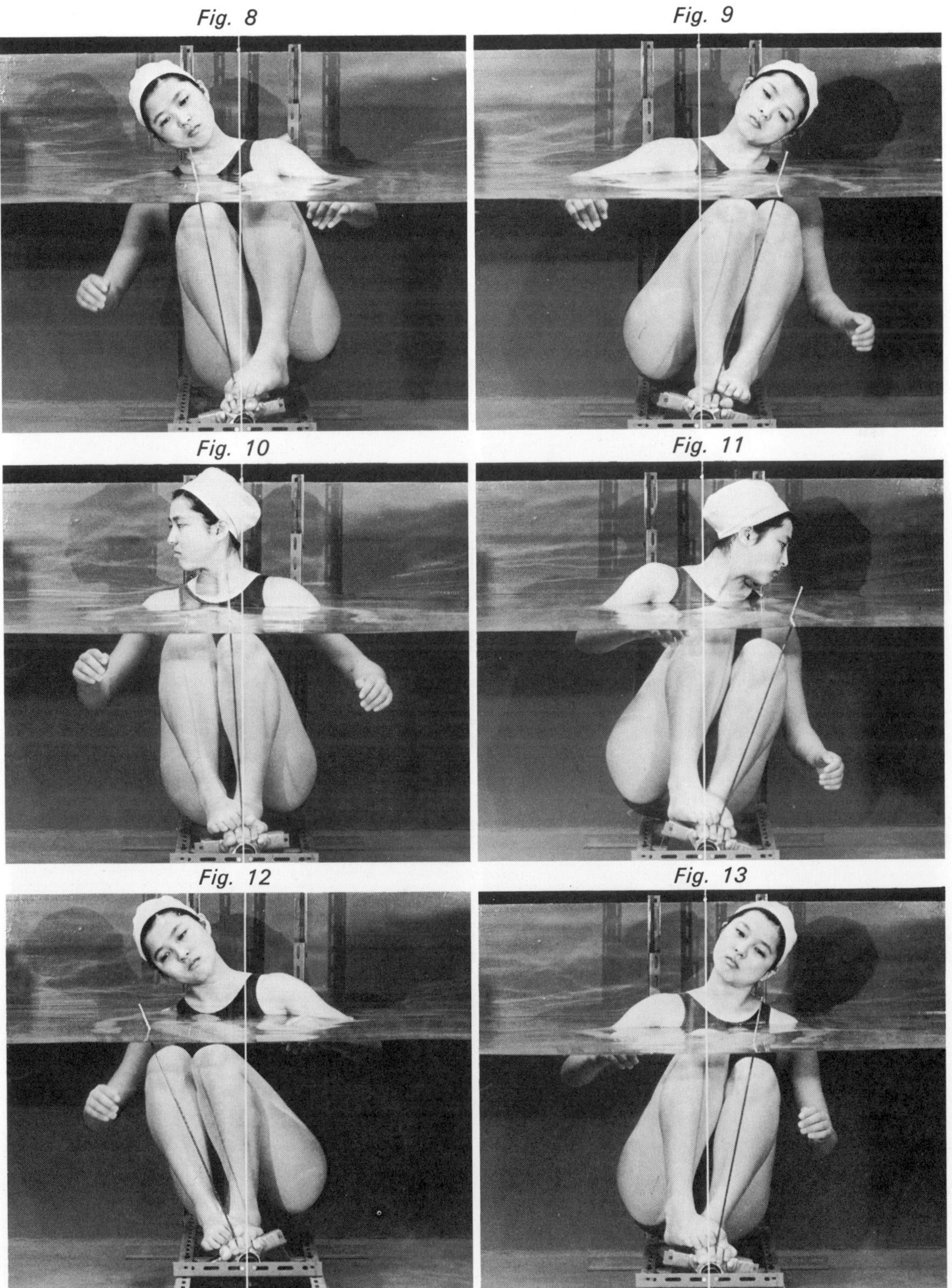

Fig. 8 *Fig. 9*

Fig. 10 *Fig. 11*

Fig. 12 *Fig. 13*

Kinesiological Response of Body to Neck Movements

With both feet used for support, the subject rotates her neck bilaterally (Figs. 14 and 15). She intentionally restrains her hips from moving as a result of rotating her neck.

After five seconds, she returns her head to face the front and releases the restraint on her hips (Figs. 16 and 17). In response to letting go of the restraint, the hips move toward the direction in which the neck had been rotated.

Using both her feet for support, the subject flexes her neck bilaterally and purposely restrains hip movement which would result from neck flexion (Figs. 18 and 19).

After five seconds, the subject straightens her neck to the upright and at the same time releases the restraint on her hips (Figs. 20 and 21). In reaction to this releasing force, the hips will move toward the direction in which the neck has been flexed.

While using first the right, and then the left foot as the support point, the model rotates her neck ipsilateral to the supporting foot while consciously restraining hip movement (Figs. 22 and 23).

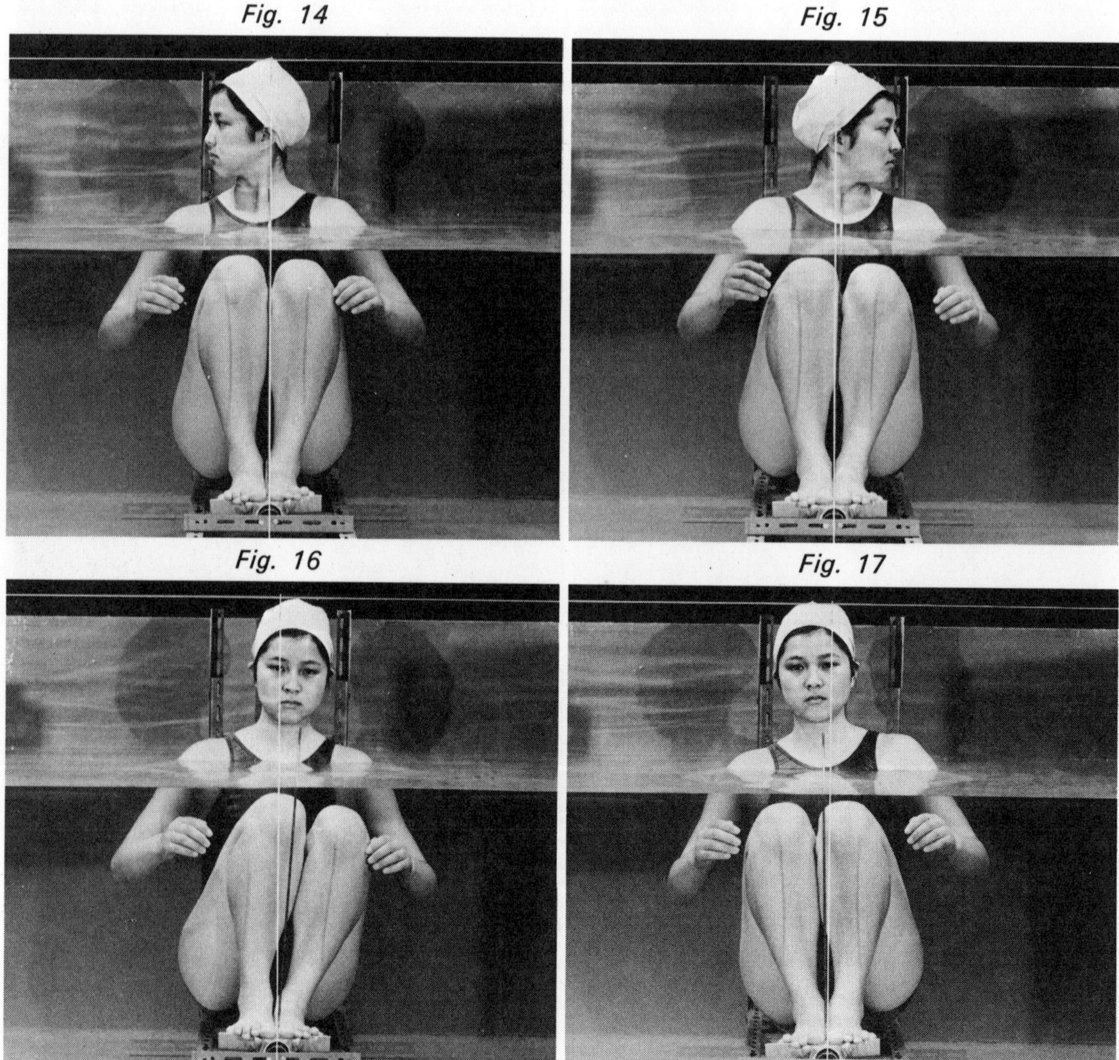

Fig. 14 *Fig. 15* *Fig. 16* *Fig. 17*

Fig. 18

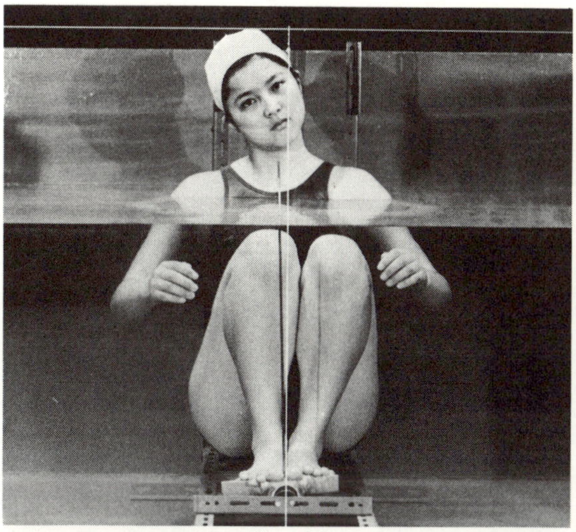

Fig. 19

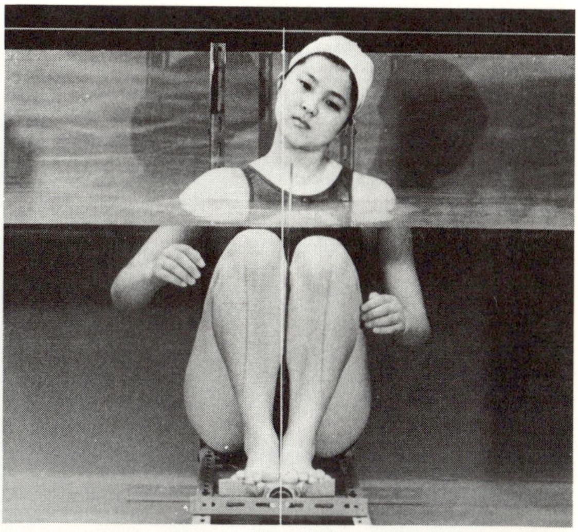

Fig. 20

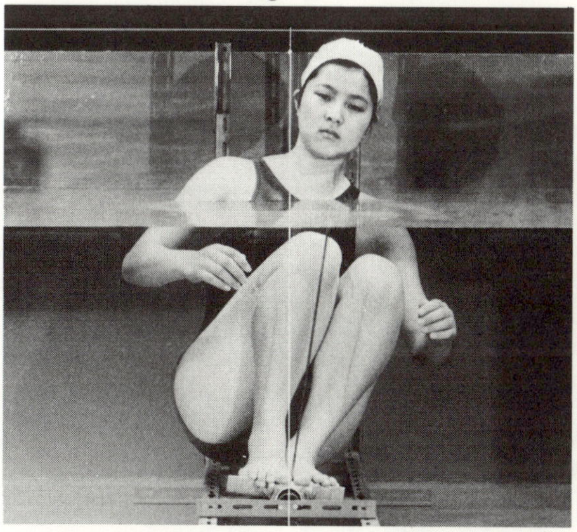

Fig. 21

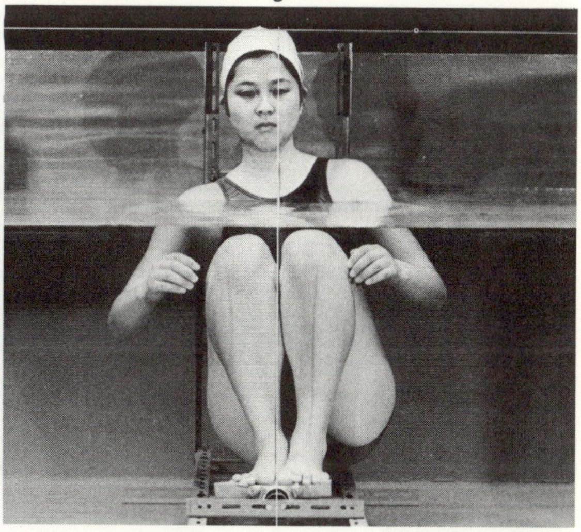

Fig. 22

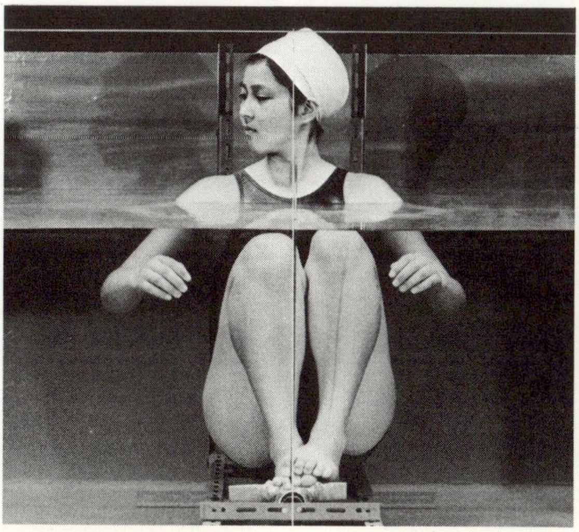

Fig. 23

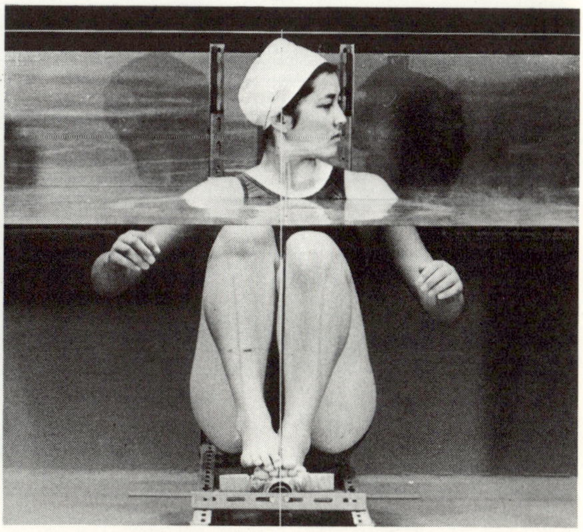

Facing forward again after five seconds and releasing the restraint kept on the hips still causes the hips to move toward the direction in which the head had been rotated (Figs. 24 and 25).

Using first the right, and then the left foot for support, the subject rotates her head contralateral to the supporting foot while consciously inhibiting hip movement (Figs. 26 and 27).

Returning the head and releasing the restraint simultaneously after five seconds still causes the

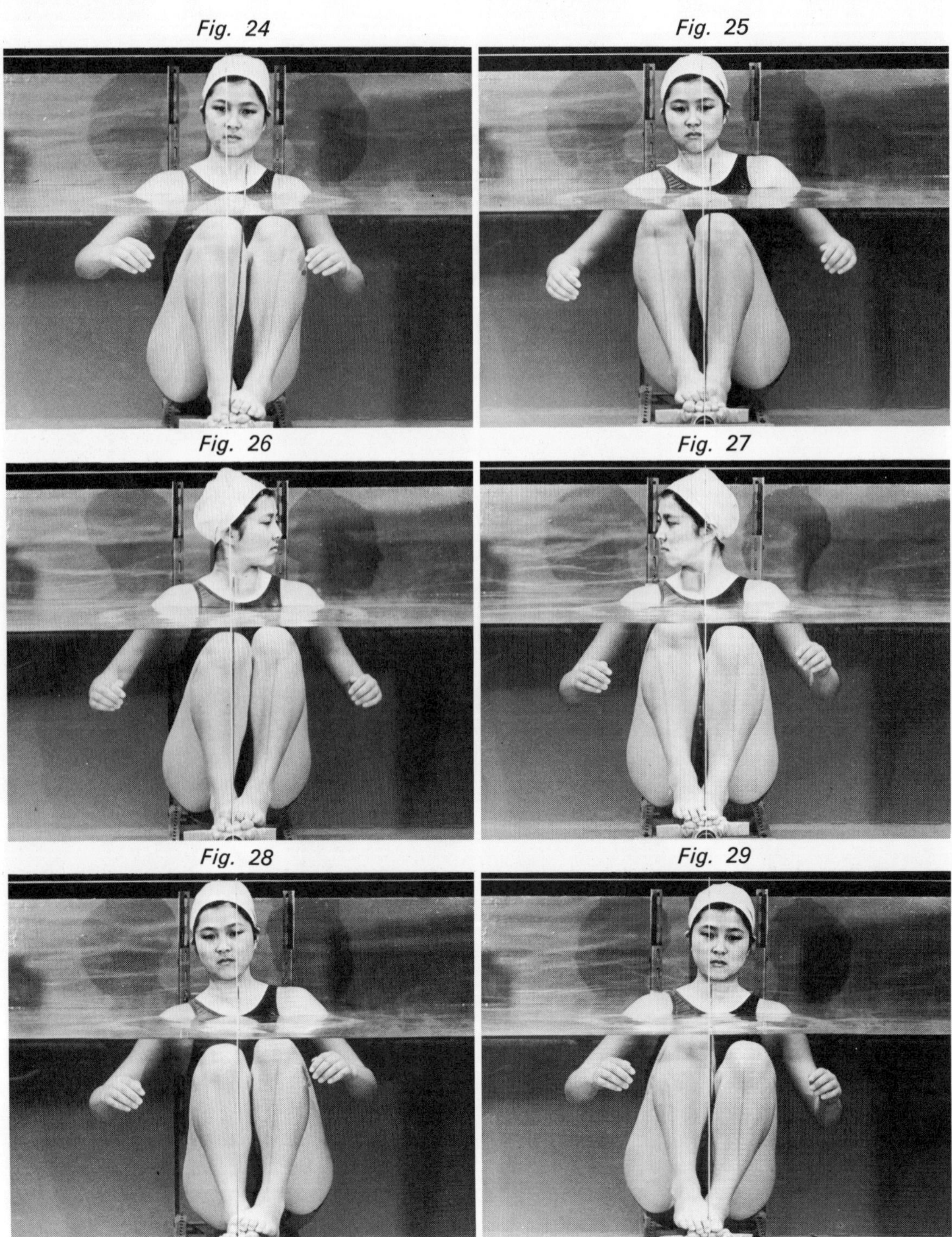

Fig. 24 *Fig. 25*

Fig. 26 *Fig. 27*

Fig. 28 *Fig. 29*

reaction in which the hips move toward the direction that the neck had been rotated (Figs. 28 and 29).

Using first the right, and then the left foot for support, the model flexes her neck to the right and consciously restrains hip movement (Figs. 30 and 31).

Regardless of which foot is used as the support point, when the neck is straightened and the restraint on the hips is released, the same reaction occurs (Figs. 32 and 33).

Using first the right, and then the left foot

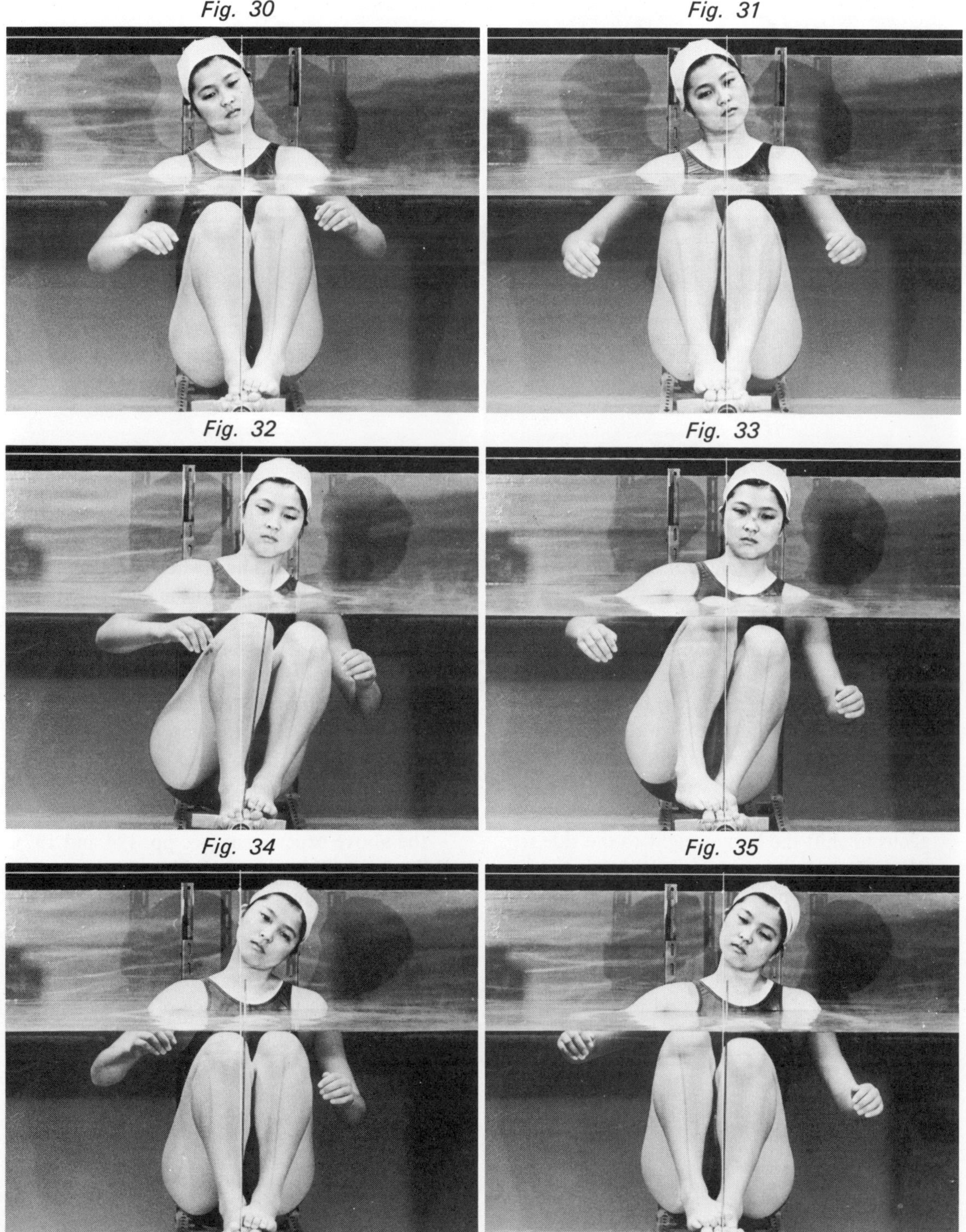

Fig. 30 *Fig. 31*

Fig. 32 *Fig. 33*

Fig. 34 *Fig. 35*

for support, the subject flexes her neck to the left while consciously restraining hip movement (Figs. 34 and 35).

In response to straightening the neck and relaxing the effort restraining hip movement, the hips move in the direction to which the neck had been flexed (Figs. 36 and 37).

Fig. 36

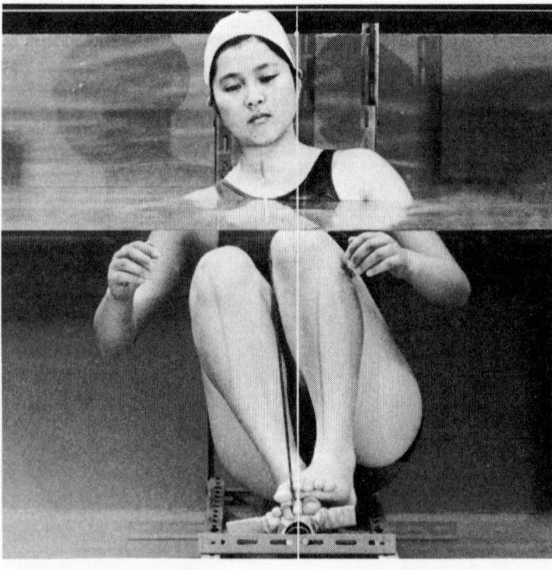

Fig. 37

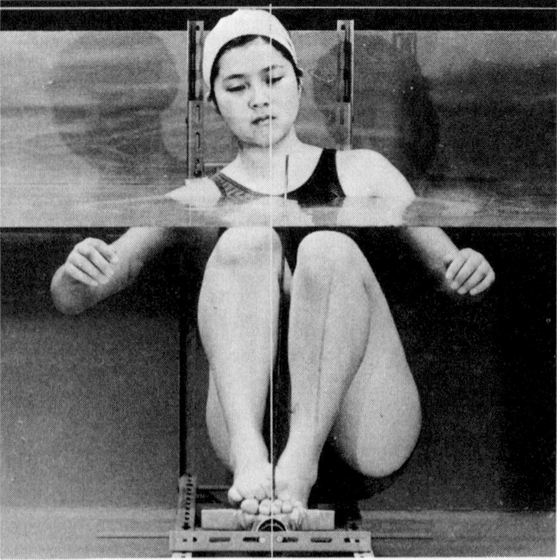

Observations from This Experiment

1. Neck rotation and the corresponding hip movement, and the angle of inclination, as well as the transfer of weight over to one foot, all appeared more smooth and substantial in Figures 6 and 11. It is clear from this that the rotation of the head to the same side of the body as the foot supporting the weight is the "easy way to move," or in this case, the easy direction in which to turn the head. In other words, this experiment provides proof that it is more advantageous to shift the body weight to the side to which the rotation is done, whether it be the rotation of the neck or of the entire body.
2. Lateral neck flexion and the corresponding hip movement, as well as the angle of inclination and the transfer of body weight to one foot, all appear smoother and more substantial in Figures 9 and 12. Accordingly, flexion of the neck to the side opposite the foot supporting the weight is the "easy way to move," or the easier direction in which to flex the neck. Thus, when the neck is flexed laterally, or when the entire body is flexed to one side, it is manifestly advantageous to place the body's weight (center of gravity) over the leg that is contralateral to the direction of flexion.
3. The importance of the proper transfer of weight during the twisting of the body in Basic Exercise 5 and during the lateral flexion of Basic Exercise 4 in Chapter 8 is proven in the above experiment (see pp. 194 and 197).
4. Figures 14 through 37 all illustrate how other body movements triggered by the rotation and flexion of the neck are restrained, and how the restraint is released after the neck is returned from flexion or rotation. The manner in which the influence of kinesiological factors are manifested in the body have been elucidated in this experiment.

6. MINOR SYMPTOMS—An Enigma to Modern Medicine

Minor Symptoms—Abnormal Sensitivity

Minor symptoms can be compared to foam which can sometimes be seen on stagnant parts of a stream. Rather than ignoring these superficial symptoms, they should be regarded as being significant indicators of a person's overall physical condition. The primary focus of diagnosis, nevertheless, must be kept on the "main stream," as the major obstructions to health need to be determined. Foam does not appear on clear running streams; when all physical mechanisms are operating as they should, no minor symptoms are present.

One's present physical state is the accumulated result of all of one's past living conditions. Concurrently, the physical state and living conditions of a person are closely interrelated. The job of a physician is to study the basic principles underlying this interrelationship. Providing instruction on healthful living should be the physician's prime responsibility. In order to fully apply the concept of the "reversibility" of a person's physical condition, physicians must first learn this principle for themselves. The study of kinesiology therefore, has truely become a field for professionals.

Reversibility of Health and Disease

There is an old saying in Oriental medicine which goes, "the superior physician cures incipient diseases while the lesser physician cures diseases after they appear." When a person's health begins to deteriorate, first abnormal sensitivity (tender spots) begins to appear, and next, functional disorders start to occur. Then the body becomes susceptible to invasions by pathogenic microorganisms and finally, gross organic disorders result. Recovery from disease occurs in reverse of the above sequence. Modern medicine concentrates on the structural changes, and the diagnostic and testing methods for this purpose have advanced to a remarkable degree, and yet, modern medicine is still reluctant to closely examine the abnormal sensitivity which accompanys disease. Health can be defined as a state of dynamic balance in the income and outgo of life energy in an individual. Human beings, in order to survive, must invariably perform a minimum of four basic functions for themselves. These four functions are respiration, injestion of nutrients, physical movements and mental activity. There are natural laws which govern each of these functions, and breaking any of these creates an imbalance. Modern medicine has largely neglected this most important point at which the imbalances first occur. To better understand this process, a more detailed examination of the physiology and morphology of the musculoskeletal system is necessary.

Physical Movement and Occurrence of Distortions

Structure of the Human Frame

If we liken the human body to a simple house, it may be illustrated as four pillars erected on four foundation stones, with crossbeams connecting the top of these four pillars, and with a roof set on top. The ceiling is held in place by cross-supports placed between the crossbeams. If this structure receives a head on one end of the roof and a tail on the other end, a four legged creature is created. The front facing triangle with the head becomes the shoulder area, and the rear triangle with the tail becomes the pelvis. The organs of this creature are contained between the roof and ceiling, and its spine is the ridgebeam. A human being is an animal similar in structure to this illustration, with the essential difference being that human beings stand erect on two legs. The most important thing about this structure is that it is capable of locomotion. When the aforementioned four basic functions go against the natural principles, the musculoskeletal system becomes distorted in form and in function.

Physiology of the Musculoskeletal System

Structural kinesiology applies to man—a mobile structure. When distortions occur in the musculoskeletal system due to some stress, abnormal tension is produced in the striated muscles connected to it. When excessive tension is created in muscles by overwork, they loose the ability to relax, causing distortions in the alignment of the skeletal structure. When such abnormal tension is allowed to persist over a long period of time, changes occur in the soft tissues surrounding these tense muscles, due to "internal pressure." When such "internal pressure" reaches a certain point, the peripheral blood vessels and nerves exhibit dysfunctions, initially in their kinesiological composition, and subsequently, in their biochemical components. The reduced circulation in the affected area also results in localized anoxia which is registered by sensory receptors as an abnormal sensation or soreness. In this manner, mechanisms triggering a series of functional disorders are set off. The exact mechanisms involved in this process have yet to be defined, but experiments on excessive stimulation of the autonomic nervous system by Réle in France, investigations related to pressure sensitive reactions by Takagi, a Japanese physiologist at Nagoya University, and studies regarding the "meridian phenomenon" by Dr. Fujita in Kanazawa, Japan, are all expected to contribute significantly to our understanding of the mechanisms involved in this process.

General Tendencies of Right Handed People

A person's body tends ot lean toward the side where the force is being exerted during physical movements and one's center of gravity usually

Fig. 1

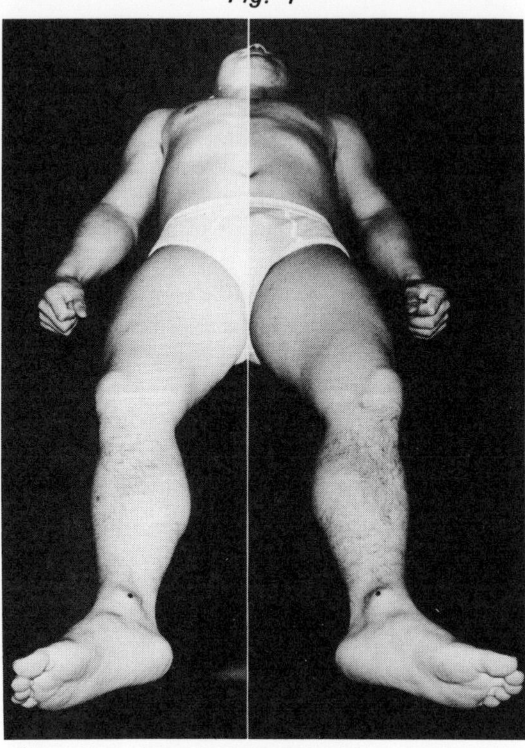

inclines in that direction. When such movements become a habit ingrained over many years, the active side of the body becomes stretched while the opposite side becomes contracted.

When the right and left legs of persons with a habit of keeping their weight on the right leg are compared at their medial malleoli, the left leg is often found to be shorter (Fig. 1). Their pelvis is inclined down to the right and the left superior anterior iliac spine is higher in most cases, than the right. Also the chest is often found to be thicker on the left side than on the right (Fig. 2). Many such persons experience discomfort on their left side. In the prone position, the ribs on the left side feel stiffer and sit higher. People with this condition have a tendency toward dysfunction of the heart and digestive system.

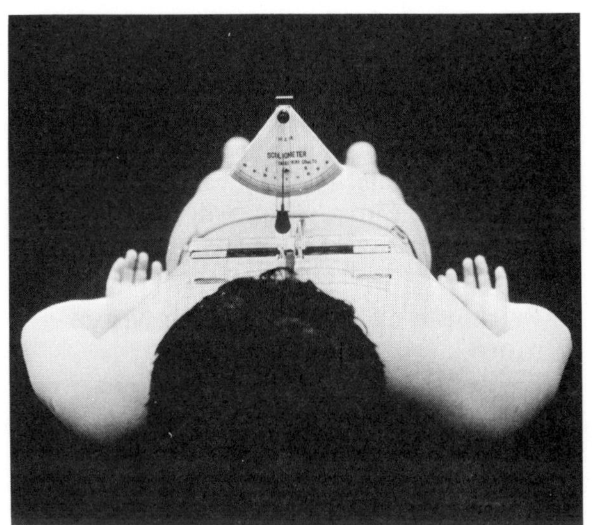

Fig. 2

Principles of Physical Movement

Principle of Movement in Linkage

Our musculoskeletal system is a mechanism controlled and coordinated by the central nervous system. When one part of the body is moved for any reason, all other parts move in linkage. It may seem like a person's finger or toe moves independently, however, if an attempt is made to move the thumb after tying it down, it becomes very apparent how sucesive joints begin to move in linkage and movement extends up the limb.

When a distortion occurs in one part of the body, other parts also become distorted in attempt to compensate for it. Conversely, to correct such distortions, the manipulation of distal parts can have positive results on another part far removed.

Principle of the Center of Gravity

All movements should ideally be performed with the lumbar vertebrae held straight and used as the axis. For this purpose, all movements must be performed with the force coming to bear on the big toe in the case of feet, and on the little finger in the case of hands. Movements performed in this manner allow for the greatest amount of efficiency and mobility with the least amount of effort, as well as being more graceful in appearance. All martial arts, dance, and many sports are based on this principle. The greater distance a pivotal point of a movement is from the center, the greater the imbalance which tends to cause distorsions. Many traditional disciplines of the Orient emphasize the importance of centering one's energy in the lower stomach; this was derived precisely from the understanding of this basic principle.

Principle of Shifting Weight

One's center of gravity (weight) must be shifted to the other side during a flexing movement, and the same side during extension or rotation movements. When this rule is not followed, not only is the movement inefficient, but distortions could result if it is forced. People involved in physical education should be well aware of this fact, and this point must be taught before anyone takes up a sport or begins an exercise program. Typically, calisthenics are performed incorrectly, especially those involving lateral flexion of the trunk.

Principle of Exhaling with Movement

Fast or powerful movements must be performed with the breath held, or while exhaling. Our nervous system and muscles do not coordinate effectively in movements performed while inhaling. In boxing matches for example, a boxer finds an opening to punch when his opponent is inhaling. Similarly, slipped disks inadvertently occur, in many cases, while one is inhaling.

Relationship of Emotions to Posture

The body assumes different postures in relation to one's mood. When a person becomes angry, his blood rises; when sad or worried, a person tends to assume a bent forward posture, and this exerts pressure on the lungs and digestive organs. When a person is striken with fear or surprise, this is said to adversely affect the kidneys in Oriental medicine. A person who is full of motivation, on the other hand, assumes a bold and upright posture.

It is not possible to induce another emotion while a person remains fixed in a certain posture. Emotions also are related to the angle or the level at which the eyes are fixed. When people are in a cheerful mood they tend to look up, while if they are depressed, they tend to look down. It is easier to concentrate when you hold a steady gaze. A person looking out of the corner of his eyes tends to be anxious and suspicious. These and many other examples from everyday observation point to the close link between emotions and one's posture.

Relationship of Diet to Health

One's diet is very much related to one's flexibility and endurance, however, discussion on this broad topic will be left to books devoted to the subject. It may be pointed out nevertheless, that imbalanced diets, habitual overeating (especially of meat), and overconsumption of white sugar are best avoided, as evidenced in recent studies. The most important thing is that everybody study what constitutes a healthy diet for themselves.

Treating Distortions in Musculoskeletal System

As pointed out earlier, when distortions occur in the musculoskeletal system, this is manifested as an abnormal posture. Localized distortions or indurations and contraction or atony results in addition to abnormal sensitivity to pressure and heat.

When a patient exhibiting such symptoms makes a movement, limitations become apparent in their ability to move completely through the normal range of motion. Such people tend to feel uneasy most of the time and find it difficult to enjoy themselves. If they are forced to make a movement in the normal range, they experience pain. This condition can be compared with a river in which the flow has become stagnant; various secondary symptoms begin to manifest themselves.

Treatments for Correcting Abnormal Morphology

Vital points, called acupuncture points, are associated with functional abnormalities and organic disorders which become manifested as abnormally sensitive areas on the skin. These points have been compiled empirically from ancient times in the Orient, and acupuncture, moxibustion and acupressure are based on this knowledge. These traditional methods of treatment are used widely today to correct physical imbalances. Other important Oriental healing arts are the *Dō-in* therapeutic exercises and the Japanese *Amma* massage techniques which were developed from *Dō-in*. Also, there are a wide variety of Western massage techniques, physical therapy and thermotherapies for correcting various physical abnormalities, and innumerable books explaining these methods are available. Many of these methods can be used to compliment Sōtai Therapy.

In all these methods which apply various forms of external stimulus to the body, first a localized abnormal area is located and then attempts are made to alleviate or correct the misalignment in the skeletal structure or to reduce abnormal tension and pressure in soft tissues to resolve distortions in the musculoskeletal system. These methods, without exception, correct distortions in an indirect way and facilitate the natural healing process.

Dynamic Treatments for Correcting Abnormal Morphology

Sōtai is a method for restoring the balance in physical form by examination of physical structure and the performance of movements based on the observation of the range of motion (mobility examination), as described in this book.

A. Passive movement

Many practitioners involved in providing such exercise or manipulation are not fully aware of the kinesiological principles involved, and therefore tend to concern themselves only with the localized and obvious distortions. *Seikotsu* (traditional bone setting in Japan) and chiropractic are among the common passive movement methods used in Japan.

B. Active movement

To succeed in this method, one must not only have a complete understanding of all the kinesiological principles, but must also be able to appy these properly.

Kinesiological Analysis

Every freely movable joint in the body has its own characteristic range of motion, and its movements can be classified into "octants" or eight kinds of motion.

These "octants" are; (1) anteflexion and dorsiflexion, (2) right and left lateral flexion, (3)

Fig. 3–a

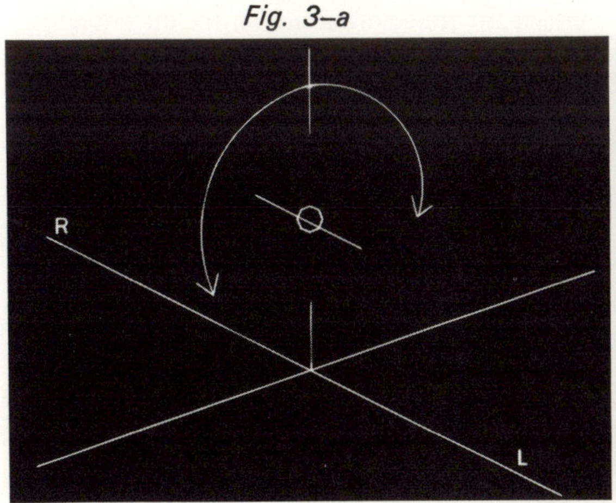

Fig. 3–b

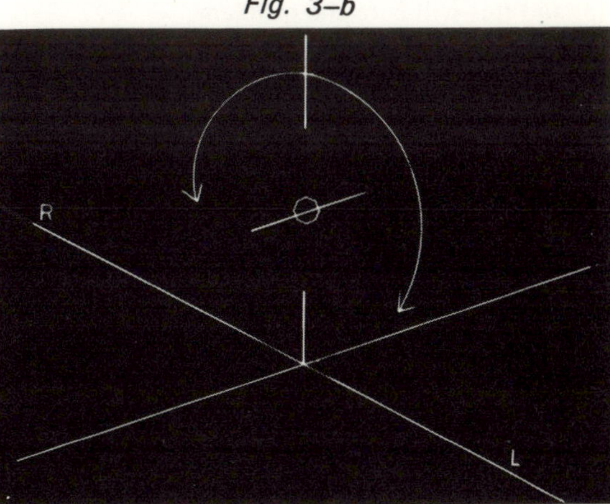

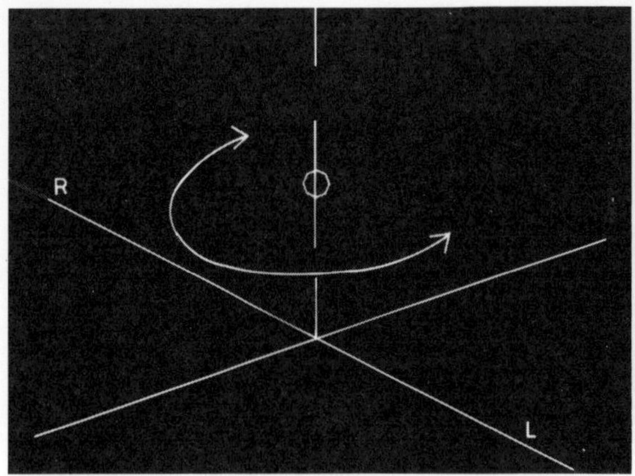

Fig. 3–c

Fig. 3–d

right and left axial rotation, and (4) contraction and extension by compressing or pulling on the joint (Fig. 3).

In joints with distortions, kinesiological analysis (referred to as mobility examination in this book) will reveal the direction and angle of the reduction in the range of motion. The motion of the abnormal joint moving back away from its maximum limit of mobility serves as the movement correcting the distortion. This may seem like an obvious point, but in fact, most everyone has failed to realize this simple point.

The author explains this principle to his patients this way: "When a movement is painful, it is just like a red light ahead; it is a warning signal to stop further movement because if continued, it could cause more complications. All one needs to do is to back the movement up, and this will cure the problem."

This corrective movement will not have the proper effect, however, unless the movement backtracks exactly on the initial course of movement. The corrective movement can be performed either actively or passively; it makes no difference. What is important, is to perform the kinesiological analysis to confirm the proper course, and to follow this precisely in reverse.

The proper corrective movement is usually pleasurable for the patient. Also, the more the corrective movement approaches the ideal, the less difference there is in the sensations produced by movements in the opposite direction. Once this principle is understood, these corrective movements can be performed by oneself (doing these movements on your own several times a day, after first checking for the comfortable direction, is like keeping up regular maintenance on a piece of machinery).

Distortions in the musculoskeletal system can be corrected by each individual. Even so, there are certain principles involved in these movements, and unless these are adhered to, there is always a danger of making a mistake and compounding the problem. Once the proper corrective movements are learned and repeated, the range of motion reduced by the physical distortion will be restored, and in turn, this increased range will have a beneficial effect on one's health.

There is no need to force movements to increase the range of motion in the direction restricted by the distortion. It is possible to increase the range of mobility of a joint by forcing it little by little over a period of time. However, any improvement is mostly a result of developing a resistance to the pain, and the "vector" of this type of increase in mobility is no different than that brought about by Sōtai movements. At present, by in large, forced movements are performed for rehabilitation and physical therapy, and not only does this demand that the patients endure a considerable amount of pain, but also it requires an undue amount of time and repetition.

Induction Technique by Active Movement

In Sōtai therapy, after the therapist locates an abnormality in one of the patient's joints, all the "octants" are checked by kinesiological analysis of four types of movement as described earlier, supporting the joint so that movement takes place only in the desired direction. In this way, the exact direction and angle of the distortion in movement becomes clear. The patient is then instructed to move the affected joint to the farthest extent comfortable, and to bring it back all the way in the opposite direction against the resistance provided by the therapist. This movement should be comfortable to perform for the patient. When the farthest point of comfortable movement is reached in the return movement, the therapist increases the resistance slightly as the patient stops the movement. Tension is held for a few seconds; then the patient relaxes all effort at once. The distortion is corrected as each component part falls back into line with the releasing action. When done correctly, the very first attempt usually proves effective.

Sōtai movements performed in the comfortable direction must be executed while the patient is slowly exhaling and as relaxed as possible. When done in this way, the principle of movement in linkage makes all the parts involved in the movement move in concert. This acts to correct the various misalignments as if they were linked together in a chain.

When this induction technique is performed on all joints with distortions, it can be seen how all movements become adjusted to the optimum angle and direction. The body *wants* to have all its parts return to the right position.

It will take some practice to become adept at performing this technique, but actually it is not very difficult. If the correction is not complete in the first attempt, the same technique should simply be repeated in a relaxed manner. Certain cases do require more time since there are differences in the history and degree of distortions.

Examination and Treatment of Minor Symptoms

It is said that the renowned physician Kiva of ancient India used a small stick like a conductor's stick to examine his patients. What could this have been used for? The difference between a distorted physique and a healthy balanced physique can clearly be seen as incongruity in the right/left, upper/lower and anterior/posterior halves of the body. One must pay close attention, because whether standing, sitting or lying down, some discrepancy is always present. This becomes apparent when two halves of the body are examined in contrast to each other. This imbalance becomes even more evident when the parts in question are moved. The kinesiological analysis must be performed in several postures so as to get the total picture.

Examination in the Supine Position

First observe the inclination or attitude of the feet and check the movement of the ankle joints (Fig. 4). Next flex the knees while keeping them together. Then place four fingers in each popliteal fossa and hold the area right below the patellas with the thumbs, checking the tendons of the flexor muscles for sensitivity by giving them a sideways snapping motion (Fig. 5). In some cases this will cause the patient to jump with pain in the popliteal region. This sensitivity is found more often on the left side.

Next, the therapist inserts both hands under the patient's hips and palpates the lateral ends of the sacrum on both sides from top to bottom (Fig. 6). Often, pressure sensitivity can

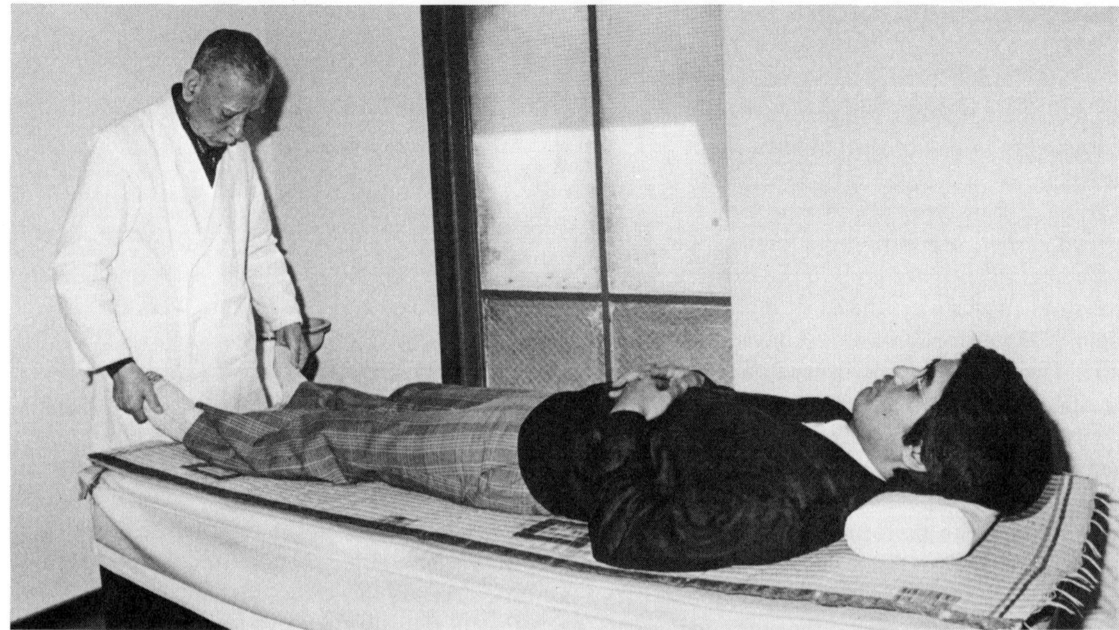

Fig. 4

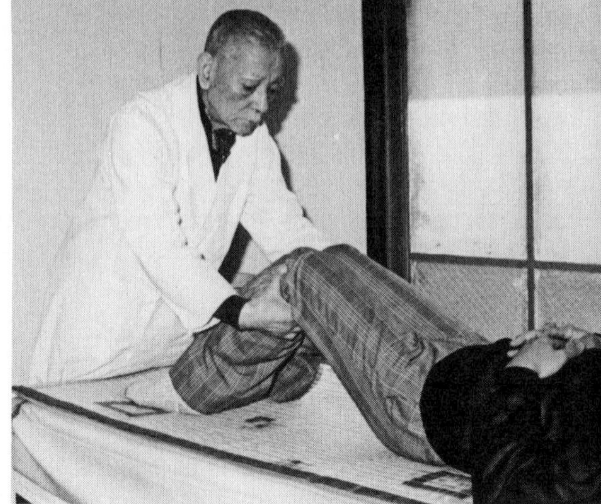

Fig. 5

be detected near the midpoint between the top and bottom end of the sacroiliac joint (close to the origin of the piriform muscles). This sensitivity is found more commonly on the left side.

The patient is instructed to keep his heel on the table while extending the distal end of the left foot raising the toes dorsally as far as they go. The therapist provides resistance by pressing down with the heel of his right hand on the foot and proximal ends of the patient's toes (Fig. 7). After holding tension for a few seconds, the patient relaxes the effort all at once allowing the left foot to fall back on the table. The pain in the popliteal region should disappear, and the sensitivity in the piriform muscle should also be gone.

If some tenderness still remains in the affected areas, have the patient bring both knees down laterally to the left until they come in contact with the table. The therapist then gives resistance to the movement of the knees going back up, placing his right hand on the outside of the knees (Fig. 8). It is permissible for the hips and back of the patient to rise slightly up off the table, and for the body to twist to some extent. Let patients move naturally according to their ability; the therapist need only provide resistance. The hypersensitivity in the piriform muscle should be gone without a trace after the routine procedure of movement against resistance, holding tension, and then releasing, is repeated a few times.

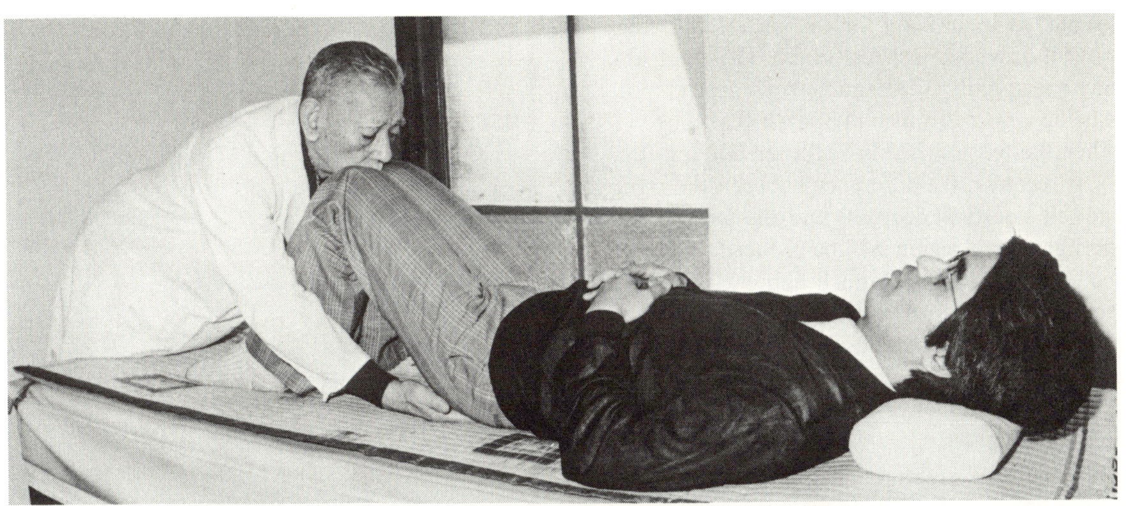

Fig. 6

Fig. 7

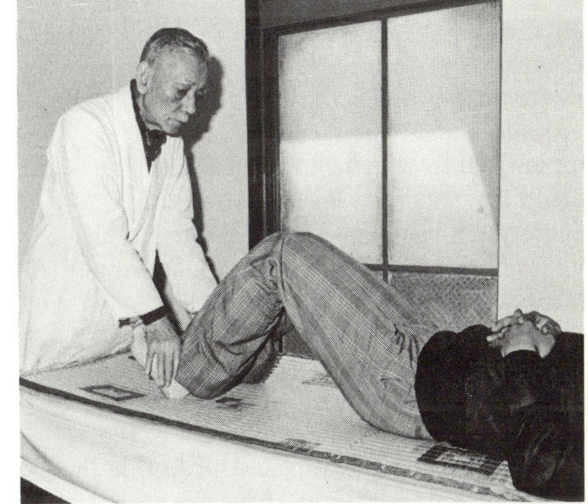

Low back pain on either side can be largely eliminated through this technique. If the first attempt is not successful, try it again. Most symptoms similar to that of a "slipped disk" will often disappear as if by magic.

Next, raise both knees flexing them and drawing them up as close to the chest as possible. When comparing the movement of the right and left legs, usually the right leg tends to be slightly less flexible. In this case, the right leg more often exhibits swelling and pain when grasped at the calf. Supporting the leg with the

Fig. 8

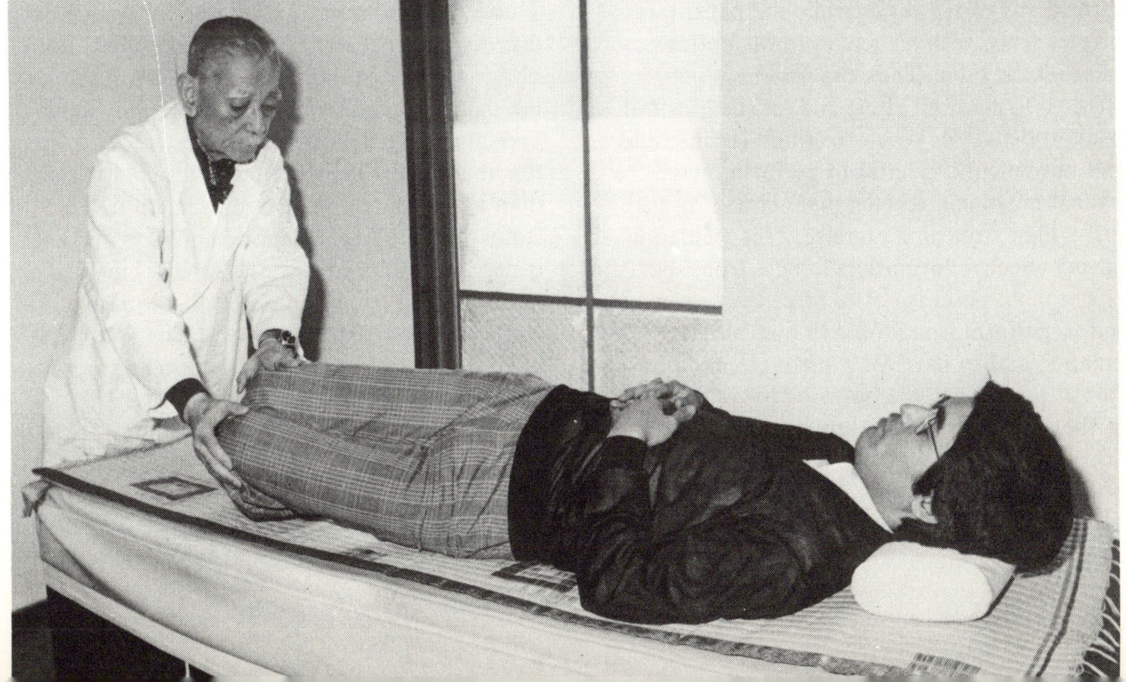

discomfort by holding the calf, have the patient move it down against resistance. The right hip may rise slightly off the table since resistance is being applied from underneath that limb. When the tension is released after holding for a few seconds, the difference between the right and left sides will decrease and the tension in the right flank region will be reduced. Also, the left leg should feel much lighter. This technique can be performed on either the right or left leg depending on the patient. This technique is effective in removing the feeling of fatigue in the lower limbs to make them feel much lighter.

The skeletal structure becomes looser as a person becomes tired. For example, the space between the tibia and fibula increases when fatigued (Figs. 9 and 10). When the above Sōtai technique is performed, relief from many gastrointestinal disorders can also be obtained, especially simple "stomach problems." It is not unusual for a patient to begin belching after a few Sōtai movements. Also quick recovery can be obtained from fatigue resulting from long walks or runs by application of this technique.

Since it is not easy for the therapist to hold the legs of the patient in the above mentioned Sōtai technique, the therapist can sit on the table in the Seiza posture at the foot of the patient. The patient then places his feet on the thighs of the therapist just above the knees (refer to p. 60, Chapter 2, Supine J-1). The legs can then be supported easily while the patient presses down with his feet until his buttocks raise off the table. Then the patient is instructed to relax all effort and let the hips fall back to the table. When the thigh is tense and this movement is painful to perform, make the patient move in a relaxed manner as if it were just a light stretching exercise. This technique is very effective for muscle fatigue from sports.

The main point is not to force the movement, but to perform it in a relaxed and pleasant manner, and to have the patient release all effort at once. Then the buttocks lift off the table in the above movement, tension in the upper abdomen decreases and discomfort in the abdominal organs is also reduced.

Fig. 9

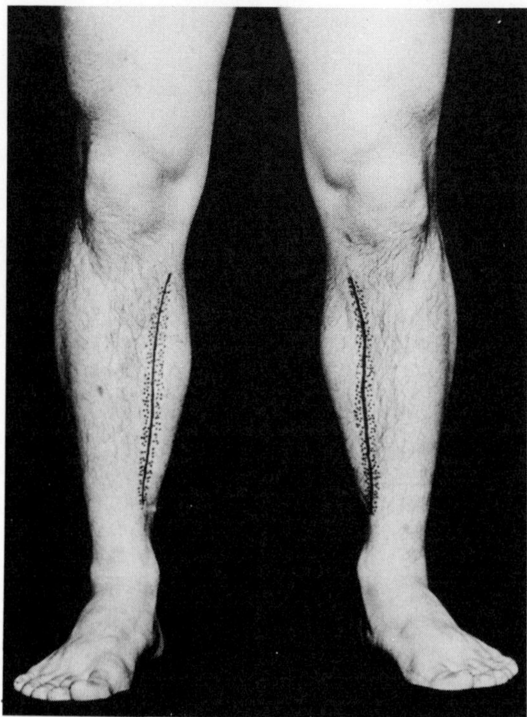

"When house calls were requested for acute abdominal pain, they often turned out to be nothing more than the retension of gas in either the transverse colon." (Roemheld: 1912)

Draw the knees about halfway up by flexing them in the supine position and raise the buttocks by placing a small cushion underneath. This reduces tension in the upper abdomen by decreasing the distance between the pubic symphysis and the xiphoid process. Next, placing the palms on the lower abdomen, apply light pressure while the patient exhales slowly from the abdomen (Fig. 11). It should take no more than a few minutes before movement in the stomach can be heard and felt. This is all that is necessary to relieve simple stomach pain; no drug need be administered. If the above method is not sufficient in removing abdominal pain, organic disorders necessitating a careful examination may be indicated.

The above example illustrates just how closely

Fig. 10

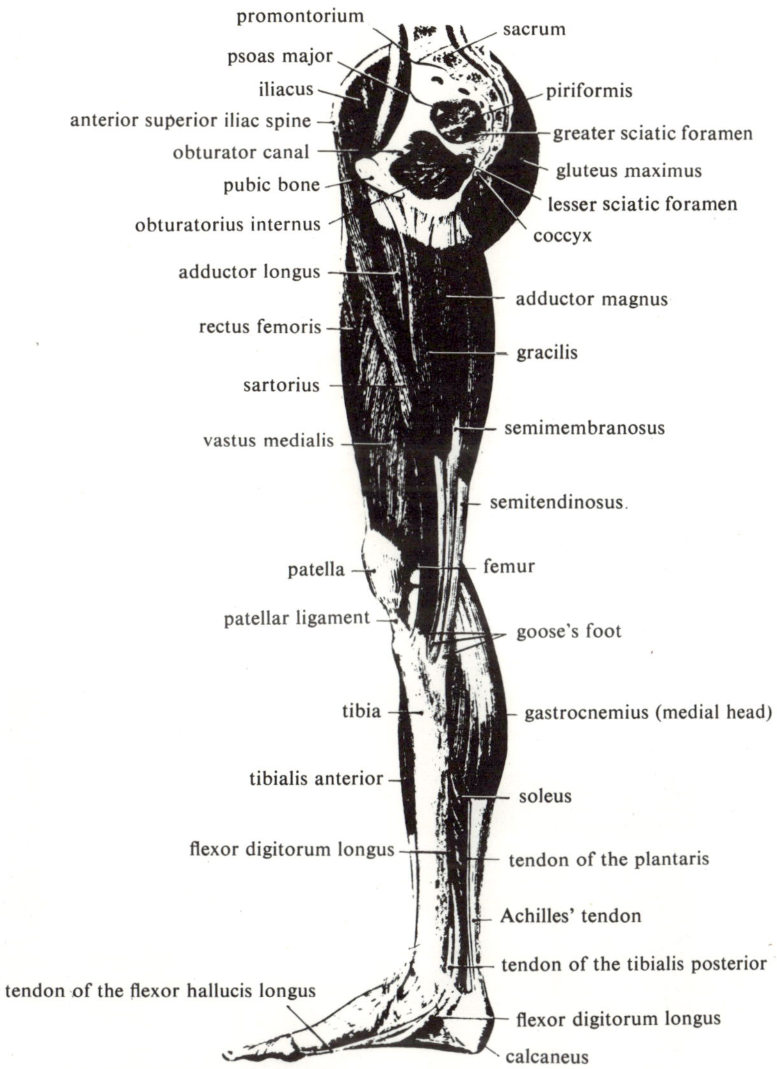

promontorium
sacrum
psoas major
iliacus
piriformis
anterior superior iliac spine
greater sciatic foramen
obturator canal
gluteus maximus
pubic bone
lesser sciatic foramen
obturatorius internus
coccyx
adductor longus
adductor magnus
rectus femoris
gracilis
sartorius
semimembranosus
vastus medialis
semitendinosus
patella
femur
patellar ligament
goose's foot
tibia
gastrocnemius (medial head)
tibialis anterior
soleus
flexor digitorum longus
tendon of the plantaris
Achilles' tendon
tendon of the tibialis posterior
tendon of the flexor hallucis longus
flexor digitorum longus
calcaneus

Fig. 11

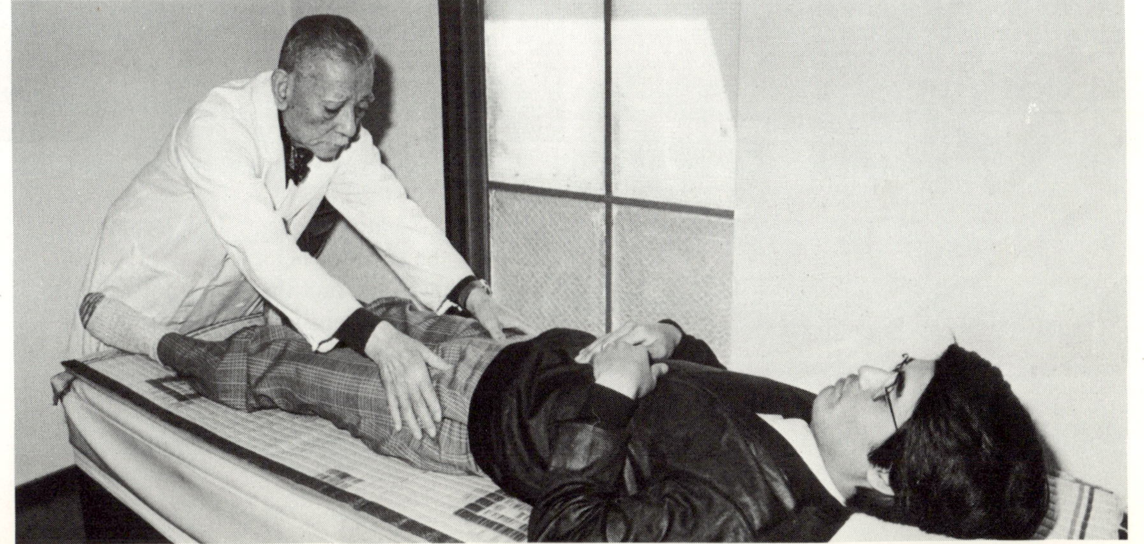

distortions in physical structure are linked with dysfunctions of internal organs. Those people who cannot seem to get rid of a cold, or who seem to have poor circulation often experience acute pain upon application of finger pressure to the left inguinal region. This hypersensitivity can be corrected by rotating the legs laterally and drawing one limb up to the side by abducting the hip joint as much as possible against resistance provided by the therapist, and holding and releasing tension in the usual manner (Fig. 12). The right hip can lift off the table, and the right knee may bend somewhat in this movement without influencing the results.

The majority of patients seem to have an excessive amount of tension in their femoral adductor muscles (Fig. 13). When this is the case, have the patient spread his knees as far apart as possible against resistance, with the knees half flexed (Fig. 14). The tension in the adductor muscles should diminish once the buttocks are allowed to fall back to the table limply, from the slightly raised position held during the Sōtai movement. This technique also has the effect of helping clear the vision. This is due to the fact that the point with the greatest pressure sensitivity on the adductor canal is also a trigger point for ocular function.

Fig. 12

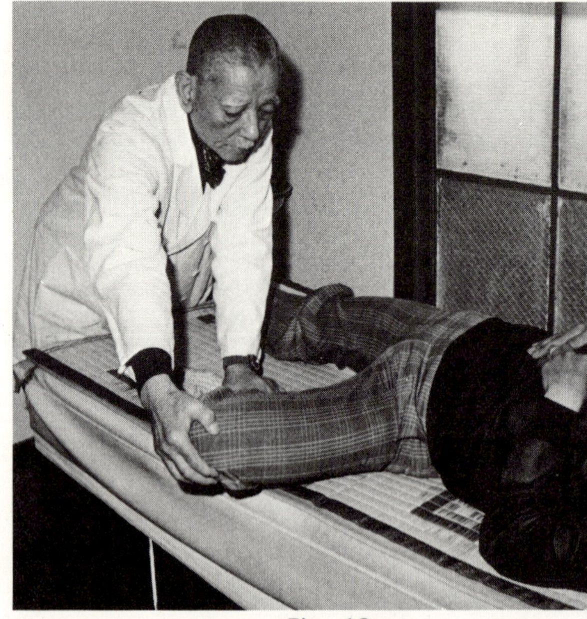

Fig. 13

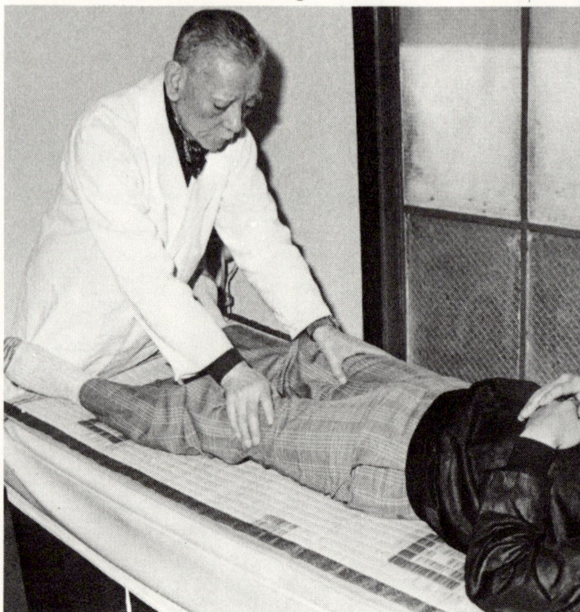

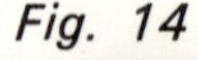

Fig. 14

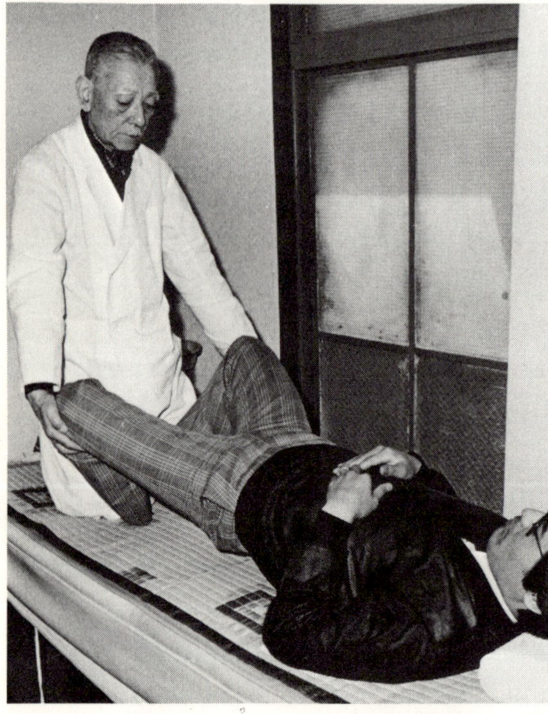

Examination in the Prone Position

As mentioned in a previous chapter, for most people, there is a tendency for their ribs to be higher on the left side when lying in the prone position, and for there to be more muscle tension on the left side than on the right. In order to balance the height of the dorsal costal arches a Sōtai movement is performed abducting the hip joint and drawing the knee up to the side against resistance (Fig. 15).

Next, the vertebrae are inspected for misalignment by palpating both sides of the spinous processes successively from top to bottom. Misalignment of a vertebra is evident when finger pressure applied to each side of the vertebra in question produces a distinctly different sensation on each side. In this case, lift the shoulders of the patient alternately from underneath while pressing on the most sensitive point along the spine. Look for the shoulder position causing the least pain at the sensitive point under pressure (Fig. 16). Then have the patient move the shoulder into this position against resistance, followed by the standard Sōtai procedure of holding tension and releasing. Repeat this technique until a noticeable change is brought about.

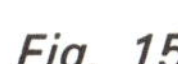

Fig. 15

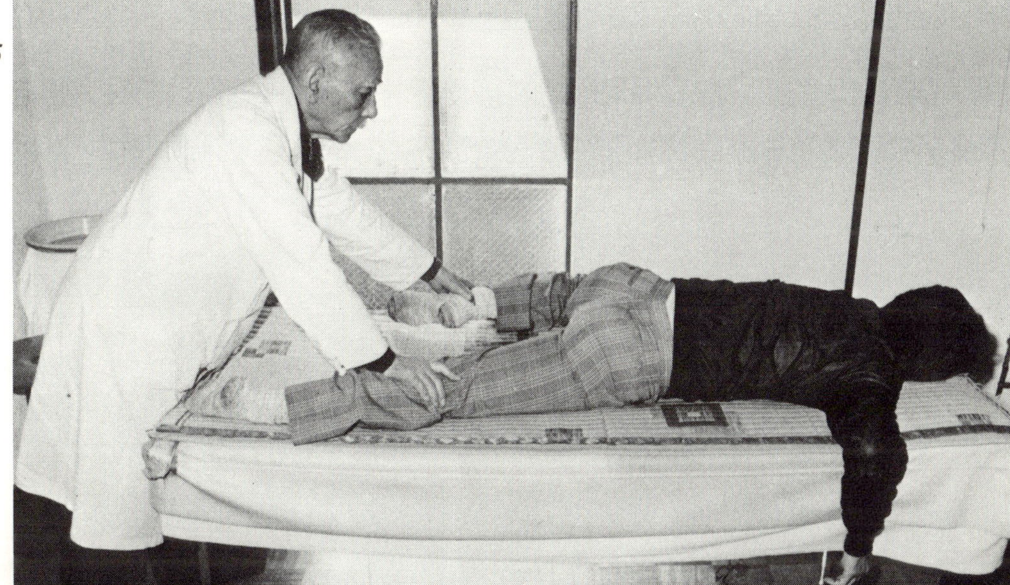

Fig. 16

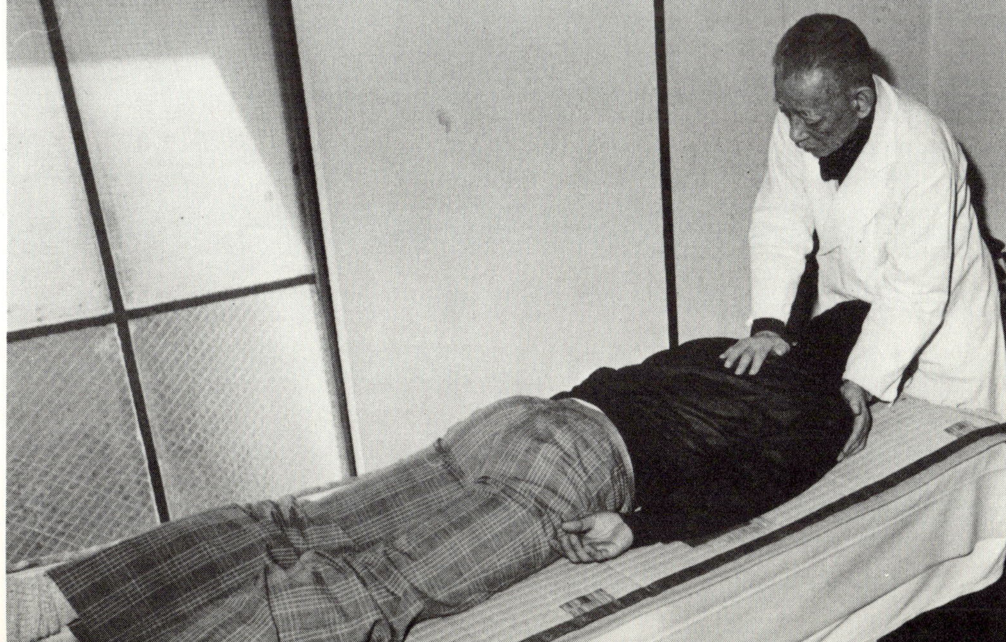

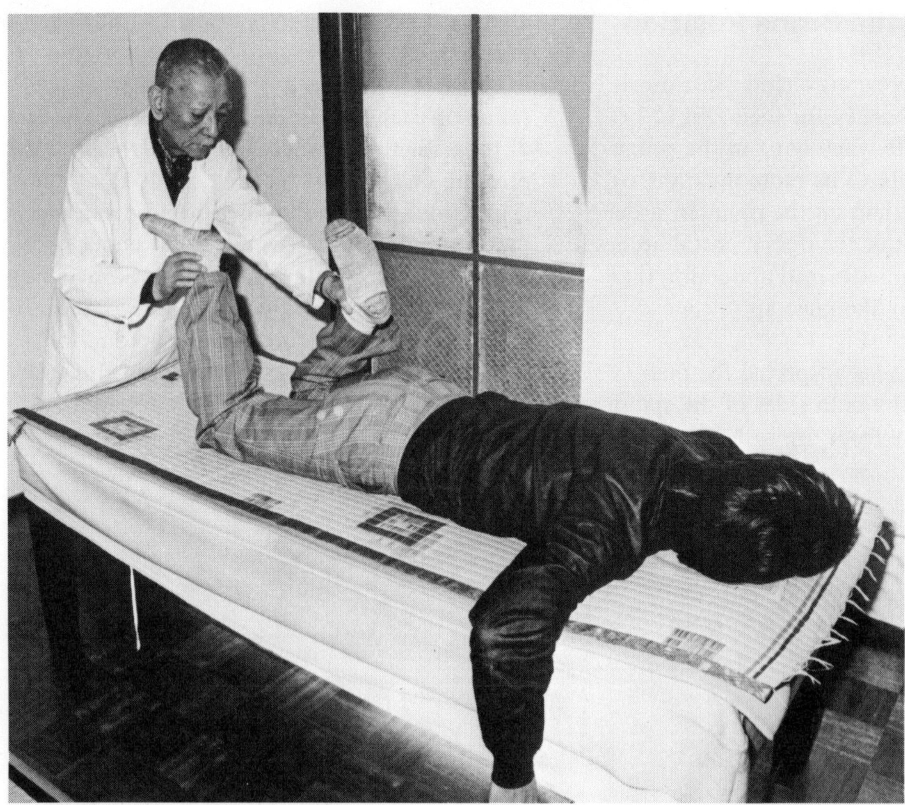

Fig. 17

Fig. 18

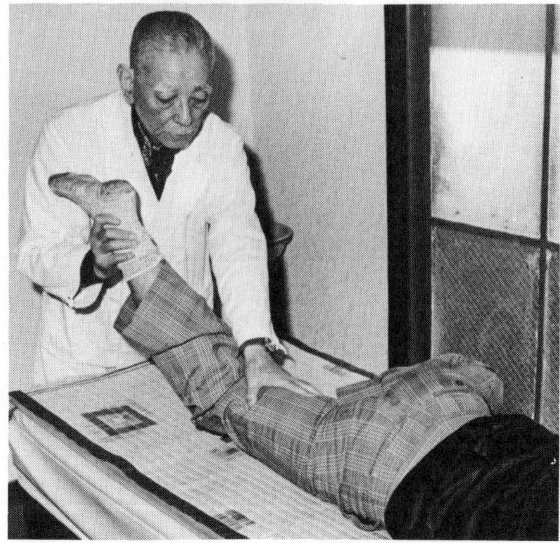

It is normal for the hips and knees to be flexible enough for the heels to reach the buttocks when pushed all the way back in knee flexion (Fig. 17). For many patients, however, their heels do not even come close to their hips. In such a case, the patient slowly extends his leg against resistance and the therapist pushes it back slightly when the patient relaxes all effort at once (Fig. 18). This should make the knees much more flexible, even to the extent of making the heels reach the hips. Repeat this technique until an appreciable change is brought about.

Examination in the Seiza and Seated Positions (feet off the floor in seated position)

Grasp the feet of the seated patient which should be hanging free, and test the movements of the ankle joint including inversion and eversion, as well as lateral and medial rotation (Figs. 19 and 20). Perform the Sōtai movements in

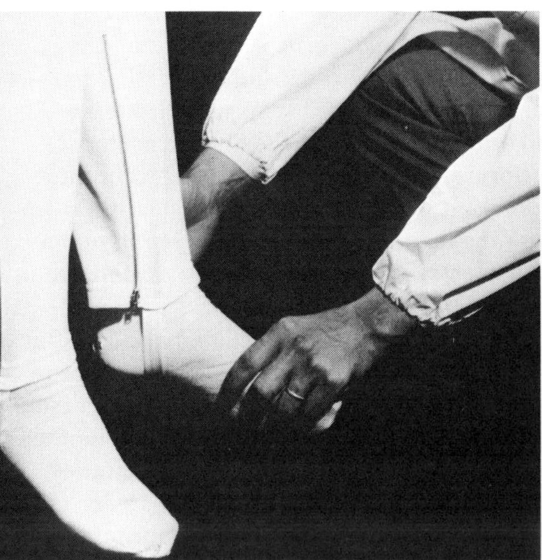

Fig. 19

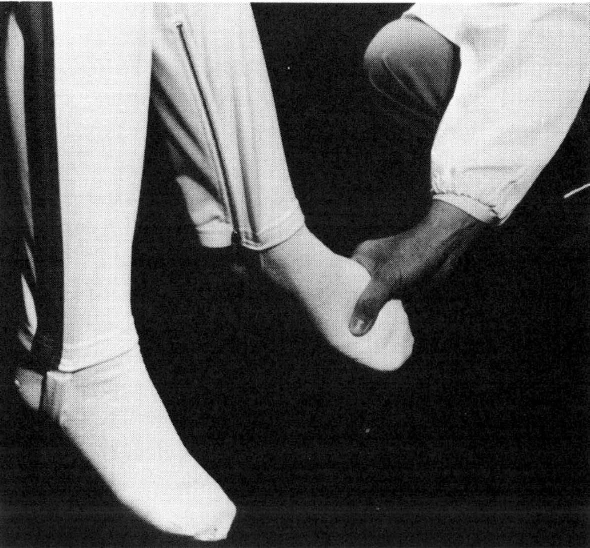

Fig. 20

the comfortable directions, repeating as necessary.

Next, test for misalignment of the lumbar vertebrae by mobility examination in both the seated and Seiza postures. When the lumbar vertebrae have a posterior curvature, this accelerates the aging process. A person's physical age, whether young or old, becomes apparent upon examination of the lumbar area. The strength and vitality of the whole body depends greatly on these vertebrae being straight and upright. The simple remedy of bending backward to correct posterior curvature is just not enough. Those persons with stooped shoulders also need a careful mobility examination and the appropriate Sōtai techniques. The mobility examination of the spine, with the patient's hands firmly clasped behind the head and the therapist holding the elbows from behind (Fig. 21) is often quite effective in correcting this condition.

There are some cases where the lower cervical or upper thoracic vertebrae protrude excessively. Such patients sometimes seem to have their head "hanging" out in front of them. This causes tension in the neck and scapular regions resulting in the hardening of those muscles, and

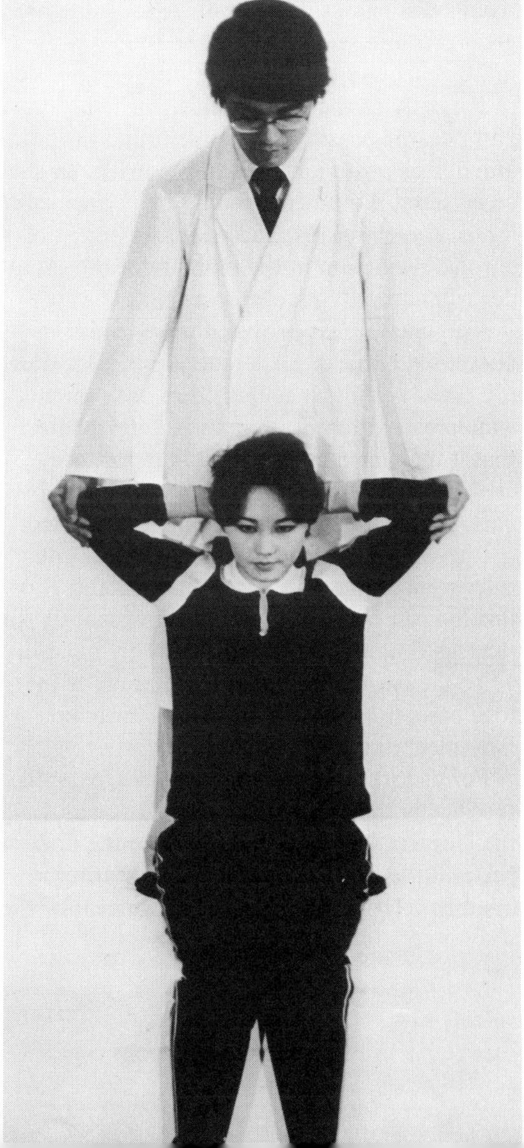

Fig. 21

often these patients complain of headaches and dizziness. In such cases, treat this condition by pressing on the thoracic vertebrae of the seated patient from above with the heel of the hand, and have the patient straighten the back against this pressure, extending the spine upward. Have the patient release effort all at once after holding tension briefly, as in other Sōtai techniques.

The shoulder joint has the greatest range of motion among all the joint of the body so it is quite difficult to determine the exact angle and direction in which the distortion exists. Kinesiological analysis of only the shoulder joint is not adequate for accurately locating the distortion. Since this joint is in kinesiological linkage with the lower half of the body, those joints of the lower extremity must also be examined carefully. In some cases, problems in the shoulder joint are alleviated just by correcting distortions in the foot. Also, sometimes great pressure sensitivity can be found in the muscles around the iliac crest on the same side of the body as the bad shoulder, or indurations and pressure sensitivity may be found in the anterior or posterior walls of the axilla. In such cases, Sōtai movements should be performed to loosen these muscles. Successful treatment of chronic restriction in the mobility of the shoulder will naturally require some time.

Acupuncture has proven quite effective in alleviating periarthritis, especially in long standing cases. Although acupuncture has become widespread in recent years, it is unfortunate that it remains mostly a technique for localized stimulation, without regard, for the most part, to the kinesiological dynamics involved.

Rheumatoid arthritis at one time was considered incurable, but given the time and effort, this too can be alleviated to a significant extent through Sōtai therapy. This naturally must involve the harmonizing and integration of the four basic functions of breathing, injection, movement and mental activity.

For distortion in the thoracic area, examine specifically the places where the ribs join the thoracic vertebrae and the sternum, and perform the mobility examination bearing in mind its relationship with the movement of the neck and shoulders.

There are some female patients of menopausal age who come to the author's clinic expressing concern that hard spots in their breasts might be cancer. When Sōtai movements are performed on such patients, paying close attention to the degree of rotation in the arms, often both the induration and pressure sensitivity in their breasts are removed. This is a technique well worth trying before going for a biopsy.

Neck pain can often be relieved at once after a careful mobility examination and the appropriate Sōtai movement on a distal part. The subjective symptoms accompanying mental illness and depression includes insomnia, dizziness, stiff shoulders, easy fatigability and anxiety. It is well known that psychosomatic problems are closely related to distortions in the musculoskeletal system, so naturally, considerable benefits can be derived from correcting these distortions. When the above mentioned complaints are assessed, most often the distortions are located around the cervical vertebrae. Headaches can be taken care of simply by performing the appropriate mobility examination and Sōtai technique. When a patient complains of dizziness, the movement of their neck must be analyzed carefully, as not all vertigo is related to dysfunctions of the inner ear. It has been substantiated by the research of a former professor at Tokushima University, Dr. Hinoki and his associates, that a relationship exists between vertigo and excessive tension of the cervical spinal muscles. As mentioned earlier, abnormal tension of the muscles exists concomitantly with misalignement in the skeletal structure. In many cases whiplash injury and slipped disks can be taken care of very simply by the examination and treatment of distortions in the musculoskeletal system. It is unfortunate that only the standard procedure of traction and wearing corsets is applied, when therapy using the appropriate Sōtai movement after a kinesiological analysis should be tried first and foremost.

Even conditions like facial palsy and trigeminal neuralgia need to be considered in light of distortions in the skull. Although the symptoms occur at the very top of the body, it is obvious that a detailed examination from the legs, or the base of the human frame, is called for. Misalignments can also occur in the cranial sutures, and this is clearly related to abnormal tension in the muscles that have their origin there.

As one illustration of a distal musculoskeletal linkage causing a physical problem, the author, when young, treated an older woman who complained of a painful area the size of a large coin on the left side of her forehead which persisted for several years despite having undergone various treatments for it. A whole variety of treatments were attempted by the author, but to no avail, until finally he decide one day to thoroughly examine this patient from head to toe. A large corn was discovered between the patient's first and second toes of the left foot. The corn was tender and the patient said it was painful when she walked. Presuming that this corn was responsible for distortions throughout her whole body, the author removed enough of the corn so that pressure no longer came to bear on it, and followed this with a series of adjustments over the patient's whole body. By the third day, the pain in the patient's head was gone without a trace. This incident caused the author to rethink his concept of the human body. Overlooking nothing more than a simple corn on the foot can sometimes cause a physician to waste a great deal of time.

Application of Kinesiology in Various Fields of Medicine

Ideally, in every healthcare specialty, treatments should be administered after first restoring the basic structural balance in the body. This holistic approach is needed in the fields of otorhinology, ophthalmology and dentistry, not to mention internal medicine, orthopedics, obstetrics and gynecology. Not only will the natural healing powers of the patient be strengthened by the therapist understanding and applying the principles of kinesiology, but remarkable clinical results should become possible.

Some older and more experienced clinicians have realized these principles on their own and treat patients for minor symptoms like stiffness in their shoulders by various manipulative techniques. Diseased conditions manifesting in the cranial area are, almost without exception, a result of distortions in the cervical vertebrae. Almost all gynecological disorders are related to distortions in the pelvic area. Even for cases of neuralgia and psychosomatic disorders, the possibility of distortions in the musculoskeletal system should not be overlooked.

In pediatrics also, exceptionally good results are possible through simple manipulation. Many ailments of infants, for instance, can be alleviated by merely tickling their sides. This is because when children are tickled, they respond involuntarily to this stimulation and change their posture in various ways. Such involuntary movement often automatically corrects distortions in an infant's physical structure and natural healing is facilitated.

Our involuntary reactions can be called a gift from heaven. Human beings instinctively want to move in the direction which makes them feel best. Our inclination is to want to move, not in an uncomfortable or a strained manner, but in this most comfortable manner. Our habitual postures during walking as well as while sleeping are a reflection of this. However, because we assume postures and make movements in our daily lives which go against basic principles of kinesiology, inevitably distortions occur. Of all human actions, going against the laws of nature is the single greatest cause of tragedy.

There is not much that can be done from outside the body to treat organic disorders affecting the central nervous system. The secondary symptoms, however, can be alleviated to a considerable extent by manipulative techniques. It is hoped that physical therapy utilizing a variety of forms of external stimulation will be developed even more in the future. To treat a patient for an ailment without correcting distortions in their frame is like bailing water with a bottomless bucket. Both physicians and researchers must strive to study the principles of motion with reverence for the laws of nature.

Daily Upkeep of the Human Frame

From all that has been detailed thus far, some understanding of the basic rules in correcting distortions should have been imparted to our readers. It really cannot be helped that some distortions in our physical frame continue to recur in our daily lives. So long as a person continues to move in ways opposed to the basic principles of movement, he or she cannot achieve mastery of any art or craft. The presence of a distortion can be found just by doing a simple mobility examination when an abnormal sensation is detected. Minor distortions can be corrected and normalized very simply by taking the time out during the course of a day to check one's own body and do some Sōtai exercises. All machines require periodic maintenance, and the human physical mechanism is no exception. The improvement and maintenance of one's own health is something for which each individual must assume responsibility. Finding the less comfortable direction of movement and doing that movement in reverse, in the more comfortable direction, is not asking too much of a person.

In order to encourage healthy breathing, one should practice abdominal breathing in bed each night before going to sleep. A minimum of ten good deep breaths moving the stomach in and out with long exhalation is recommended. This breathing must be practiced every night until one is able to take only two or three breaths per minute without discomfort.

The macrobiotic guideline advising intake of vegetables, grain and animal food in the same proportion as the ratio of incisors, molars and canine in our teeth, is a good rule of the thumb for a healthy diet. We should respect the traditional wisdom regarding our diet and health which considers our body and the earth to be one inseparable whole. The ideal thing is for each individual to learn exactly what is necessary and sufficient for his own nutrition. One would be surprised at how little food it really takes to stay healthy. The most important thing is not how much food, but how well the food is chewed and digested.

For our mental health, keeping a positive and optimistic outlook in life is the best medicine. This can be done by preeminently directing our thoughts toward the pleasant, beautiful and joyous things around us, and by being thankful for those good things in life and verbalizing one's delight and joy. One need not even pay any attention to negative things and events which cannot be changed, much less talk about such unpleasant things. The heart turns in the direction of the words we speak; this is the principle governing our mental health. So keep in mind that your words are like the steering wheel of your destiny.

Our feet are at the very foundation of our physical structure. Therefore our toes are of special importance, and so assuming the Seiza posture can be beneficial. This type of sitting is done correctly by folding the legs underneath you and sitting squarely on your soles. Movement of the spine, such as dorsiflexion and anteflexion, right and left lateral flexion, as well as rotation in both directions, can be done in the Seiza posture everyday to locate the presence of discomfort or lack of ease in movement. The Sōtai movement is the comfortable movement done in the opposite direction to correct the situation. A person who does not have the slightest bit of tenderness in the soles of their feet when pressing strongly between its joints with the thumbs, may be considered to be in good health.

It is not good for a therapist to become overly concerned about the exact location of the abnormal sensitivity when attempting to correct distortions. The location of sensitivity in relation to the actual distorsion and to the central nervous system is analogous to the images projected on to a screen by a slide projector. The images or "shadows" appear in certain areas of the screen because of the slide (distortions) located between the projecting light and the screen. The picture changes every time the slide is changed. It is pointless to chase just these "shadows" on the screen. Let it suffice to say, abnormal sensitivity is produced far more often by imbalances in myogen (a spontaneously coagulable muscle protein—the slide) than by that in neurogens (a transmitter substance— the screen).

The author of this book took up general medical practice in his late twenties abruptly after having worked for a time as a researcher in neurophysiology. Since that time he has treated thousands of patients for a wide variety of complaints. During these long years of clinical practice, he has had the opportunity of reviewing the viability of the various traditional healing practices which abound in Japan. He finally came to the conclusion that there was a common thread which ran through all of them. Although such healing methods were practiced without awareness of this, in most cases they relied on some form of external stimulation to adjust a person's physical structure.

The technique of backtracking a movement in the comfortable direction and instantly releasing effort when the movement reached its end was developed in the 1920's by Michio Takahashi, the founder of the Seitai school. This discovery is worthy of special note in the annals of medical history.

Health is the natural result of right living. This must be something done for oneself, rather than being something provided by others. This very understanding is what makes it possible for people to really improve their health. Yoga and many other schools have been teaching similar approaches for thousands of years, but there is no specific mention of the principles of kinesiology (movement) as described in this book. It is hoped that a more complete understanding of all methods of healing will be gained through the approach offered here.

7. SŌTAI EXERCISES—Active Movement in the Comfortable Direction

In our daily lives we all have various ingrained patterns of movement such as lifting objects, or reaching out with the arms, or stretching the back. Among these movements, those which cause the body's center of gravity to shift forward (stoop) seem to be the greatest in number. There is a natural principle of movement which dictates that, for such forward movement to be stabilized and maintained, one must necessarily be able to perform bilateral movement (lateral flexion and rotation) with some stability. The bilateral movements which stabilizes anterior and posterior movements will be presented in this chapter. These exercises are basic active movements which can be performed alone.

Foot Stretch in Seiza Posture

One assumes a sitting posture similar to the Seiza posture with the buttocks resting on the heels and the knees on the floor. The feet should be spread apart no wider than the hips. The bottom of the toes should contact the floor by stretching into dorsiflexion.

The feet are rotated from the posture of Figure 1 and the hips are slowly brought down into the positions shown in Figures 2 and 3. After deciding which direction is easier to move

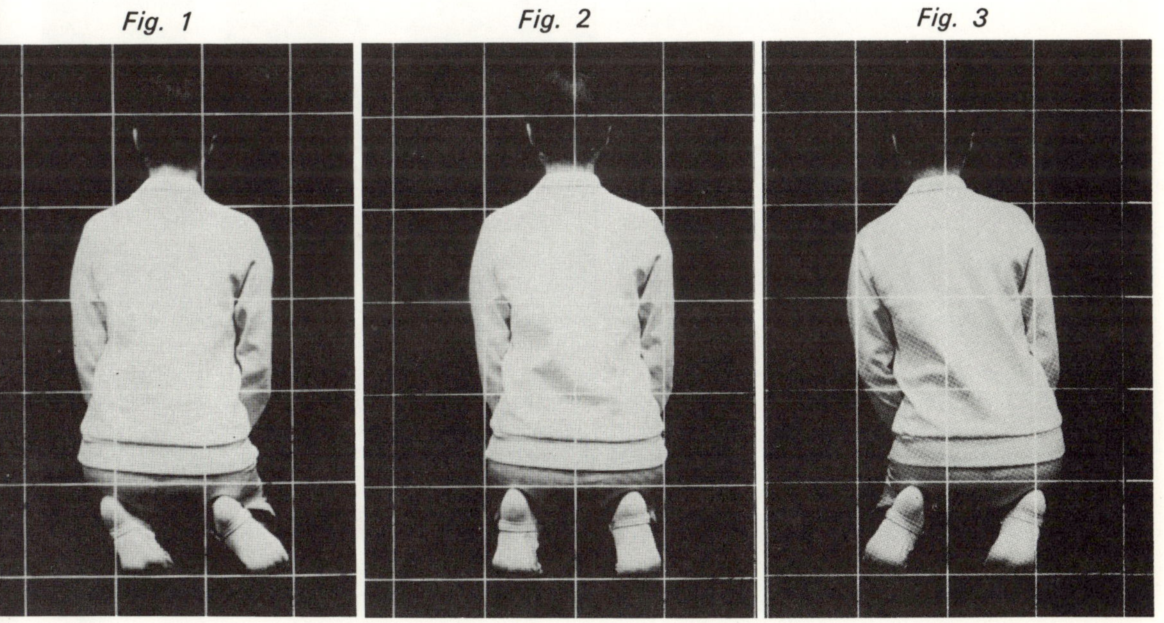

Fig. 1 *Fig. 2* *Fig. 3*

in, this movement is repeated three or four times. When there is no discernable difference to either side, the movement can be performed several times on both sides. (The grid lines on the figures are to show more distinctly the manner and extent of hip motion.)

It would be ideal if a person could acquire a habit of doing this exercise every morning. This exercise may initially prove painful, especially at the toes, however, discomfort can be gradually eliminated through repetition until the exercise can be performed without effort. Deminishing of pain is a sure sign that the first steps toward health are being made. (This exercise is ideal for those persons seeking relief from chronic shoulder tension and low back pain.)

Foot Stretch on All Fours

This position is assumed by placing the hands on the floor with the fingers spread wide apart, from the posture shown in Figure 2. The hands are placed apart the width of the shoulders, in front of the knees at the most comfortable place (Fig. 4). Without lifting the buttocks off the heels, the upper torso is turned posterolaterally as if turning to look behind (Figs. 5 and 6). After gaining some practice, one can turn as to look at the hips. This movement also should be repeated several times in the comfortable direction. This should take no more than thirty seconds. This exercise also may prove to be painful for the toes, but gradual reduction in this pain is an indication that one is on the road to health.

Fig. 4

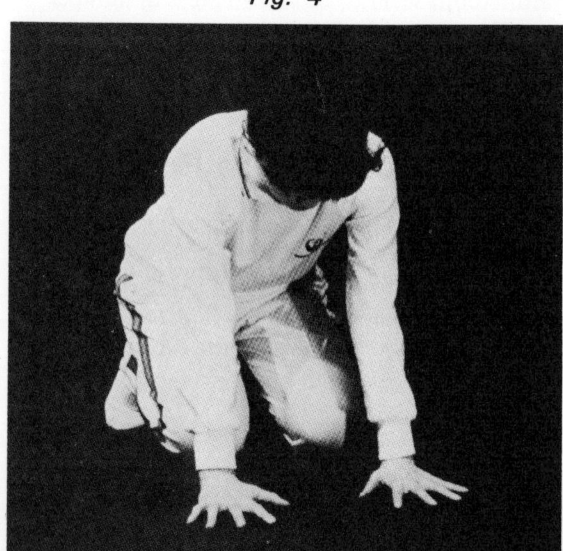

Fig. 5

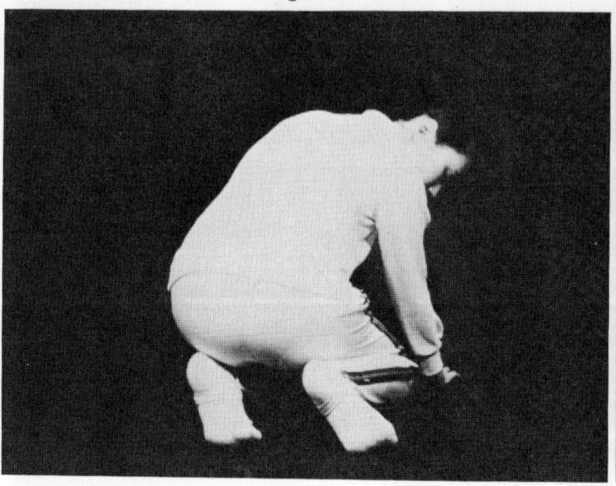

Fig. 6

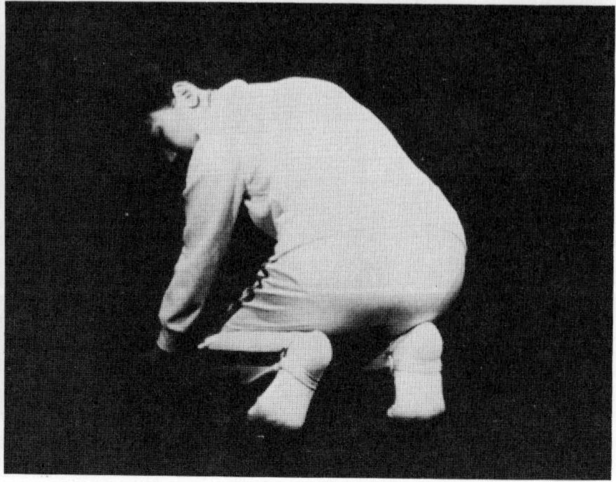

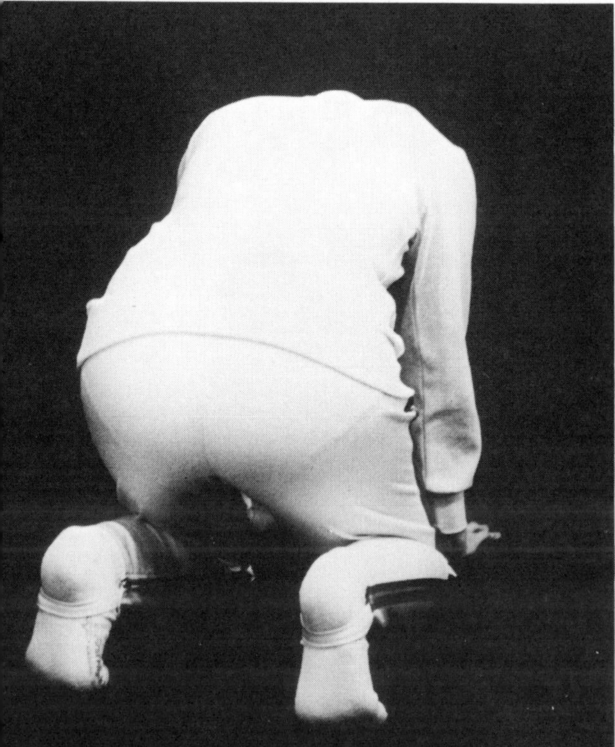

Fig. 7

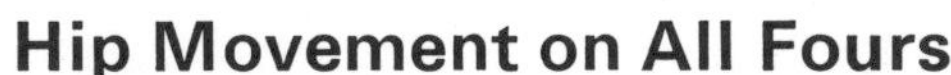

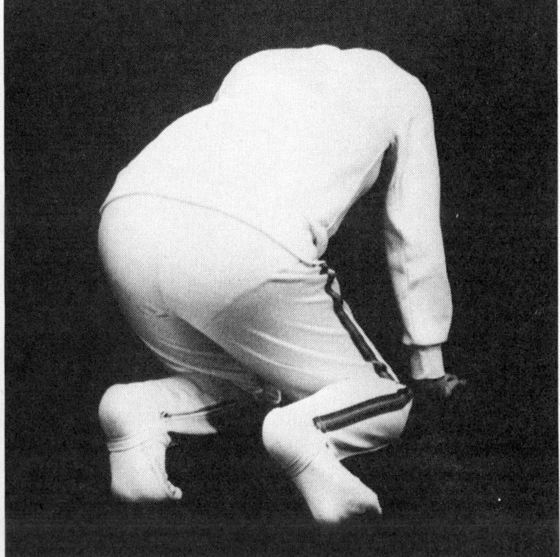

Fig. 8

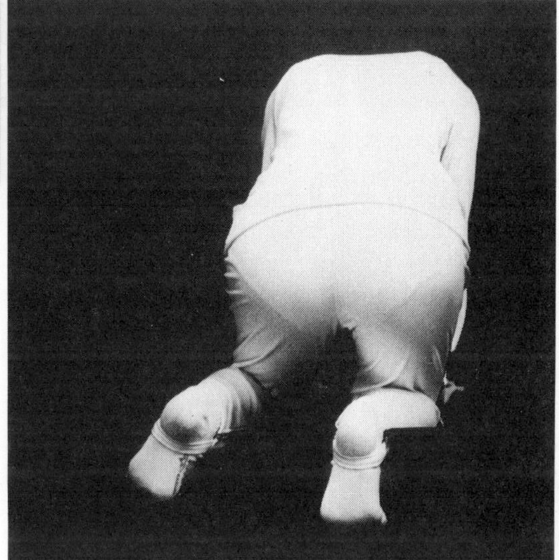

Fig. 9

Hip Movement on All Fours

From the posture shown in Figure 4, the hips are raised off the heels as shown in Figure 7. The hips are then alternately turned to each side (Figs. 8 and 9). Since the hips are freer than in the preceding exercises, their movement can be greater. If more discomfort is experienced when moving to one side than the other, cease movement in the less limber direction and move the hips several times in the direction of least discomfort.

After movement several times in the comfortable direction, again move toward the less comfortable side to check for improvement. One will usually notice that the movement has become easier. (Absolutely avoid all movements which are a strain or excessively painful.)

The posture shown in Figure 10 is assumed by firmly planting the hands and feet on the floor. The fingers must be spread apart and the hips should be held at a height which allows the hands and feet to remain in steady contact with the floor. Keeping the feet flat on the floor,

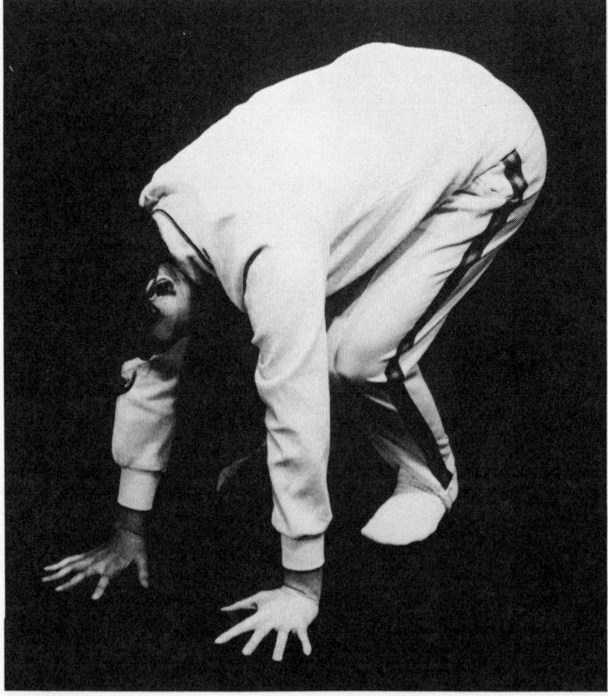

Fig. 10

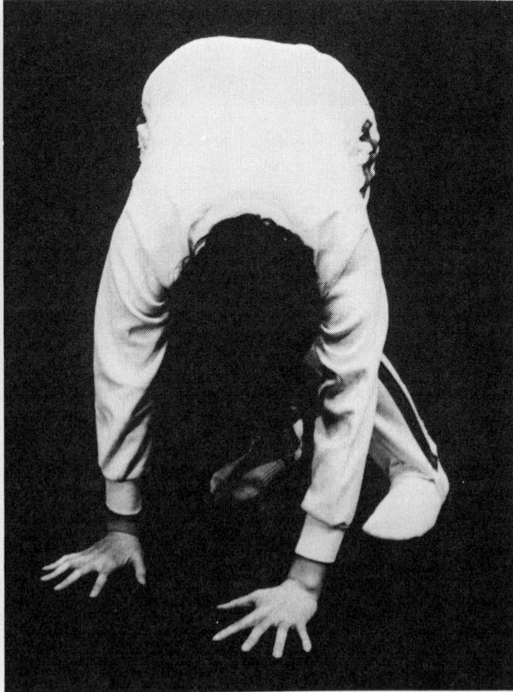

Fig. 11

the hips are turned alternately to each side to compare the ease of movement in each direction (Fig. 11). If movement to the right and left can be performed with equal ease, the movement can be repeated several times in both directions. When one direction proves more difficult to move in, slowly move in the opposite direction three or four times.

Flexion and Lateral Elevation of Knees.

Lying prone, flex the knees alternately and draw one knee up part way to the side (Figs. 12 and 13). The head may be turned in the most comfortable direction.

When no discomfort is experienced in the movements of preceding exercise, alternately draw the knees farther up to the side (Figs. 14 and 15).

Persons who can raise their knees this far without any discomfort can be regarded as having a passing mark (Figs. 16 and 17). Those persons experiencing greater discomfort when drawing up one knee as opposed to the other, this movement should be repeated three or four times on the side which proves with greater ease. (This exercise is effective for cases of low back pain.)

Note: This is the same active movement presented on page 79. When someone is available, the Sōtai movement on page 78 is recommended. For other active movements which can be performed alone, refer to the explanations in Chapter 2 and the exercises in the following chapter.

Fig. 12

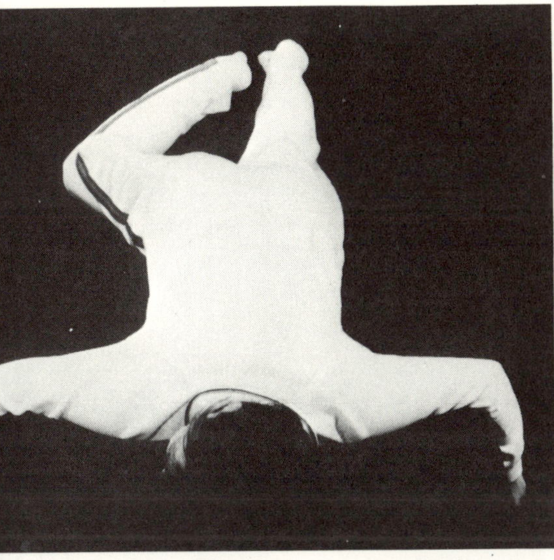

Fig. 13

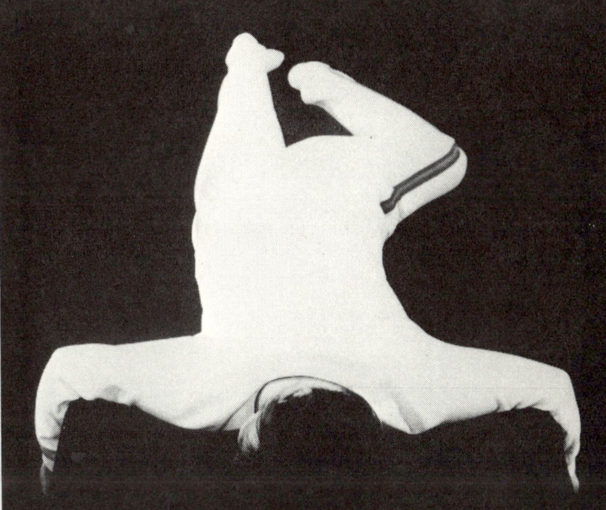

Fig. 14

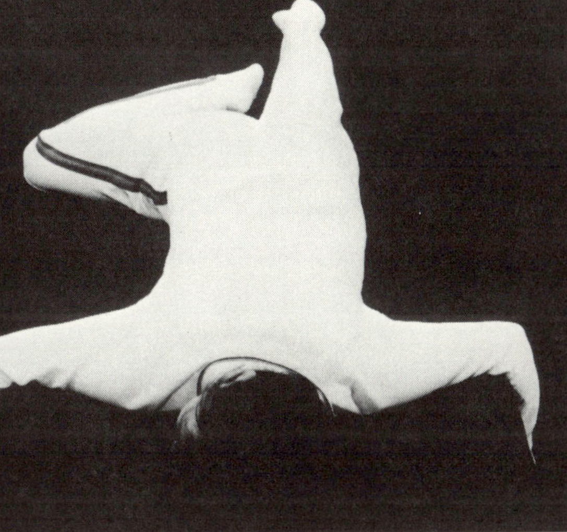

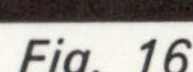

Fig. 15

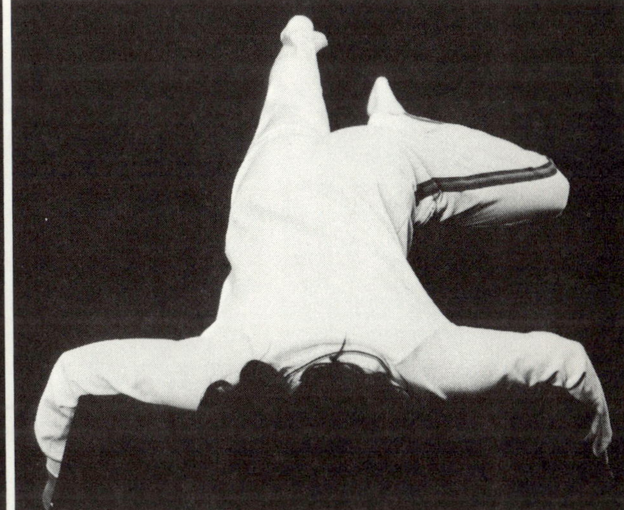

Fig. 16

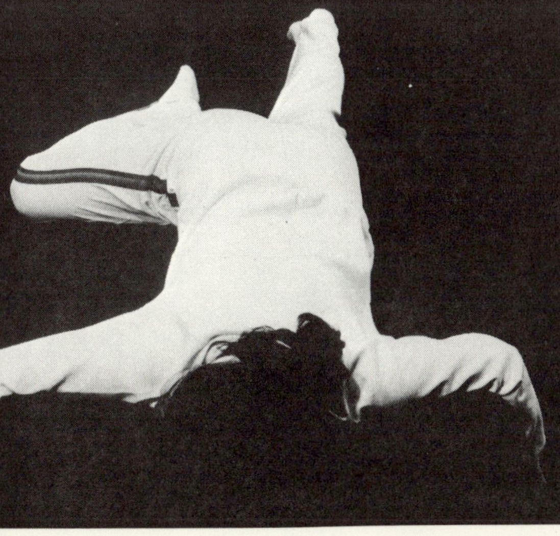

Fig. 17

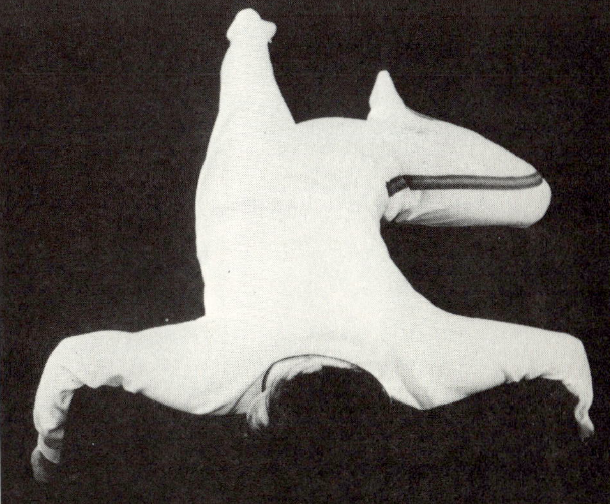

8. EXERCISES APPLYING KINESIOLOGICAL PRINCIPLES

The basic exercises presented in this chapter are for building and maintaining health—a prerequisite for a happy life. The simple rule to be followed in all of these exercises is to relax the body as completely as possible and move while exhaling the breath. These exercises can be readily performed by any person, young or old, any time and any place.

When the body is moved slowly during exhalation, only the very minimum of energy is required. To move slowly, as described before, implies a rate at which a person's hand immersed below the surface of water can move without disturbing the surface.

There is no need in these exercises to match the rhythm of another person. Even if ten people start a movement together, they should complete it each in their own time. The important thing is to follow one's own pace and move in a relaxed manner while exhaling.

It is also important to remember that when making bilateral (right and left) movements one often finds, upon careful consideration, that there is a direction in which the movement can be made with greater ease compared to the other direction. If this is the case, one should proceed by performing the movement in the easy direction two or three times. Any movement which causes difficulty, discomfort, or pain should be absolutely avoided.

If a person does strenuous exercises or sports with a substantial bilateral difference, the likelihood of a negative outcome is only too obvious. Hard physical exercise should only be done after making movements in the direction of comfort and attaining a functional balance so that movement in the difficult direction can be performed with maximum ease.

In this section, the laws of physical movement will be outlined in practical terms in six Basic Sōtai Exercises.

Fig. 1

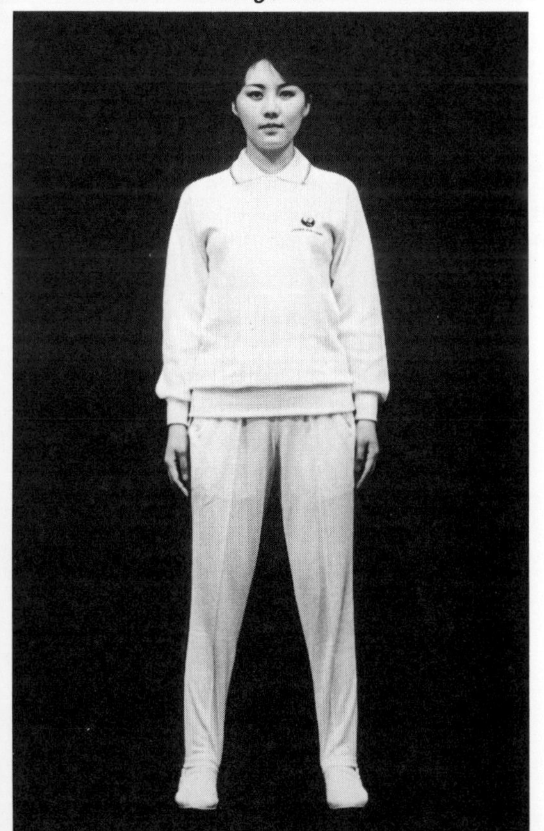

Basic Exercise 1—*Abduction of arms to horizontal*

Basic posture (natural stance): The feet are placed apart about the width of the hips, and are kept parallel to each other (Fig. 1). A relaxed and stable stance is assumed by drawing the chin in slightly and straightening the back. The line of vision is concentrated on one point straight ahead.

This posture is the initial position for the Basic Exercises 1, 3, 4, 5, and 6 (the best width for the foot stance is the greater of either the width of the hips or the shoulders).

Place the feet parallel to each other (so that imaginary lines drawn from the center of the heel to between the first and second toes are parallel) and plant the soles down evenly to achieve a balance in distribution of body weight (Fig. 2).

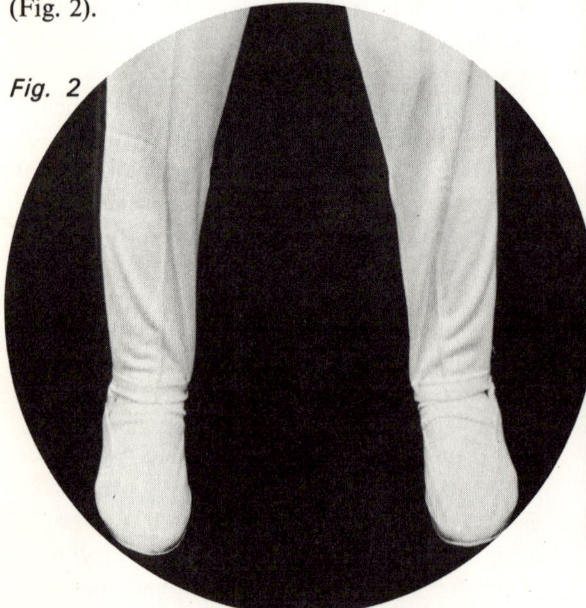

Fig. 2

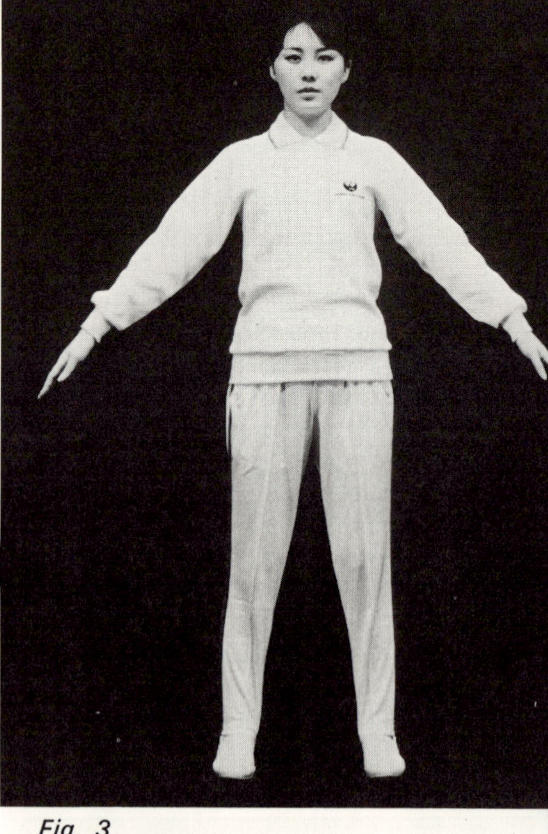

Fig. 3

After stilling the mind, assume the natural stance shown in Figure 1 and inhale deeply into the abdomen. Then slowly raise both arms to the side while exhaling quietly (Fig. 3).

Exhalation of the breath and raising of the arms should be synchronized so that the arms reach horizontal just as exhalation is complete (Fig. 4).

After breathing in and out once in this position, the arms are suddenly dropped as the breath is exhaled (Fig. 5). This movement is repeated three to five times. Even five slow repetitions should take no more than eighty seconds.

When the arms are abducted, it is possible to analyze bilateral imbalances by kinesthetically determining which arm is more difficult to raise. (Figure 6 as an example, has the patient with more difficulty on the left side).

When a situation like that in Figure 6 arises, the following steps may be taken to correct the imbalance.

1. After shifting the center of gravity to the leg ipsilateral to the arm which is more difficult to abduct, both arms are raised evenly (weight shifted left in Figure 7).
2. If the arms still cannot assume a horizontal position, Basic Exercises 4 and 5 can be performed before returning to Basic Exercise 1.
3. The weight may be shifted over to the left leg (in this example) when the arms begin their abduction.

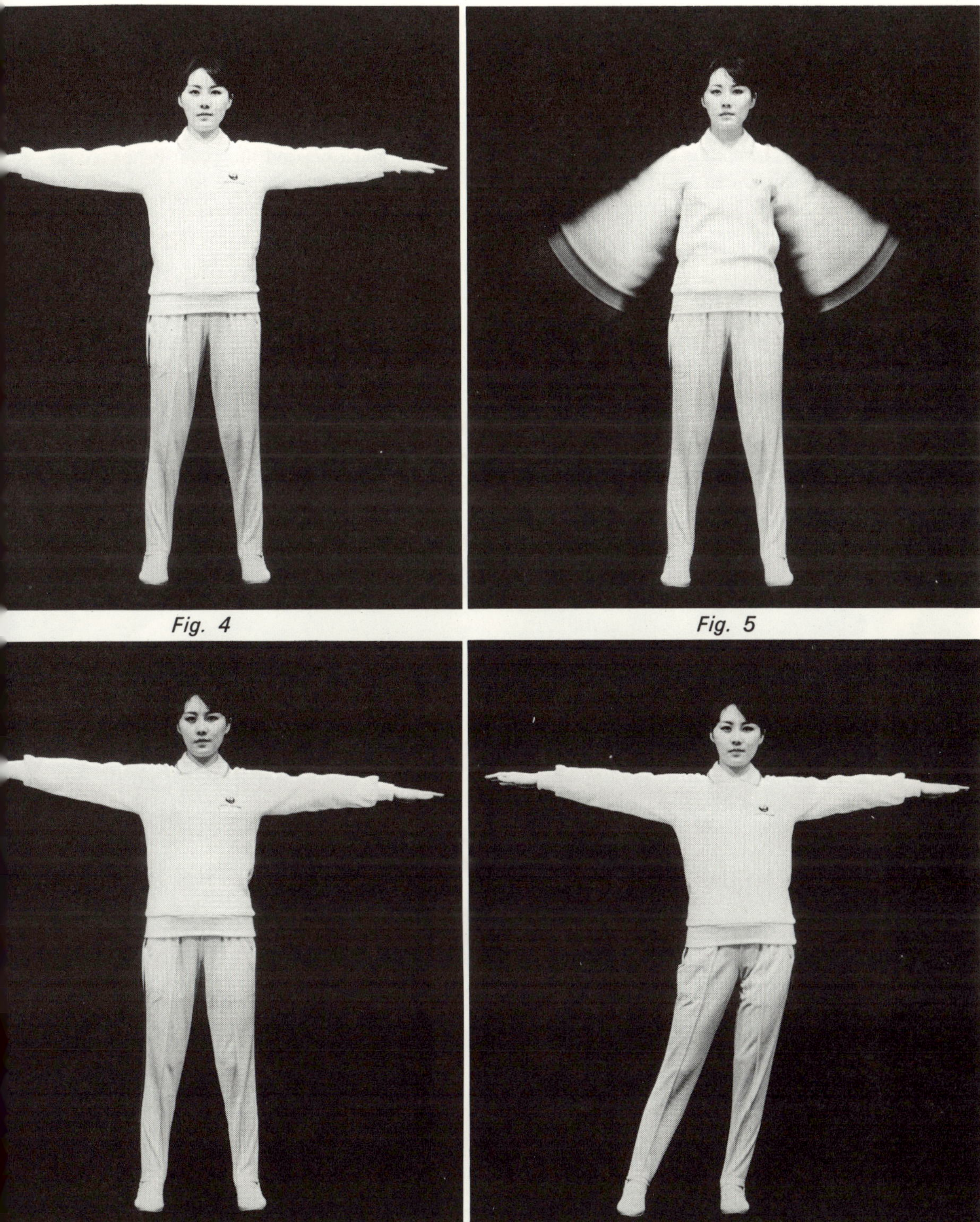

Fig. 4

Fig. 5

Fig. 6

Fig. 7

Basic Exercise 2—*Marching in place*

The line of vision is concentrated on a point directly ahead, and the feet are placed evenly together (Fig. 8). The chin is drawn in slightly and the back is straightened. It is best if the patient can assume this erect stance easily and naturally.

As stationary marching steps are begun, the hips are flexed until the thighs become perpendicular to the torso (Fig. 9). These steps must be executed with vigor so that the entire sole of each foot meets the floor at once. At first, the range of the arm swing forward should reach shoulder height, and backward, only as far as they swing naturally.

When the patient becomes accustomed to the arm motion, then the arm swing may be increased up to eye level (Fig. 10). Arm swings much beyond this point is not recommended since it can create torsion which is undesirable. (In this marching exercise, the sole of one foot should meet the floor completely before the other foot is lifted. This serves to keep the center of gravity stable.)

Although this movement is repeated up to thirty times, the total time expended should be less than forty seconds. If more time than this is taken, the movements no longer resemble marching steps because the motion of each leg becomes isolated from the other.

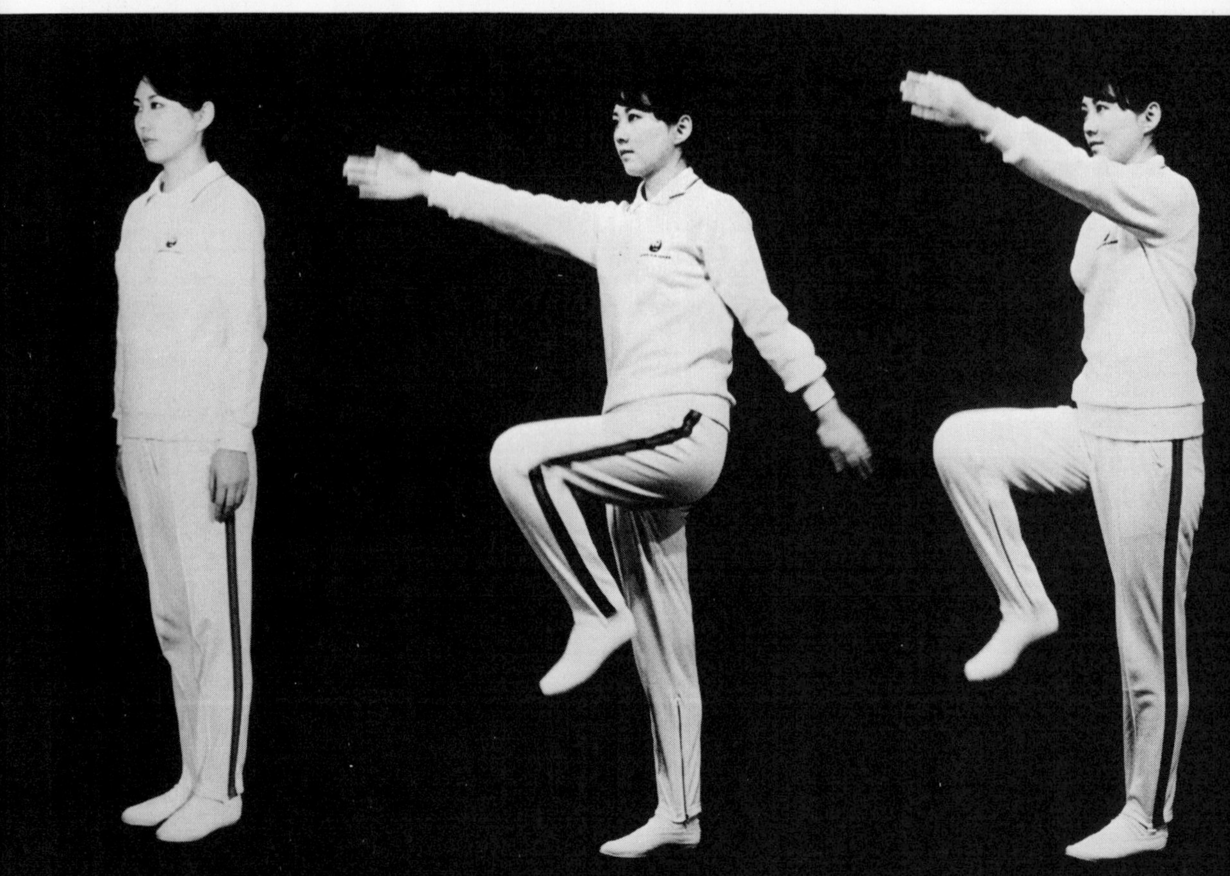

Fig. 8 *Fig. 9* *Fig. 10*

Basic Exercise 3—*Anterior and posterior flexion*

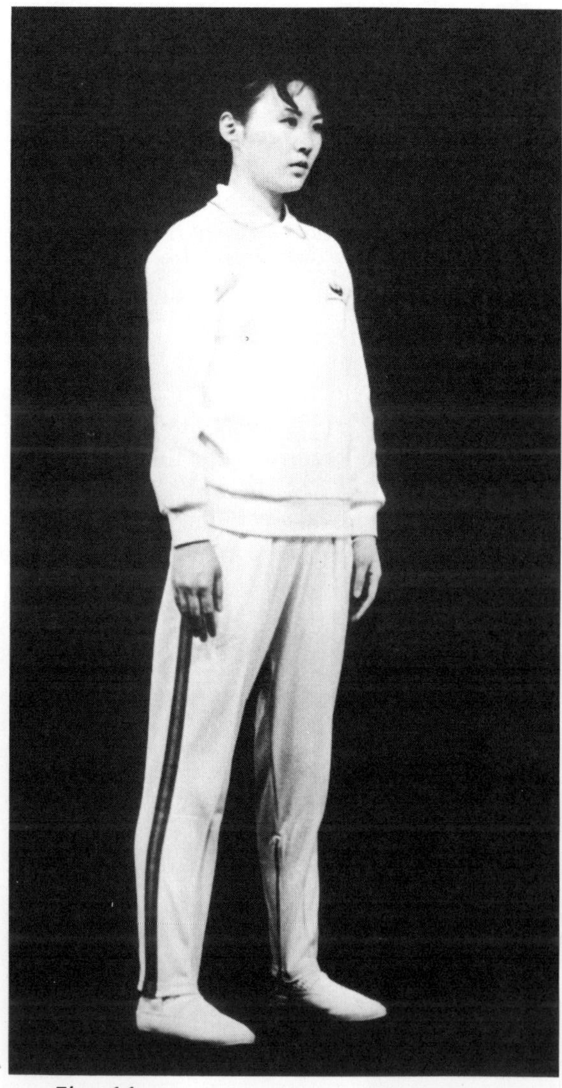

Fig. 11

Assume the natural stance of Basic Exercise 1 in a relaxed manner and inhale the breath into the lower abdomen (Fig. 11).

After releasing all tension from the head, neck, and shoulders, slowly lean forward while exhaling. letting the arms hang down limply (Fig. 12).

Fig. 12

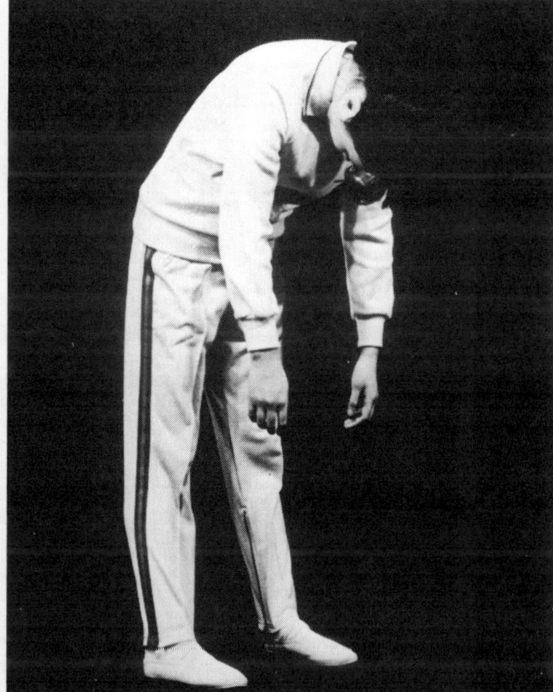

Continue with the forward trunk flexion while breathing out until the trunk is bent forward fully (Fig. 13). It is most desirable that the completion of the forward bending movement coincide with the end of the exhalation. Take one full breath after reaching the fully bent position.

Fig. 13

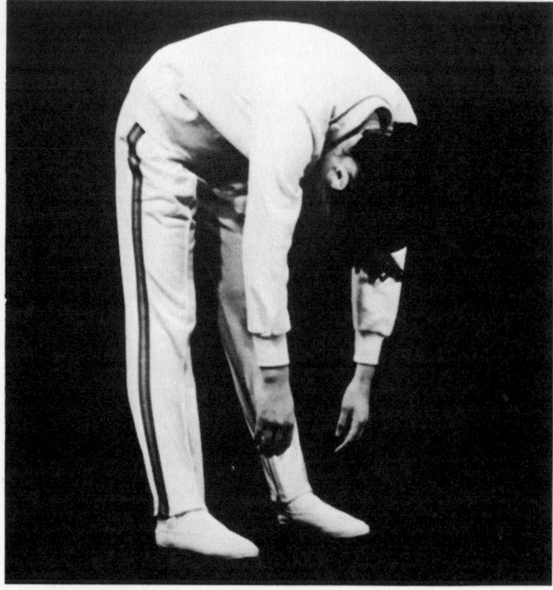

Fig. 14

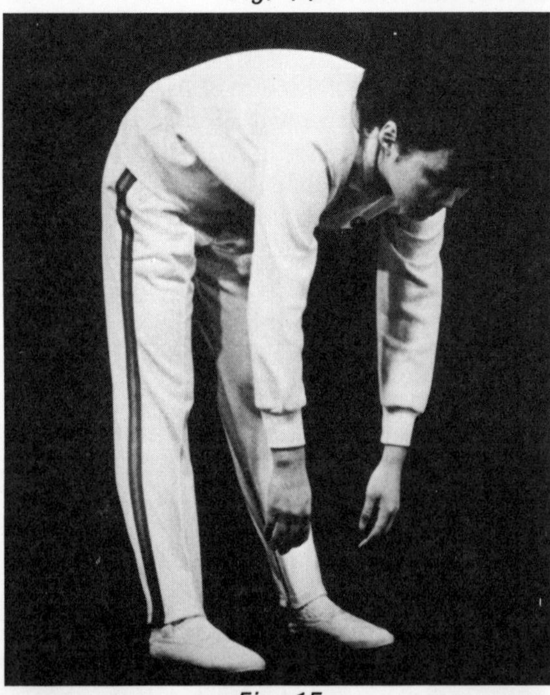

Fig. 15

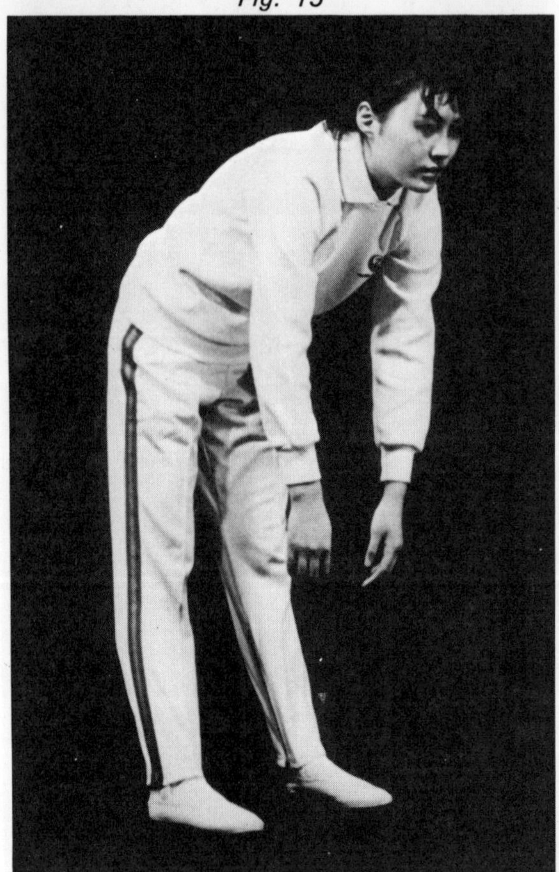

The forward flexion should be stopped immediately if any tension or strain is felt in the back or the legs. Such painful sensations are the body's way of warning that one must not go any further. It is important not to cause undue strain, so movement beyond the point of discomfort should be absolutely avoided.

Before beginning to return back to the upright position from the forward bend, first extend the neck (lift the face up) so as to move one's center of gravity backward (Fig. 14).

While exhaling, keeping the head uplifted, slowly return to the upright position as if drawing the waist forward (Fig. 15).

The last portion of the breath is exhaled as the return movement is completed (Fig. 16). One full breath is taken in this position.

Next, placing the hands upon the hips for stability, arch the body backward while exhaling (Figs. 17 and 18). As in the case of the forward bend, the backward bend must be stopped

Fig. 16

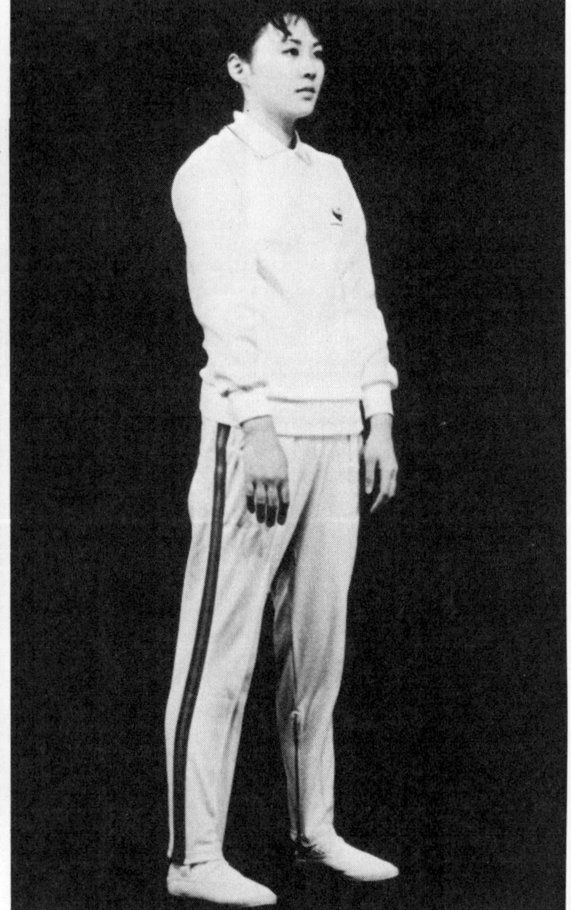

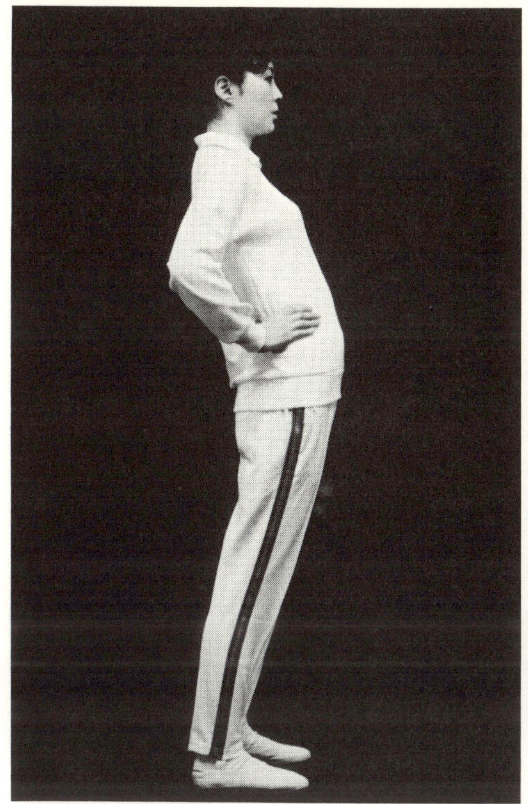

Fig. 17

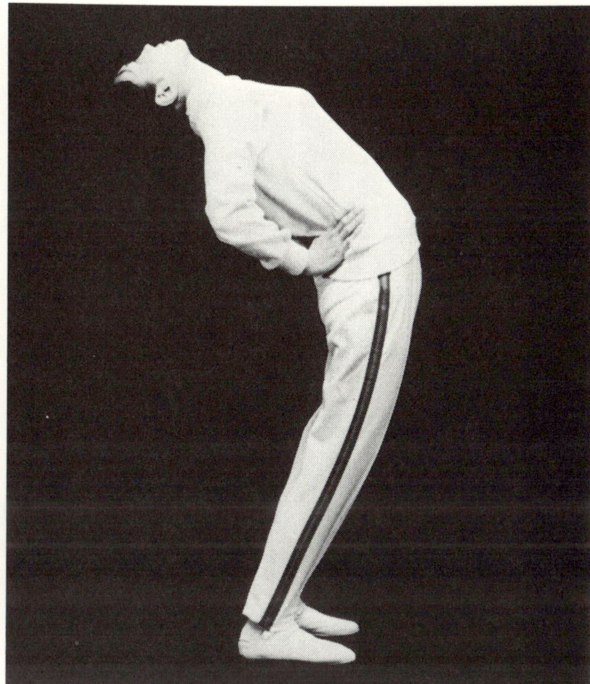

Fig. 18

just before the onset of discomfort or pain. After completing one breath in the back bend position, slowly return to the upright position while exhaling (Fig. 19).

The following steps are suggested for those persons who are unable to perform the forward flexion movement smoothly:

1. The hips can be moved back and forth.
2. The patient may begin by stretching backward very gently two or three times before attempting the forward bend.
3. Basic Exercise 5 can be done prior to attempting the forward bend.

Even people whose bodies lack flexibility will find that performing this exercise each morning continuously for a month enables them to touch the floor with their fingertips. However slowly the exercise is done, the three to five repetitions should require no more than three minutes. The forward bend may be accomplished with more comfort and ease if the hips are drawn backward during the movement.

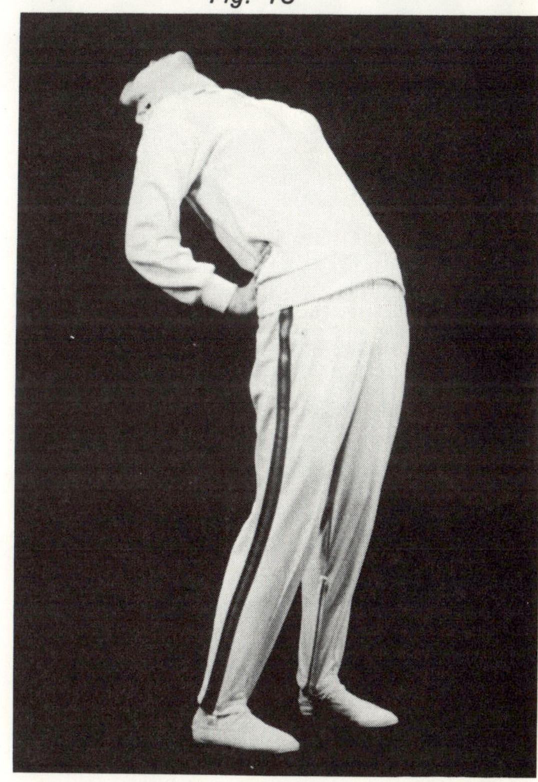

Fig. 19

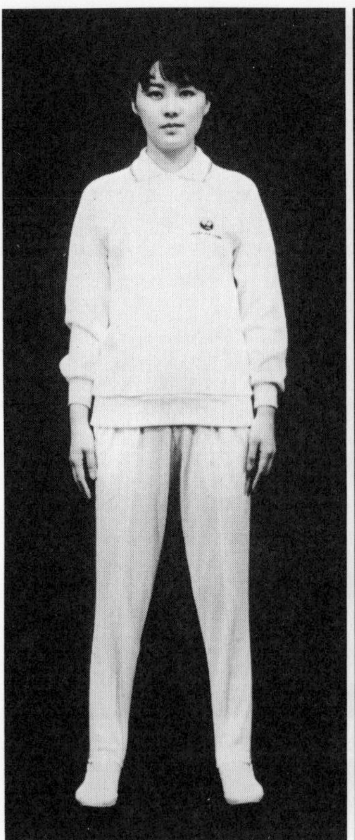

Fig. 20

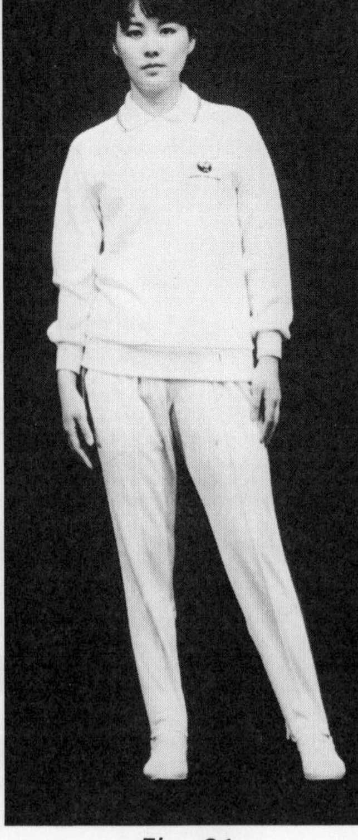

Fig. 21

Basic Exercise 4—*Bilateral flexion*

The natural stance of Basic Exercise 1 is assumed in a relaxed manner, and the breath is drawn into the abdomen (Fig. 20).

The upper body and hips are shifted to the right while exhaling, setting the center of gravity over the right leg (Fig. 21). (Just moving the hips to the right does not properly shift the center of gravity.)

Then, the hips are pushed out to the right as the upper body is simultaneously inclined to the left (Fig. 22). (Inclining the upper body to the left and shifting the hips to the right, while very similar, is not appropriate.)

When lateral flexion to the left is accomplished by shifting the center of gravity com-

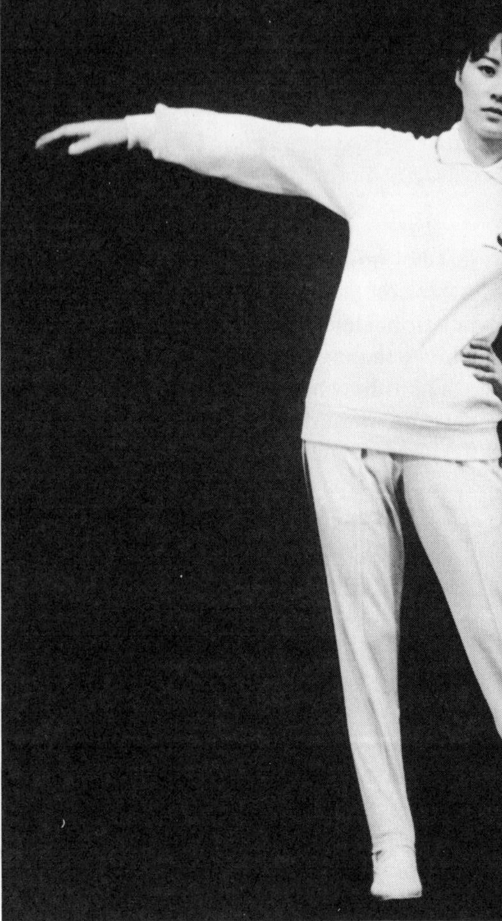

Fig. 22

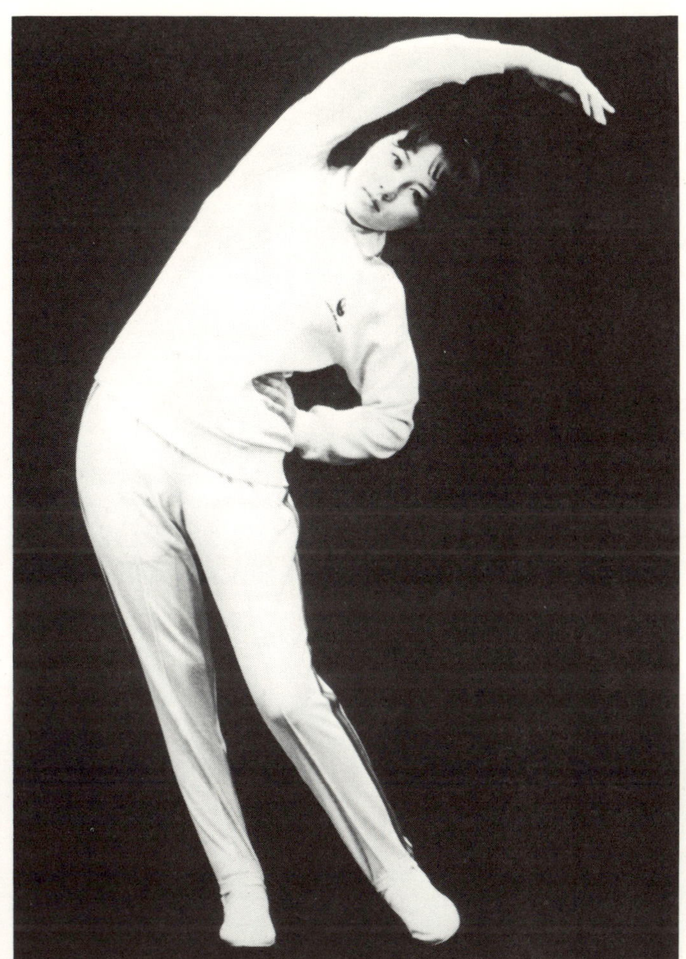

Fig. 23

pletely over to the right leg, the right foot is planted firmly on the floor (Fig. 23). The left foot is relaxed and the knee bends forward slightly and the heel raises off the floor. The left hand serves to stabilize the center of gravity, while the right hand aids the lateral flexion movement. One full breath is taken in this position. The body is then slowly returned to the straight position while exhaling. The return movement of the arms, hips, and upper body must be made simultaneously.

To properly transfer one's weight over onto one leg, the upper body and waist should be shifted to one side together (Fig. 24).

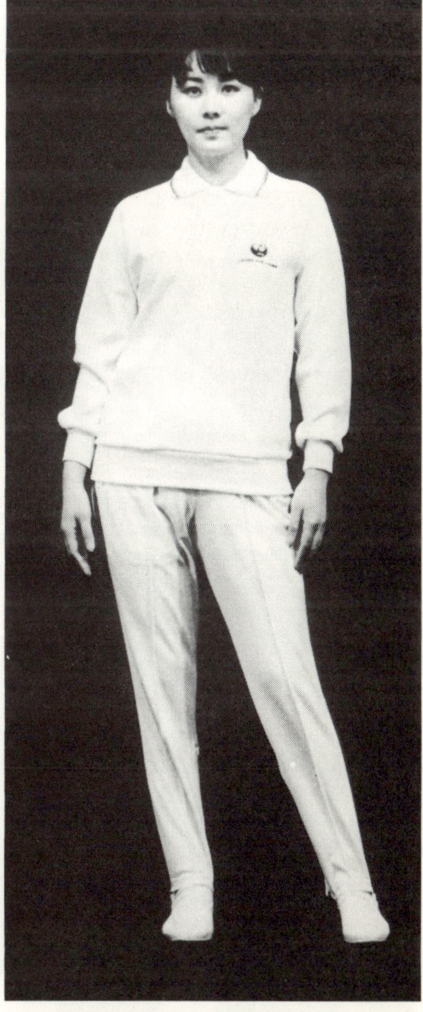

Fig. 24

The left hand can be placed on the waist when moving the upper body and hips together to the left (Fig. 25).

Just pushing the hips farther to the right after completely shifting one's weight on to the right leg will produce lateral flexion to the left (Fig. 26).

Also, just placing both hands on the waist and pushing the hips from side to side while exhaling can produce beneficial results. This exercise is good for those persons unable to raise their arms completely.

This exercise is normally repeated three to five times bilaterally, but if flexion toward one side produces discomfort or tension, the patient may first bend to the opposite side two or three times. After this, flexion can be performed to both sides much smoother and with greater ease.

Fig. 25

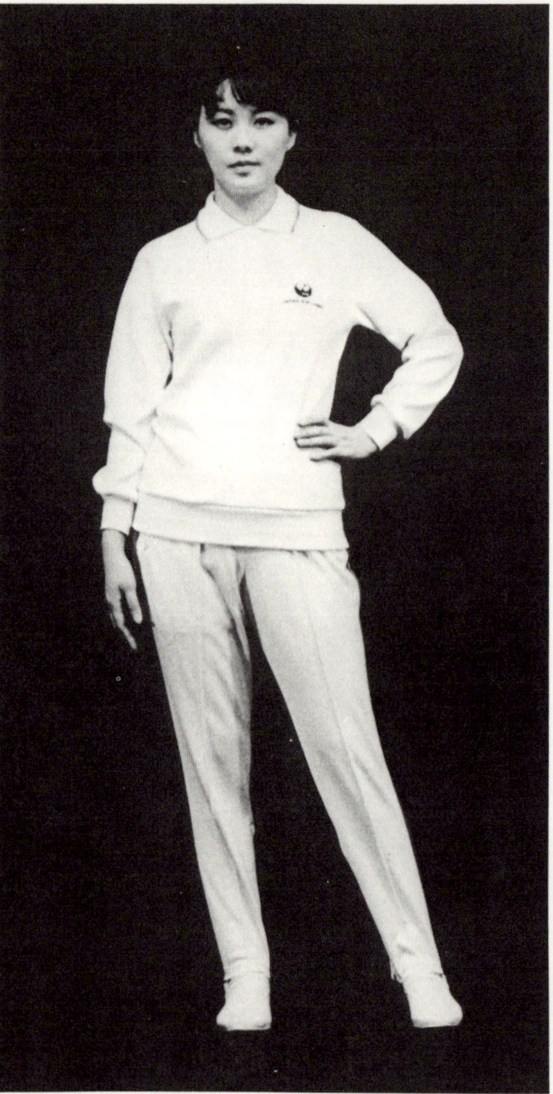

Fig. 26

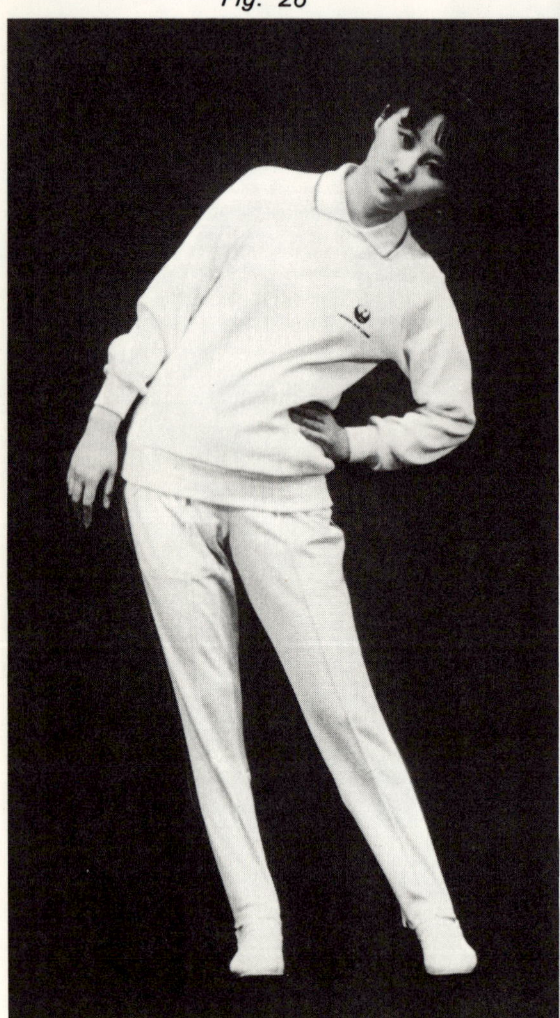

It is important that the sole of the foot holding the body's weight be planted squarely on the floor. The essential principle to be kept in mind when performing this type of movement is to make sure that the weight is shifted to the side being extended (opposite side from flexion). This crucial point for correct movement is often left unexplained even in special exercise programs.

Basic Exercise 5—*Bilateral rotation*

Assume the natural stance of Basic Exercise 1 (Fig. 27). Relax and draw a deep breath into the abdomen.

While exhaling, slowly transfer the body weight over to the right foot and twist the body to the right (Fig. 28).

Both arms are raised slowly while continuing to twist to the right and shifting the body weight over to the right foot (Fig. 29).

The body's weight is transferred completely over on to the right foot, and the arms, face and eyes, as well as one's attention are pointed

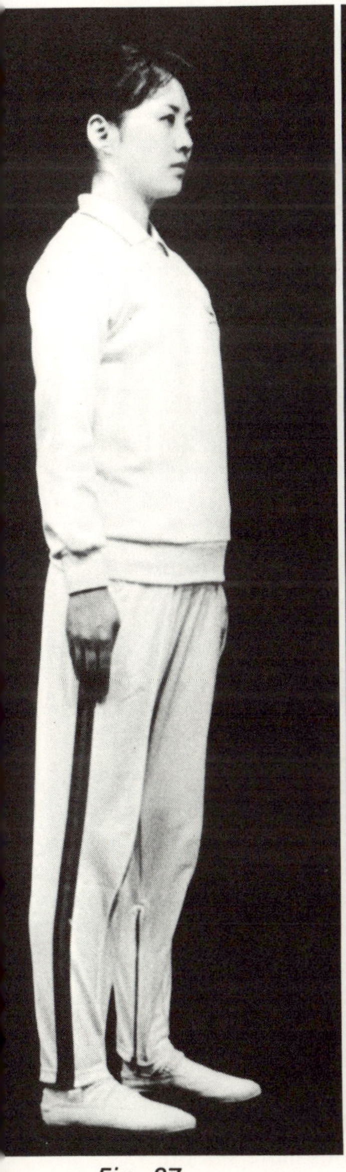

Fig. 27

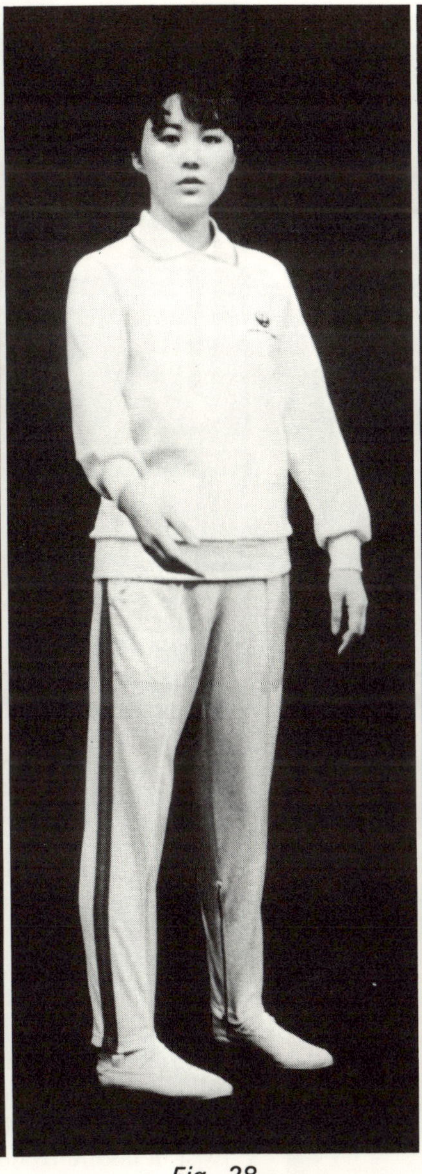

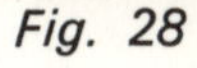

Fig. 28

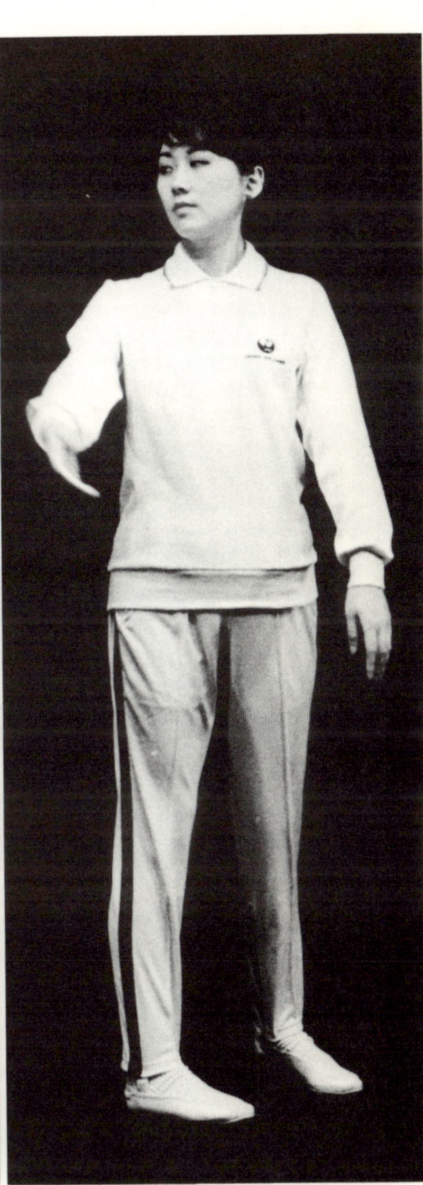

Fig. 29

in the right posterolateral direction (Fig. 30). A full breath is taken in this position. Then while exhaling, slowly return to the original stance.

It is of paramount importance that the right foot holding the body weight contact the floor squarely without budging. The left leg, on the other hand, is relaxed without any weight on it, so the heel rises off the floor and the toes remain barely in contact (Fig. 31).

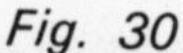
Fig. 30

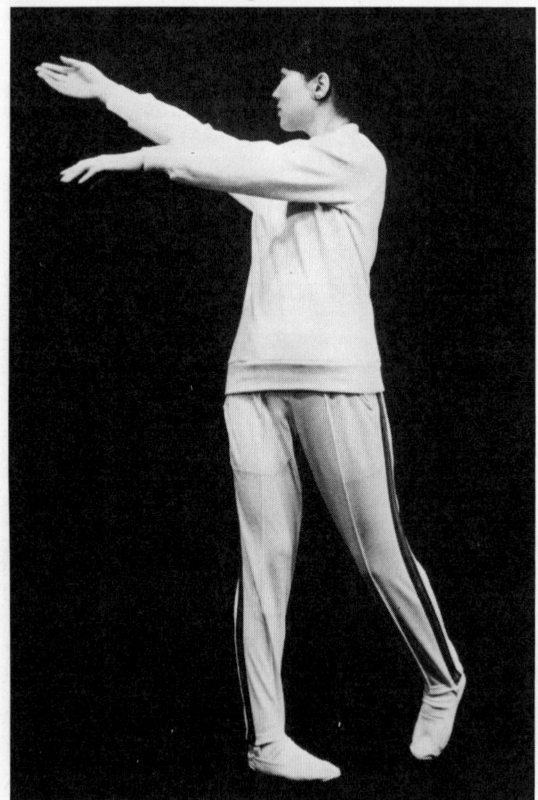

Fig. 31

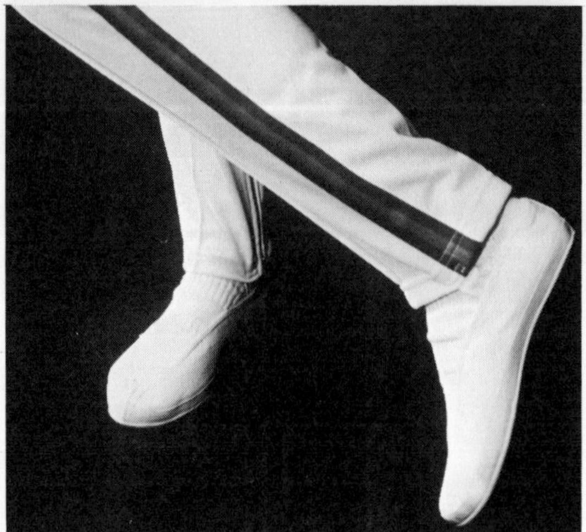

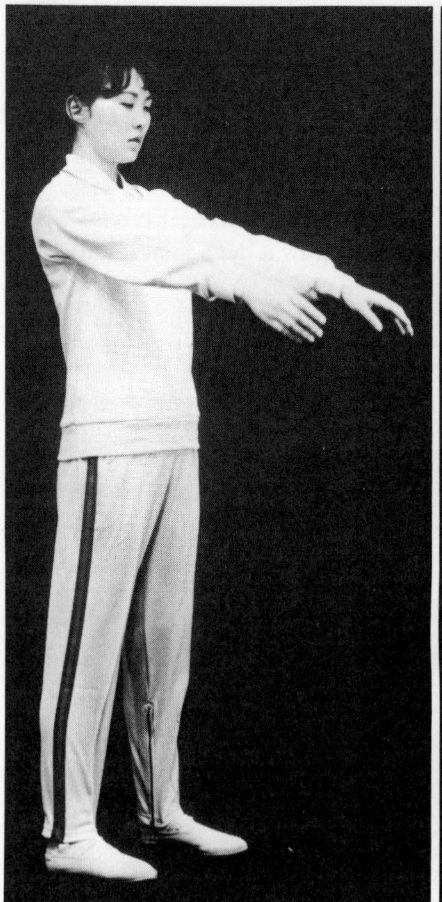

Fig. 32

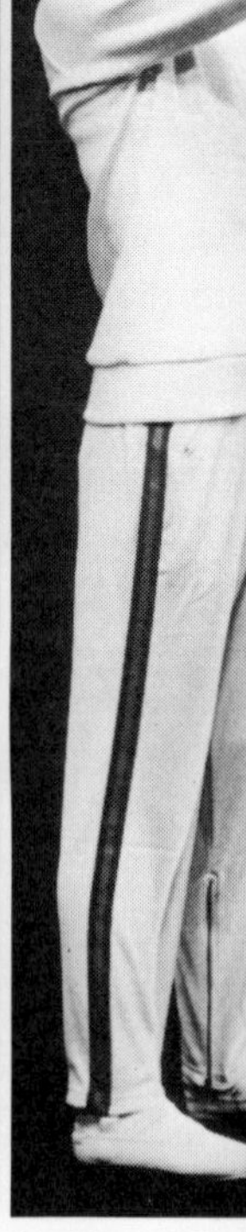

Fig. 33

The movement of the arms following the twisting of the body, aid in the rotation movement and help maintain the center of gravity. The arms may be raised to chest height prior to beginning the rotation movement (Fig. 32).

It is also possible to raise the hands as far up as eye level, and then to slowly twist the body while exhaling (Figs. 33 and 34). Initially, however, it is usually easier to rotate the trunk with the arms raised to a height lower than the shoulders.

Although this exercise is normally repeated three to five times, if turning in one direction should prove to be more difficult, uncomfortable, or painful than the other direction, one can twist in the easier direction two or three times first. It should then become possible to twist in both directions more smoothly.

When rotating the body to the right, it is

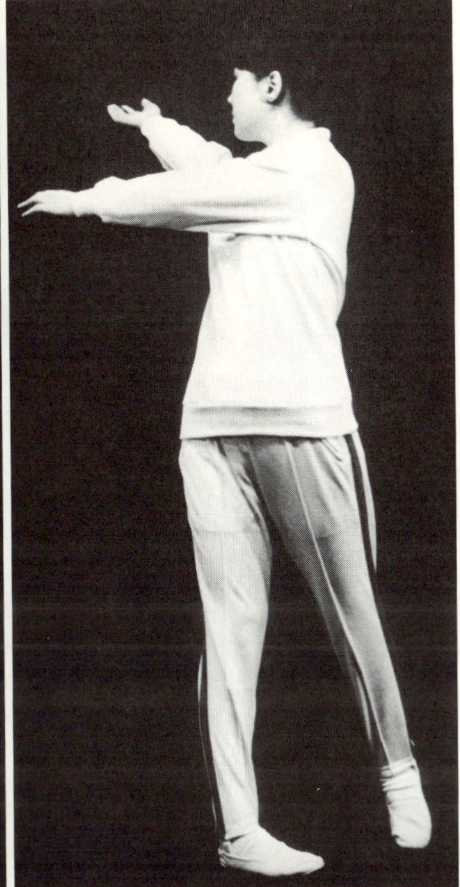

Fig. 34

helpful to hold the right hand with the palm facing upward and the left hand with the palm facing downward. The exact opposite holds true when rotating to the left.

The most important principle to be kept in mind when doing this type of exercise is that one's weight must always be shifted over to the side to which the body is turning.

Basic Exercise 6—*Body extension*

The natural stance of Basic Exercise 1 is assumed and the breath is drawn into the abdomen (Fig. 35).

While exhaling, stand up on the toes and draw the arms up in front of the body (Fig. 36). All these movements must be made simultaneously.

Standing still higher up on the toes, raise the arms high above the head (Fig. 37). The fingertips should also be fully extended. Keeping steady in this posture, take a full breath. Then let the breath out all at once and allow the arms and heels to drop back down. Repeat this exercise three to five times.

After learning this exercise, each person can modify it slightly, such as by standing up on the toes first, and then raising the arms (Fig. 38).

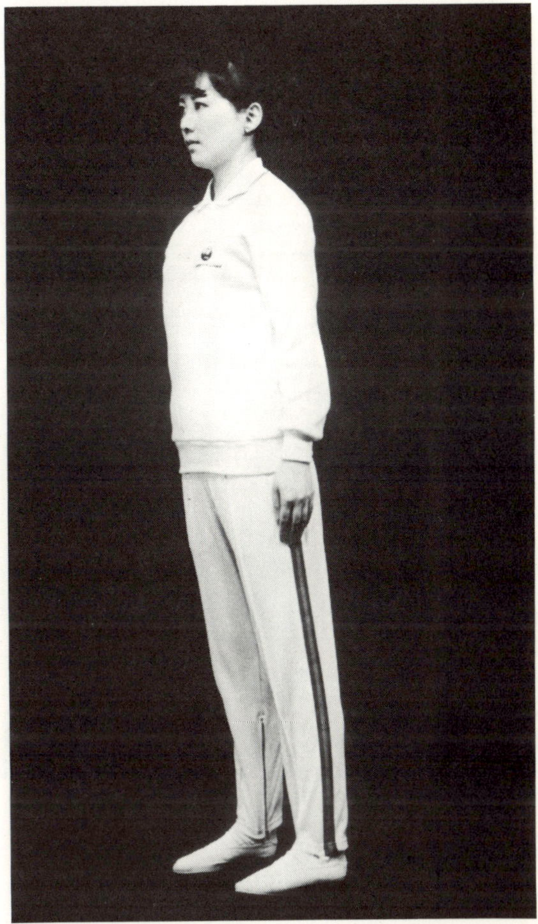

Fig. 35

Note: There are several ways in which the arms may be raised in this exercise.

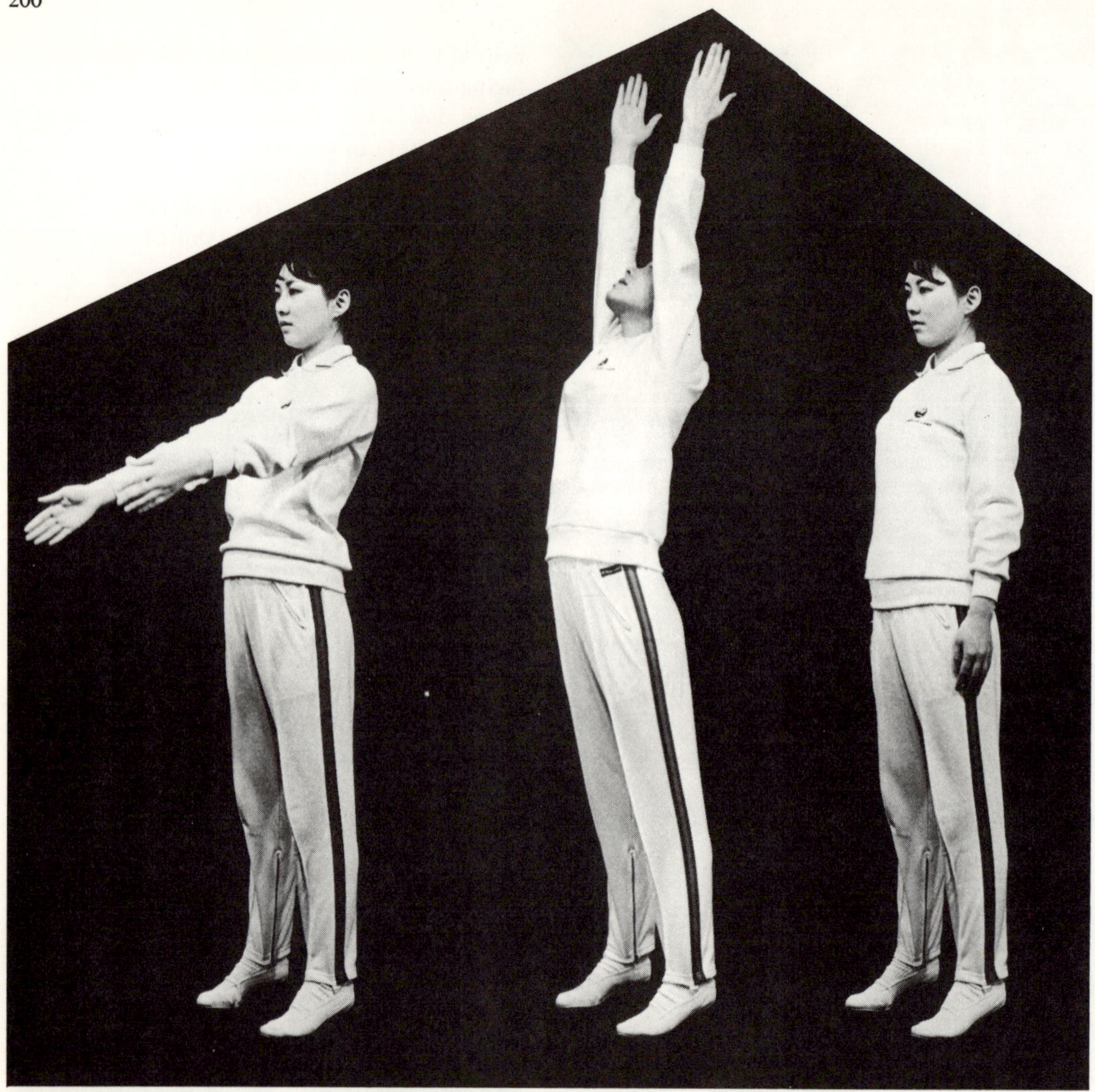

Fig. 36 *Fig. 37* *Fig. 38*

1. Raising the arms in front of the body
2. Raising the arms laterally
3. Raising the arms anterolaterally (forward diagonal)

The important points to remember when doing this exercise are:

1. Move slowly while exhaling the breath.
2. Take one full breath after your body is fully extended.
3. Let the breath out and relax the body and return to the original position all at once.

9. SŌTAI TREATMENT ACCORDING TO SYMPTOMS

Many types of complaints can be alleviated by performing a combination of up to ten Sōtai movements from out of the twenty-eight basic techniques and sixty procedures (including that of the supine, prone and seated postures as well as the palpation and mobility examinations). Discomfort can be eliminated completely by repeating these combinations two or three times a day.

Discomfort and abnormal sensations can occur anywhere in the body, and usually slight amounts of discomfort are ignored, but when this develops into acute pain or functional disabilities it becomes cause for concern. Furthermore, if the cause of such impediment cannot be identified, it can become a real source of anxiety.

The initial occurrence of abnormal sensations or discomfort is simply the warning signal of the body (to bring it to a person's notice) and one need not be worried about serious complications. If warning signals like this are repeatedly ignored, however, the unfortunate result may be a "writ of summons" (need of medical attention) and at times may result in serious illness.

Sōtai therapy is not a disease specific symptomatic method of treatment. One cannot, for instance, ask for a Sōtai technique for curing liver diseases. In fact, if there are ten patients with liver problems, all with different complaints, a combination of Sōtai techniques to alleviate discomfort in each case would result in ten different combinations.

Of the patients visiting Dr. Hashimoto's Onkodo Clinic in Sendai, more than half have made their rounds of numerous hospitals and have undergone a host of tests and examinations, and have received some type of medical diagnosis. Some of these patients have changed hospitals every six months to a year, moving from hospital to clinic like a bird in migration, trying every type of therapy available including acupuncture, moxibustion, chiropractic and massage. These patients come labeled with medical diagnoses which are varied and numerous. Below are a representative sample of the diseases and symptoms;

> headache, heaviness of head, asthenopia, nasal obstruction, rhinitis, tinnitus, hearing impairment, insomnia, neurosis, autonomic nervous dysfunction, Basedow's disease, trigeminal neuralgia, facial palsy, stomatitis, whiplash injury, neck strain, cervico-brachialgia, stiff shoulders, anemia, hypotension, hypertension, tracheitis, asthma, bronchitis, lobar pneumonia, cardiac insufficiency, ventricular hypertrophy, arteriosclerosis, gastritis, gastric catarrh, gastroptosis, gastric ulcer, gallstones, cholecystitis, chronic hepatitis, liver cirrhosis, renal disease, mastitis, rheumatoid arthritis, gout, lumbago, sciatica, herniation of intervertebral disk, diabetes, climacteric disorders, prostatic hypertrophy, menstrual disorders, constipation, diarrhea, hemorroids, feeling cold, breech baby, sterility, lupus erythematosus, epilepsy, Meniere's syndrome.

Even if each patient had only one of these diseases or symptoms listed above, this would amount to at least 54 patients for which no less than 700 Sōtai movements would be required. There are, of course, movements utilizing a common technique, and these can be combined to be effective in each case. There are common Sōtai techniques which can be used to alleviate different symptoms, for example, those of all ten of the aforementioned hypothetical patients with liver diseases. This division of symptoms into ten categories for a combination of techniques can be thought of as the equation giving the greatest common denominator for each symptom group.

Notes concerning this chapter

1. One Sōtai routine should consist of no more than three repetitions of each Sōtai movement (excessive repetition can cause fatigue and may produce negative results). The Sōtai treatment can be given two or three times a day.
2. All Sōtai movements should be performed paying close attention to breathing and timing.
3. Using these examples of combinations as reference and choosing Sōtai techniques in accordance with each patient's condition makes a more versatile approach possible by broadening the range of practical application.

Sōtai for Correcting Physical Imbalances without Regard to Specific Symptoms (Basic Forms)

1) Minor Imbalances

These Sōtai movements can be performed where ever mobility examination reveals differences in kinesthetic sense between the right and left sides of the body, or where presense of minor discomfort indicates the existence of slight irregularities in the body. Since there are only eight "octants" or movements possible to a joint, mobility diagnoses can be performed quickly and easily. And although the number of possible movements is limited, they are also capable of correcting great imbalances and eliminating discomfort.

This combination of movements can be performed alone using intrinsic force, so it may also be practiced as a personal exercise regimen. This normalizes sensitivity in the knee, lumbar, thoracic and cervical regions.

Sōtai Therapy

1. Supine G-1 (p. 45)
2. Supine H-1 (p. 50)
3. Supine K-1 (p. 64)
4. Prone A-2-a (p. 75)
5. Prone A-2-b (p. 76)
6. Seated D-1 (p. 100)
7. Seated D-2 (p. 102)
8. Seated E-1 (p. 102)
9. Seated E-2 (p. 105)

2) Large Imbalances

This combination of Sōtai techniques may be used to alleviate symptoms when the body is showing distinct signs of an imbalance. Also, performing these movements even though no signs of physical imbalances are present can be beneficial since these comprise the core group of movements—the very minimum needed to achieve a balanced and truly healthy body.

Sōtai Therapy

1. Supine G-1 (p. 45)
2. Supine H-1 (p. 50)
3. Supine H-2 (p. 52)
4. Supine J-1 (p. 60)
5. Supine K-1 (p. 64)
6. Supine L-1 (p. 67)
7. Supine L-2 (p. 68)
8. Supine M-1 (p. 69)
9. Supine N-1 (p. 72)
10. Prone A-2-a (p. 75)
11. Prone A-2-d (p. 75)
12. Prone D-1 (p. 86)

13. Seated A-1 (p. 90)
14. Seated D-1 (p. 100)
15. Seated D-2 (p. 102)
16. Seated E-1 (p. 102)
17. Seated E-2 (p. 105)
18. Seated I-1 (p. 118)

Headache, Heaviness of Head, Migraine, Nasal Obstruction, Facial Palsy, Insomnia, Neurosis, and Depression Due to Hypertension, Common Cold or Hangover

Discomfort occuring in the head and facial areas often originate in the cervical region. In fact, it is a tenent in Sōtai Therapy that removing perssure sensitivity and indurations in the neck muscles often relieves the chief complaint of the patient. Nevertheless, since pressure sensitivity and indurations in the neck are usually linked to, or otherwise arise as a result of distortions in other parts of the body, it is still necessary to perform Sōtai over the entire body.

Sōtai Therapy

1. Supine B-3 (p. 34)
2. Supine D-1 (p. 38)
3. Supine G-1 (p. 45)
4. Supine H-1 (p. 50)
5. Supine J-1 (p. 60)
6. Supine K-1 (p. 64)
7. Supine L-1 (p. 67)
8. Supine L-2 (p. 68)
9. Supine M-1 (p. 69)
10. Prone A-2-a (p. 75)
11. Prone A-2-b (p. 76)
12. Prone A-2-d (p. 77)
13. Prone B-1 (p. 80)
14. Seated A-1 (p. 90)
15. Seated B-4 (p. 97)
16. Seated D-1 (p. 100)
17. Seated D-2 (p. 102)
18. Seated E-1 (p. 102)
19. Seated E-2 (p. 105)
20. Seated F-1 (p. 107)
21. Seated I-1 (p. 118)
22. Seated I-4 (p. 121)

Note:

- Give special attention to the cervical and upper thoracic vertebrae.
- Perform following Sōtai with special care:
  Supine G-1, M
  Prone A-2
  Seated A, E-1 and 2, I-1 and 4
- Examples of Sōtai combination (routines)
  1) Seated B-1 (p. 93) and 4, A; Supine G-1, H-1, K, M
  2) Prone B-1; Seated B-1 and 4, A, D-1 and 2; Supine G-1, H-1, M

Asthenopia (Flickering, Astringency, Hyperemia and Sensation of Foreign Object in Eye; Reduction in Field of Vision), Deteriorating Eyesight

Back in 1935, while examining a patient who complained of sensations of having a foreign object in an eye, Dr. Hashimoto came across an extremely sensitive point on the liver meridian. He provided acupuncture stimulation at this point, whereupon the unpleasant sensation in the eye disappeared all together. Upon further clinical study, Dr. Hashimoto found that acupuncture stimulation of the adductor muscles of patients complaining of deteriorating eyesight, flickering, astringency and hyperemia of the eyes often resulted in dramatic improvement and restoration of visual acuity. In even got to a point where his patients would request that they be given this treatment again since it worked so well. Based on this experience, Dr. Hashimoto named a new acu-point, "Sei-gan" (clear eyes).

Subsequently, by testing many types of Sōtai techniques to find the one that would best reproduce the effects of acupuncture stimulation at this point (to relieve tension in the adductor muscles), Dr. Hashimoto finally arrived at Sōtai technique Seated I-1 (p. 118).

Similar results are also obtainable by applying finger pressure to the most sensitive point on the adductor muscles at the medial side of the thigh (usually located one third the distance from the knee to the pubis). Steady pressure should be exerted for about thirty seconds on the area within a one centimeter radius of the point (pressure stimulation for over sixty seconds is not recommended as this could prove excessive).

Sōtai Thearpy

1. Supine G-1 (p. 45)
2. Supine H-1 (p. 50)
3. Supine H-2 (p. 52)
4. Supine I-1 (p. 55)
5. Supine J-1 (p. 60)
6. Supine L-1 (p. 67)
7. Supine L-2 (p. 68)
8. Supine M-1 (p. 69)
9. Prone A-2-b (p. 76)
10. Prone A-2-d (p. 77)
11. Prone B-1 (p. 80)
12. Prone B-2 (p. 82)
13. Prone C-1 (p. 84)
14. Seated B-1 (p. 93)
15. Seated B-2 (p. 94)
16. Seated C-1 (p. 98)
17. Seated E-1 (p. 102)
18. Seated E-2 (p. 105)

Note:

- Perform the movements to relax muscle tension in adductor canal.
- Perform following Sōtai with special care:
  Supine G-1, H-1, I-1, M
  Prone B-1 and 2
  Seated E-1 and 2
- Examples of Sōtai combinations (routines)
  1) Seated B-1 and 2; Supine G-1, H-1, M; Prone B-1 and 2, A-2-b and d
  2) Supine G-1, H-1, I-1, M; Seated B-1 and 2

Whiplash Injury, Neck Strain, Pain and Heaviness in Neck

A form of neck strain commonly known as a "crick in the neck" is often experienced early in the morning upon arising with neck pain and limitation of head movement. Whiplash injury occurs as a result of sudden impact from the rear. Neck pain and loss of mobility can also result from facing a particular direction (or maintaining an awkward posture) for extended periods. The pain and discomfort which the patients complain of in these cases are usually located in the cervical region, but detailed mobility examination often reveals that the physical distortions responsible for the discomfort are to be found elsewhere. Since the human body is like a "mobile building" which is dependent on the legs for locomotion, an important rule in Sōtai is to perform the palpation and mobility examinations, as well as the corrective movements, from the feet first. The Sōtai techniques for the neck should come last.

Since restrictions in neck mobility are often

present in cases of whiplash injury and neck strain, the Sōtai combinations have been separated into three groups:

A. For cases of severe pain or restriction in mobility
B. Additional techniques for when pain has subsided and mobility is restored
C. For patients who are capable of doing Sōtai movements on their own

Sōtai Therapy

Case A:

1. Supine B-1 (p. 32)
2. Supine B-2 (p. 33)
3. Supine B-3 (p. 34)
4. Supine C-1 (p. 36)
5. Supine G-1 (p. 45)

Case B:

1. Supine H-1 (p. 50)
2. Seated B-1 (p. 93)
3. Seated D-1 (p. 100)
4. Seated D-2 (p. 102)

Case C:

1. Supine E-1 (p. 42)
2. Supine H-1 (p. 50)
3. Prone A-2-d (p. 77)

Note:

- Give special attention to the upper thoracic and lumbar vertebrae, as well as the sacral area.
- Perform following Sōtai with special care:
  Supine B-1 and 3, G-1, H
  Prone A-2
  Seated D-1 and 2
- Examples of Sōtai combinations (routines)
  1) Seated B-3 (p. 95) and 1; Supine G-1, H-1, Seated D-1 and 2
  2) Supine E, G-1, H-1; Seated B-3 and 1, D-1 and 2

Pain of Shoulder, Elbow and Arm; Cervico-brachialgia, Shoulder Stiffness, Frozen Shoulder and Arthritis

Regardless of what the patient may believe, frozen shoulder (scapulohumeral periarthritis) in advanced ages never occurs all of a sudden. It always results from a gradual accumulation of abnormal sensations and tension (warning signals) in one's legs, lower back and side. The 99 percent of the therapists who treat shoulder problems become preoccupied with treatment of the localized pain and restriction in mobility, thus usually limiting themselves to symptomatic treatment, but this can hardly be called adequate. Piecemeal treatments ignoring the chain-reaction principle whereby distortions in other parts of the body cause pain and restrict the mobility of the shoulder joint, can be compared to a parent indulging a spoiled child by giving candy every time he cries.

Sōtai Therapy

1. Supine G-1 (p. 45)
2. Supine H-1 (p. 50)
3. Supine H-2 (p. 52)
4. Supine J-1 (p. 60)
5. Supine M-1 (p. 69)
6. Supine N-1 (p. 72)
7. Prone A-2-b (p. 76)
8. Prone A-2-d (p. 75)
9. Prone B-1 (p. 80)
10. Prone B-2 (p. 82)
11. Prone C-1 (p. 84)
12. Prone D-1 (p. 86)
13. Seated B-2 (p. 94)
14. Seated B-4 (p. 97)
15. Seated E-1 (p. 102)
16. Seated E-2 (p. 105)
17. Seated F-1 (p. 107)

18. Seated G-1 (p. 110)
19. Seated G-2 (p. 113)
20. Seated H-1 (p. 116)

Note:

- Give special attention to the following areas when treating respective parts.
  Shoulder—around iliac crest (flank)
  Arm—suprascapular area
  Elbow—infrascapular area
- Perform following Sōtai with special care:
  Supine G-1, H, N
  Prone B-1 and 2, C-1
  Seated B-2 and 4, G-1 and 2, H
- Examples of Sōtai combinations (routines)
  1) Seated B-2 and 4; Supine G-1, H-1, M; Prone B-1 and 2, A-2-b and d
  2) Seated B-2 and 4; Supine G-1, H-1; Seated F, G-1 and 2, H

Wrist Pain (Tendovaginitis) and Edema of Hands (Heart, Liver or Kidney Condition)

For some people the sensation of grasping with their hands feels different in the morning than in the evening. It cannot be said which sensation is the more normal one during grasping, but in either case, it is a fact that such differences do occur. In such a case, the sensation of grasping and opening the fingers of the right and left hands should be compared. Grasping and opening movements should be performed two or three more times with the hand that can grasp with the greatest ease. Other types of hand exercise ideal for this condition are the clasping together of the fingers of both hands and also rolling a couple of walnuts around in the hand.

Sōtai Therapy

1. Supine G-1 (p. 45)
2. Supine H-1 (p. 50)
3. Supine L-1 (p. 67)
4. Supine L-2 (p. 68)
5. Prone A-2-b (p. 76)
6. Prone A-2-e (p. 78)
7. Prone D-1 (p. 86)
8. Seated B-1 (p. 93)
9. Seated B-2 (p. 94)
10. Seated A-1 (p. 90)
11. Seated D-1 (p. 100)
12. Seated D-2 (p. 102)
13. Seated G-1 (p. 110)
14. Seated J-1 (p. 121)
15. Seated J-2 (p. 123)
16. Seated J-3 (p. 124)

Note:

- Give special attention to infrascapular area and rotation of arms and fingers (specific technique not covered in this manual).
- Perform following Sōtai with special care:
  Supine G-1, H-1
  Prone A-2, D
  Seated G-1, J-1, 2, and 3
- Example of Sōtai combinations (routines)
  1) Perform only the movements in the seated posture
  2) Supine G-1, H-1; Seated A, D-1 and 2, G-1, J-1, 2, and 3
  3) Supine G-1, H-1; Prone A-2-b and e, D; Seated A, D-1 and 2, J-1, 2, and 3

Pain and Heaviness in Back (Heart, Liver, Gallbladder, Kidney and Stomach Conditions), Hump Back, Palpitation, Shortness of Breath

Since all organs in the body are innervated by spinal nerves, it is only natural that reactions to diseases in these organs should appear around the thoracic and lumbar vertebrae. Often doctors and therapists, and even patients speak in terms of problems in a particular organ causing back pain or stiff shoulders. Most often this is not the case at the onset of the pain or discomfort (except where drugs are administered). It could be the case after some time elapses and the pain and discomfort become chronic. This is evidenced by the fact that at the incipient stages of pain and discomfort, even the most rigorous lab tests using the newest of techniques will not reveal any organic pathology. The initial sensation of discomfort is a warning signal that a distortion has occured somewhere in the body. Such distortions may either be hidden or conspicuous. The real relationship between sensations of discomfort and organic disorders comes after the initial symptoms of distortion are ignored and functional disorders arise. This eventually progresses to organic disorders which in turn amplifies the pain reaction in various parts of the body.

Sōtai Therapy

1. Supine G-1 (p. 45)
2. Supine H-1 (p. 50)
3. Supine H-2 (p. 52)
4. Supine K-1 (p. 64)
5. Supine M-1 (p. 69)
6. Prone A-2-a (p. 75)
7. Prone A-2-c (p. 77)
8. Prone A-2-d (p. 77)
9. Prone A-2-e (p. 78)
10. Prone B-1 (p. 80)
11. Prone C-1 (p. 84)
12. Prone C-2 (p. 85)
13. Prone D-1 (p. 86)
14. Seated A-1 (p. 90)
15. Seated B-2 (p. 94)
16. Seated D-1 (p. 100)
17. Seated D-2 (p. 102)
18. Seated F-1 (p. 107)
19. Seated I-1 (p. 118)
20. Seated I-4 (p. 121)
21. Seated I-5 (p. 121)

Note:

- Give special attention to anteflexion, dorsiflexion, rotation and extension of spine.
- Perform following Sōtai with special care:
  Supine G-1, H, K, M
  Prone A-2, C-1 and 2
  Seated A, D-1 and 2, I-1 and 4
- Example of Sōtai combinations (routines)
  1) Seated A, D-1 and 2, F, I-1 and 5
  2) Supine G-1, H-1, K, M; Prone A-2-b and d; Seated A

Low Back Pain (Lumbago, Menstrual Cramps), Sciatica, Herniation of Intervertebral Disks, Scoliosis, Constipation, Diarrhea, Heaviness and Chilling of Lower Back (Colds and Fatigue)

Low back pain is so common it seems that even those who have never had stiff shoulders have experienced low back pain at one time or another. There are those who wake up in the early hours of the morning with low back pain, and these people loose sleep because of this pain.

This low back pain occurring before dawn has been compared to that of a nagging toothache, and seems to be unbearable for anyone. It is easy to understand how low back pain can be so distressing because the waist area is a crucial part of the human body where one's weight and movements are balanced out above and below.

When Sōtai movements are performed with people having scoliosis, their spine often begins to straighten out. Although the spine may not completely return to normal, its abnormal curvature should decrease to some extent. Sudden low back pain such as the so-called "slipped disk" is a result of accumulated distortions in the body due to improper shifting of body weight (use of legs) in movement. It is therefore important that one pay closer attention to shifting the body weight in the right way.

Sōtai Therapy for Back Pain (A) —for sudden low back pain (e.g., slipped disks)

1. Supine E-1 (p. 42)
2. Supine G-1 (p. 45)
3. Supine H-1 (p. 50)
4. Supine J-1 (p. 60)
5. Supine B-1 (p. 32)
6. Prone B-2 (p. 82)
7. Prone A-2-a (p. 75)
8. Prone A-2-b (p. 76)
9. Prone A-2-d (p. 77)
10. Prone A-2-e (p. 78)
11. Prone C-1 (p. 84)
12. Seated A-1 (p. 90)
13. Seated D-1 (p. 100)
14. Seated D-2 (p. 102)
15. Seated I-1 (p. 118)
16. Seated I-2 (p. 118)
17. Seated I-4 (p. 121)

Note:

- Give special attention to movement of waist and shifting weight.
- Perform following Sōtai with special care:
  Supine G-1, H
  Prone A-2, C
  Seated D-1 and 2, I-1 and 4
- Examples of Sōtai combinations (routines)
  1) Seated A, D-1 and 2, I-1, 2, and 4
  2) Supine G-1, H-1; Seated A, D-1 and 2
  3) Supine G-1, H-1; Prone B-1 and 2, A-2

Sōtai Therapy for Back Pain (B) —for chronic cases of low back pain

1. Supine B-1 (p. 32)
2. Supine B-2 (p. 33)
3. Supine B-3 (p. 34)
4. Supine B-4 (p. 35)
5. Supine C-1 (p. 36)
6. Supine E-1 (p. 42)
7. Supine G-1 (p. 45)
8. Supine H-1 (p. 50)
9. Supine H-2 (p. 52)
10. Supine J-1 (p. 60)
11. Supine K-1 (p. 64)
12. Supine M-1 (p. 69)
13. Prone B-1 (p. 80)
14. Prone B-2 (p. 82)
15. Prone A-2-a (p. 75)
16. Prone A-2-b (p. 76)
17. Prone A-2-c (p. 77)
18. Prone A-2-d (p. 77)
19. Prone A-2-e (p. 78)
20. Prone C-1 (p. 84)
21. Prone C-2 (p. 85)
22. Prone D-1 (p. 86)
23. Seated B-1 (p. 93)
24. Seated B-3 (p. 95)
25. Seated B-4 (p. 97)
26. Seated C-1 (p. 98)
27. Seated A-1 (p. 90)
28. Seated D-1 (p. 100)
29. Seated D-2 (p. 102)
30. Seated I-1 (p. 118)
31. Seated I-4 (p. 121)
32. Seated I-5 (p. 121)

Note:

- Give special attention to movement of waist and shifting weight.

- Perform following Sōtai with special care:
  Supine B-1, 2, and 3, C-1 and 2 (p. 37), G-1, H-1
  Prone A-2, B-1 and 2
  Seated B-2 and 4, D-1 and 2, I-1, 4, and 5
- Examples of Sōtai combinations (routines)
  1) Seated A, D-1 and 2, I-1, 4 and 5
  2) Seated B-1 and 3, A; Supine G-1, H-1; Prone B-1 and 2, A-2
  3) Supine B-1 through 4, G-1, H-1; Prone B-1 and 2, A-2; Seated B-1 and 3, A, D-1 and 2

Sōtai Therapy for Back Pain (C) —active movement exercises for the patient

Each Sōtai movement listed here in the Supine and Prone postures *must be performed slowly while exhaling the breath.*

1. Supine H-1 (p. 50)—Take the raised knee down the right and left alternately. When pain results when turning the knees beyond a certain point on both the right and left sides, perform the movement five times in each direction to the point just before the pain starts. (*Time required:* 1½ to 2 minutes)

   After this, straighten out the knees and rest for about a minute, and then repeat the movements three more times.
2. Prone A-2-d (p. 77)—Draw the leg which does have pain, three times up to the side. (*Time required:* about 1 minute) When both legs cause pain, without forcing it, perform this movement with the leg that gives the least pain.

Fatigue, Pain and Edema of Legs (Diabetes, Liver Cirrhosis; Kidney and Heart Conditions)

If subject A and B walk the same distance under the same conditions and only A complains of fatigue, then clearly A's legs and body are weaker than that of B. Our legs are supports which hold the body from underneath, so if they become weak the pelvic region is immediately affected and subsequently the whole body begins to weaken. It is up to the individual whether to first strengthen the legs through exercise, or to do this after performing Sōtai movements to restore the balance and normalize abnormal sensitivity.

The calves of some women can be made about a centimeter thinner just by performing the right Sōtai technique, but what is more important is to determine the cause of why they got so big in the first place. When observing women walking in high heeled shoes for example (with Japanese), an unstable gait is common with the body stooped forward and without full extension of the knees, and this is a cause of undue strain. This is like knowingly perpetuating low back pain, poor circulation and menstrual problems.

Concerning diabetes, it is written in texts of Oriental medicine that a reaction appears on the anterior tibial area of the leg. In such cases Sōtai technique Supine J (p. 60) is often effective.

Sōtai Therapy

1. Supine B-2 (p. 33)
2. Supine B-4 (p. 35)
3. Supine C-1 (p. 36)
4. Supine G-1 (p. 45)
5. Supine H-1 (p. 50)
6. Supine J-1 (p. 60)
7. Supine K-1 (p. 64)
8. Supine L-1 (p. 67)
9. Supine L-2 (p. 68)
10. Supine M-1 (p. 69)

11. Prone A-2-b (p. 76)
12. Prone A-2-d (p. 77)
13. Prone B-1 (p. 80)
14. Prone B-2 (p. 82)
15. Prone C-1 (p. 84)
16. Seated B-2 (p. 94)
17. Seated B-3 (p. 95)
18. Seated B-4 (p. 97)
19. Seated A-1 (p. 90)
20. Seated C-1 (p. 98)
21. Seated C-2 (p. 99)
22. Seated D-1 (p. 100)
23. Seated D-2 (p. 102)

Note:

- Give special attention to extension of leg.
- Perform following Sōtai with special care:
  Supine G-1, J
  Prone A-2
  Seated B-2, 3, and 4
- Examples of Sōtai combinations (routines)
  1) Supine B-2 and 4, C-1, G-1, H-1, J-2; Prone B-1 and 2; Seated B-3 and 4, C-2
  2) Seated B-3 and 4, C-2; Prone B-1 and 2, A-2

Knee Pain

Balance in the human frame is maintained at the key points of the feet, knees, pelvis and neck. The knees are especially important in maintaining the forward and backward balance. Therefore, for people who have large distortions in their physical makeup, the knees tend to become over burdened, and functional disabilities begin to occur. Even those of advanced age whose backs are extremely bent can usually walk with relative ease, so long as their knees are capable of straightening completely. Neck movements also come easily for such people. The human body is a mechanism linked together from top to bottom and any distortions are transferred from one end to the other. Imbalances are compensated for only through the body's functional dynamics. Which is to say, those who complain of knee pain almost always have discomfort in other parts of their body as well. It is important to pay attention so as not to overlook associated distortions.

Sōtai Therapy

1. Supine B-1 (p. 32)
2. Supine B-3 (p. 34)
3. Supine G-1 (p. 45)
4. Supine F-1 (p. 44)
5. Supine H-1 (p. 50)
6. Supine J-1 (p. 60)
7. Prone A-2-b (p. 76)
8. Prone A-2-d (p. 77)
9. Prone A-2-e (p. 78)
10. Prone D-1 (p. 86)
11. Seated B-1 (p. 93)
12. Seated B-2 (p. 94)
13. Seated B-3 (p. 95)
14. Seated C-1 (p. 98)
15. Seated C-2 (p. 99)
16. Seated D-1 (p. 100)
17. Seated D-2 (p. 102)
18. Seated E-1 (p. 102)
19. Seated E-2 (p. 105)
20. Seated F-1 (p. 107)

Note:

- Give special attention to the rotation of the ankle and hip joints. (When knee is swollen and full of fluid, it proves more effective when Sōtai is performed after it is drained.)
- Perform following Sōtai with special care:
  Supine B-1, 2 and 3, F, G-1
  Prone A-2
  Seated B-1, 2 and 3, D-1 and 2
- Be sure to exercise due caution in the Sōtai techniques Seated C-1 and 2.
- Examples of Sōtai combinations (routines)
  1) Supine B-3, F, G-1; Seated B-1 and 2, C-2
  2) Seated B-1 and 2, C-2; Supine F, G-1; Prone A-2

AFTERWORD

Medical science today has become extremely complex and incomprehensible to the layman. Although medicine has become scientifically advanced, it is still at a loss to cure many diseases. The expression modern medicine or Western medicine are not apt descriptions of medicine as it is practiced today. When this cosmopolitan medicine is compared to natural medicine, it can be called artificial medicine. Nevertheless, natural medicine itself is very vaguely defined and is quite complicated in actual practice. Many methods have been advocated as being natural, resulting today in a whole myriad of natural approaches to health. Yet there does not seem to be one approach among these that is positively effective in every case.

Personally, having studied and practiced chiropractic for almost ten years in the United States, I recognized the importance of natural medicine involving not only manipulation but a wider range of holistic approaches. Coming back to Japan, I have met many practitioners of various types of natural healing methods, but Dr. Keizo Hashimoto among them stands out as an especially remarkable figure. His approach to health was just the kind of natural physiotherapeutic method I had been looking for. Dr. Hashimoto arrived at the principles of *Sōtai Therapy* after trying out a whole array of natural approaches himself. The thinking behind Sōtai is exceedingly simple, all one needs to is "return to what is natural." What this means is that to become free of pain, one must move away from pain toward comfort. And people can actually do this for themselves by performing a series of movements which allows a person to "escape" from pain. All movements we make are variations on the eight basic types of movement described in this book, and the natural power to heal oneself is enhanced by moving in the direction which comes the easiest for a person.

All disease is cured by the power of nature. God is the only one who can heal wounds; all man can do is bandage the wound. Man possesses the great power of nature which is capable of righting itself. The key in any form of therapy is how to draw forth this great power of nature to effect a cure. Dr. Hashimoto explains the essential functions of man as being breathing and injection plus mental and physical activity. His patients are encouraged to bring a balance in their lives through proper breathing and eating and wholesome physical and mental activity. There are chiropractors in the United States which advocate therapy for bringing a balance in a triangle with the three sides of mind, nutrition and structure. It is clear that Sōtai Therapy which adds the element of movement, or balance through motion, is invaluable in facilitating the natural healing powers of nature.

Therefore, there is great meaning in making this method known throughout the world, and I am very happy that this book on Sōtai Therapy is being published in English to become available all over the world. There may be some problems which remain in reaching a complete understanding of Sōtai through this book alone. Therefore, thought is being given to other means of enabling a better understanding of Sōtai Therapy in the future. I sincerely hope that as many people as possible gain true health through this book to enjoy their life to the fullest.

KENZO KASE D.C.

INDEX